Low GI Eating Made Easy

Other books in the Low GI series

The Low GI Diet
The Low GI Diet Cookbook
The Low GI Life Plan
The Low GI Guide to the Metabolic Syndrome and Your Heart
The Low GI Guide to Managing PCOS
The Low GI Shopper's Guide to GI Values
The New Glucose Revolution
The New Glucose Revolution & Children with Type 1 Diabetes
The New Glucose Revolution & Healthy Children
The New Glucose Revolution & Losing Weight
The New Glucose Revolution & Sports Nutrition
The New Glucose Revolution for People with Diabetes

Low GI Eating Made Easy

Dr Jennie Brand-Miller
and Kaye Foster-Powell
with Philippa Sandall

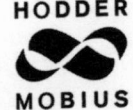

HODDER
MOBIUS

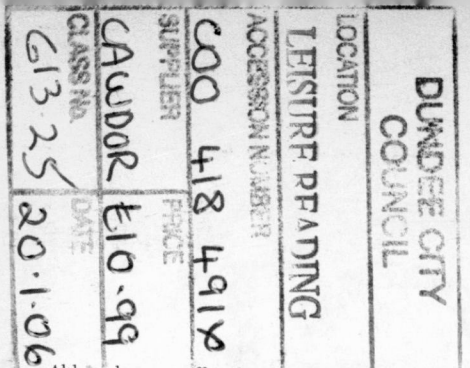

Although every effort has been made to ensure that the contents of this book are accurate, it must not be treated as a substitute for qualified medical advice. Always consult a qualified medical practitioner. Neither the authors nor the publisher can be held responsible for any loss or claim arising out of the use, or misuse, of the suggestions made or the failure to take medical advice.

First published in Great Britain in 2005 by Hodder and Stoughton
A division of Hodder Headline

The right of Prof. Jennie Brand-Miller, Kaye Foster-Powell, Philippa Sandall to be identified as the Authors of the Work has been asserted by them in accordance with the Copyright, Designs and Patents Act 1988.

A Mobius Book

1

A CIP catalogue record for this title is available from the British Library

ISBN 0340896000

Typeset in Berkeley Book by Palimpsest Book Production Limited, Polmont, Stirlingshire

Printed and bound in Great Britain by
Clays Ltd, St Ives plc

Hodder Headline's policy is to use papers that are natural, renewable and recyclable products and made from wood grown in sustainable forests. The logging and manufacturing processes are expected to conform to the environmental regulations of the country of origin.

Hodder and Stoughton Ltd
A division of Hodder Headline
338 Euston Road
London NW1 3BH

Contents

PART 1

Understanding
low gi eating

Understanding the GI helps you choose both the right amount of carbohydrate and the right type of carbohydrate for your long-term health and wellbeing.

'JUST TELL ME WHAT TO EAT!'

These days, working out exactly what you should be eating can be confusing. There are so many people and organisations – particularly the media – with an opinion on the best diet, whether it be low carb, low fat, high protein or any number of fad ideas, that wading through it all seems like mission impossible.

Once upon a time it seemed simple – you just cut down on bread and potatoes if you wanted to lose weight. Then they said fat was the problem and you should eat more 'complex' carbs. Now there are the best-sellers telling you to banish carbs altogether – not just refined sugar, but starch too. And we won't even start on grapefruit diets or soup diets . . . So, who is right? What should you eat?

First of all, we human beings are individuals. Being fussy about food doesn't stop with childhood. When it comes to meal times each one of us has likes and dislikes. We are influenced by the traditional foods, recipes and dietary customs of our family background, and, in addition, some of us have special health requirements that govern what we should or shouldn't eat. That's why one diet or set of food rules can't possibly apply to everybody. When you pause to think about it, the one-diet-fits-all notion doesn't make any sense at all.

There are, however, certain important characteristics of the foods we eat that make some better for us than others. The GI, or glycaemic index, is one of those characteristics – one for which we are still learning the relevance to our health. What we do know is that many of the world's traditional staple foods are low GI, which means that they form the basis of a healthy, flexible, diet, whoever you are and wherever you live. A low GI diet is a way of eating long term that suits everybody, every day, every meal.

The fuels we need for good all-round nutrition and wellbeing

Our bodies run on fuel, just like a car runs on petrol. In fact, our bodies burn a special mix of fuels that come from the protein, fat and carbohydrate in the food we eat for breakfast, lunch and dinner and the snacks we enjoy in between.

Every day (several times a day) we need to top up our 'tank' with the right balance of these fuels.

So, the first step in answering the question 'But what should I eat' is to take a closer look at these fuels – where we find them and what they do.

> You can read this book from beginning to end if you want to, or just flick through and pick up any tips or ideas that take your fancy.

PROTEIN – KEEP IT LEAN

We need protein to build and maintain our body tissues. Foods rich in protein include:

- lean meat (beef, pork, lamb)
- skinless poultry
- fish and seafood
- eggs
- low fat dairy foods such as cottage cheese, skimmed milk and low fat yoghurt
- pulses including beans, chickpeas and lentils and soya products such as tofu and calcium-enriched soya beverages
- nuts

Protein is also a satiating nutrient. Compared with fat and carbohydrate, eating protein will make you feel more satisfied and keep those hunger pangs at bay between meals.

Meat, fish, seafood and poultry are the richest sources

> ### Protein and GI
>
> With the exception of pulses (beans, peas and lentils), and milk and yoghurt, protein foods such as meat, chicken, fish and eggs don't contain carbohydrate, so they do not have GI values.

of protein. As long as you trim the visible fat and avoid high fat creamy sauces, batter and pastry or crumb coatings you can basically eat lean protein as much as you like – but you will probably find there are natural limits on how much of these foods you wantto eat.

Because your body can't stockpile extra protein from one day to use up the next, you need to eat it every day. By including a protein-rich food with every meal, you can also help satisfy your hunger between meals.

Protein plus micronutrients

Protein foods are excellent sources of micronutrients such as iron, calcium, zinc, vitamin B12 and omega-3 fats.

- Lean red meat is the best source of iron you can get.
- Fish and seafood are important sources of omega-3 fats.
- Dairy foods supply the highest amounts of calcium.
- Eggs are great sources of several essential vitamins and minerals including vitamins A, D and E and B-group vitamins, in addition to iron, phosphorus and zinc.
- Pulses (beans, peas and lentils) are nutritional powerpacks – high in fibre, a valuable source of carbs, B vitamins and minerals and potent phytochemicals.
- Nuts are one of the richest sources of 'good fats' and the anti-oxidants vitamin E and selenium.

Protein: the bottom line

Keep your protein lean and eat according to your appetite.

> ### Watch the fat when cooking. Opt for:
>
> - grilling
> - barbecuing
> - pan-frying
> - stir-frying
> - baking or roasting
>
> Be wary of coatings such as breadcrumbs, batter or pastry. You'll end up with something that could have a high GI and is most likely high in fat too.
>
> ### When choosing from menus, hold back on:
>
> - crumbed schnitzel or rissoles
> - crumbed or battered fish and seafood
> - meat and chicken pies
> - tempura

FOCUS ON THE GOOD FATS

We now know that a low fat diet is not necessarily the only way to eat for weight loss or overall health. Our bodies need a certain amount of good or unsaturated fat (think nuts, seeds, olive oil and avocados) to function properly and thrive. Good fats:

- provide us with essential fatty acids that form our cell membranes
- help us absorb the fat-soluble vitamins A, D, E and K
- form part of our body's hormones
- provide insulation
- help us absorb some anti-oxidants from fruit and vegetables
- help to make food taste better

The problem with fat is the amount we eat, sometimes without realising it. Fat provides lots of calories – more

Essential fatty acids

Your body actually requires some types of fats – called essential fatty acids – which can't be manufactured by your body and must be obtained through your diet. The best sources are:

- seafoods
- polyunsaturated oils
- linseeds
- mustard seed oil
- rapeseed oil

than any other nutrient per gram. This may be great for someone who's starving, but it's a real disadvantage to those of us who already eat too much. The main form in which our bodies store those extra calories is, you guessed it, fat.

The most concentrated sources of fat in our diets are butter, margarines and oils. While it's easy to reduce your fat intake when you can see it, it's difficult with the concealed fats in foods such as cakes, biscuits, crisps and muffins, regular pop corn or a packet of instant noodles. That's why it's important to read the labels on food packaging.

It's not just the quantity of fat in your diet you have to think about – the type of fat can make a big difference to your health and your waistline. Focus on including the good fats in your diet and minimising foods that are high in saturated fat and trans fatty acids.

While a low fat diet is recommended for weight loss, this doesn't mean a no fat diet. Studies show that some fats, particularly those found in fish, nuts and olive oil, are beneficial in reducing abdominal fat when included as part of a weight loss diet.

Health tip:

When shopping, look for products low in saturated fat, rather than just low fat products. The saturated fat content should be *less than 20 per cent of the total fat.*

Choosing the good fats

Emphasise the following mono- and polyunsaturated fats in your diet:

- olive and rapeseed oils
- mustard seed oil

- margarines and spreads made with rapeseed, sunflower or other seed oils
- avocados
- fish, shellfish, prawns, scallops, etc.
- walnuts, almonds, cashews, etc.
- olives
- muesli (not toasted)
- linseeds

Giving bad fats the flick

Minimise saturated fats and oils including:

- fatty meats and meat products – e.g. sausages, salami
- full fat dairy products – milk, cream, cheese, ice-cream, yoghurt
- coconut and palm oils
- crisps, packaged snacks
- cakes, biscuits, slices, pastries, pies, pizza
- deep-fried foods – fried chicken, chips, spring rolls

A word of warning

Some high fat foods – chocolate, nuts, sausages, pizza, crisps and ice-cream – have low GI values. When you are choosing low GI foods, you're after low GI carbs, not high fat foods.

Fat: the bottom line

Focus on monounsaturated and omega-3 fats for long-term health.

CARBOHYDRATE – IT DOESN'T MAKE SENSE TO LEAVE IT OUT!

Carbohydrate is a vital source of energy found in all plants and foods such as fruit, vegetables, cereals and grains. The simplest form of carbohydrate is glucose, which is:

- a universal fuel for our body cells
- the only fuel source for our brain, red blood cells and a growing foetus
- the main source of energy for our muscles during strenuous exercise

So, it *really* doesn't make sense to leave carbs out!

If you were thinking about trying a low carbohydrate diet, here's just some of what you'll be missing out on:

- vitamin E from wholegrain cereals
- vitamin C from fruits and vegetables
- vitamin B6 from bananas and wholegrain cereals
- pantothenic acid, zinc and magnesium from wholegrains and pulses
- anti-oxidants and phytochemicals from all plant foods
- and fibre which comes from all the above, and *doesn't come from any animal food*

 ## Health tip:

Forget about simple and complex carbohydrates. Think in terms of low GI and high GI.

How your body revs on carbs

When you eat foods such as bread, cereals and fruit, your body converts them into a sugar called glucose during digestion. It is this glucose that is absorbed from your intestine and becomes the fuel that circulates in your blood stream. As the level of blood glucose rises after you have eaten a meal, your pancreas gets the message to release a powerful hormone called insulin. Insulin drives glucose out of the blood and into the cells. Once inside, glucose is channelled into various pathways simultaneously – to be used as an immediate source of energy or converted into glycogen (a storage form of glucose) or fat. Insulin also turns off the use of fat as the cell's energy source. For this reason, lowering insulin levels is one of the secrets to life-long health. However, cutting carbs is not the answer.

What we now know is that not all carbs are created equal. In fact, they can behave quite differently in our bodies. The glycaemic index or GI is how we describe this difference, ranking carbs (sugars and starches) according to their effect on blood glucose levels. After testing hundreds of foods around the world, scientists have found that foods with a low GI will have less of an effect on blood glucose levels than foods with a high GI. High GI foods will tend to cause spikes in your glucose levels whereas low GI foods tend to cause gentle rises.

> ### The 'carb in'/'carb out' balance
>
> The body attempts to maintain a balance between 'carb in' (the carbs you get from food) and 'carb out' (the carbs you burn for energy). If you deliberately avoid eating carbohydrate but maintain your normal activity, you are likely to eat more calories than you need as your body drives you to eat more in search of the 'carb deficit'.

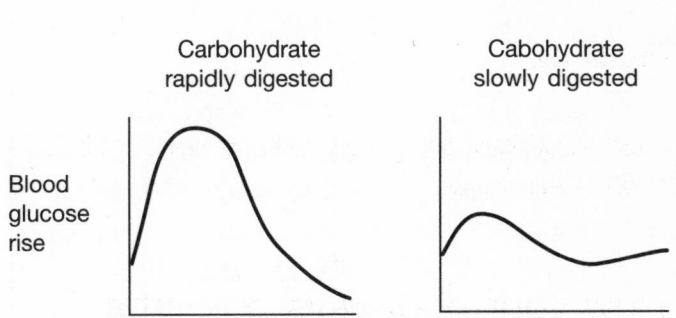

Carbohydrate rapidly digested

Cabohydrate slowly digested

Blood glucose rise

- High GI foods such as white bread, potatoes, jelly beans and cornflakes are converted to glucose quickly.
- Low GI foods such as rolled oats, apples, pasta and yoghurt are converted to glucose slowly.

Our diet these days tends to be dominated by high GI refined and processed carbohydrates – white bread, biscuits, light crispy cereals, crackers, crisps, doughnuts, cakes, and so on. Eating more of these refined carbs means we are eating less traditional starchy foods such as truly wholegrain bread (e.g. pumpernickel), fruit, porridge oats, cracked wheat (bulghur and tabbouleh), barley, dried peas, beans and lentils. These low GI foods are not only digested more slowly, they are also richer in micronutrients than their high GI counterparts.

Carbs: the bottom line

Carbohydrate is the mostly widely consumed substance in the world after water – it's cheap, plentiful, sustainable and the basis for a healthy diet. Choosing delicious, safe and satiating low GI carbs reduces your day-long insulin levels more effectively than any other single dietary change.

Taste test

Try this simple test for yourself. Take a bite of fluffy white bread and keep it in your mouth for two minutes. What's left? Virtually nothing – the enzymes in your mouth have made short work of it. Now take a cooked (al dente) pasta shell (or other shape) and hold it in your mouth. After two minutes, you'll find you still have a clearly defined piece of pasta left. That's because the carbohydrates in the pasta are resistant to enzyme action. So it is with all the starches in low GI foods.

Yesterday, today and tomorrow . . .

About 10 000 years ago, when humans moved from hunting and gathering to farming, our diet was very different from what it is today, and it suited our bodies just fine. We ate a fair bit of meat and seafood, plenty of vegetables and fruits, tree seeds such as nuts and pulses and coarsely ground cereal grains. We may not have had any labour-saving devices, but preparation was pretty uncomplicated – we ground the grains between stones and cooked food over an open fire. This meant we digested and absorbed food slowly and the blood glucose rise after meals was gradual and prolonged.

That all changed with the 19th-century industrial revolution which brought prosperity and radical inventions – and a fundamental shift in our diet. We began to eat much more refined carbs and far fewer beans and pulses. And we tucked into sponge cakes and fluffy white breads all made with the powdery white flour that the high-speed roller mills were able to produce. We now know that this shift has triggered a string of unintended health effects, many of which are beginning to reach epidemic proportions. This new diet meant the blood glucose rise after a meal was higher and more prolonged, making the pancreas produce more insulin.

Traditional diets all around the world contain slowly digested and absorbed carbohydrate – foods we now know have a low GI. Today we eat more carbohydrate in the form of refined sugars, starches and cereal products. These high GI carbs have been shown to spike insulin levels, which can promote hunger and, over the long term, may increase the rates of obesity and other chronic diseases of ageing.

SO WHAT DOES GI HAVE TO DO WITH YOU?

Eating a lot of high GI foods can put pressure on your health because it pushes your body to extremes. This is especially true if you are overweight and sedentary. In the same way that the stormwater pipes of a city are over-loaded after a heavy downpour, your body's glucose response mechanisms are stretched after a load of quickly digested carbs.

Switching to eating mainly low GI carbs that slowly trickle glucose into your blood stream keeps your energy levels perfectly balanced and means you will feel fuller for longer between meals. The whole idea is to replace highly refined carbohydrate such as white bread, sugary treats and crispy, puffed cereals with less processed carbs such as wholegrain bread, pasta, beans, fruit and vegetables.

Only foods containing carbohydrates can have their GI measured. And although the GI applies to the carbo-hydrate, its 'value' – high or low – is influenced by how it is packaged in the food, including the presence of protein, fat and water.

 ## Health tip:

High GI foods eaten with low GI foods score somewhere in between, so there's no need to completely avoid eating high GI foods like baked potatoes. Just include some low GI foods at the same meal. You can live with a low GI diet – it's all about moderation.

GI – whoever thought of that?

It all began with researchers trying to discover the best foods for people with diabetes. The aim was to find out which carbohydrates raised blood glucose the least. Scientists found that when people ate a specified portion of ice-cream it raised their blood glucose just as much as the portion of potato did. Up till then everyone with diabetes was being told to avoid all sweets. Everyone just assumed that 'simple' sugar would raise their blood glucose more than bread and potatoes. These days we know the GI of hundreds of foods from studies all around the world. In Part 3 (page 101), you can check out the top 100 low GI foods.

Not so long ago we believed complex, starchy carbohydrates such as bread and potato were more slowly absorbed than the simple, sugary carbohydrate in cakes, biscuits, jams and honey. In learning about the GI of foods we've realised that this isn't true. Foods such as pasta and grain bread are off limits in many low carb fad diets – but it's precisely these carb foods that fill us up and give us energy. All you have to do is look for the low GI types.

Health tip:

When shopping and planning meals, choose smart carbs, the low GI ones that produce only gentle rises in blood glucose and insulin levels because they are slowly digested. Lowering insulin levels is the secret to long-term health.

Crisps vs chocolate bar

Which is better for your blood glucose? Most people with diabetes would see the chocolate bar as taboo, but by measuring the blood glucose rise after different foods scientists have proved this to be unfounded. Crisps and chocolate have an almost identical effect on blood glucose. *Why?*

The carbohydrate in chocolate is sucrose, which is 50 per cent fructose (which has little effect on blood glucose levels) and 50 per cent glucose (high GI), giving it a medium GI overall. In crisps the carbohydrate is cooked (swollen) starch, which is readily digested to yield 100 per cent glucose molecules. Therefore, fully cooked starch has twice the impact on blood glucose levels as the same quantity of sugar.

WHAT ARE THE BENEFITS OF LOW GI EATING?

Low GI eating has science on its side. It's not a diet. There are no strict rules or regimens to follow. It's essentially about making simple adjustments to your usual eating habits – such as swapping one type of bread or breakfast cereal for another. You'll find that you can live with it for life. Low GI eating:

- reduces your insulin levels
- lowers your cholesterol levels
- helps control your appetite
- halves your risk of heart disease and diabetes
- is suitable for your whole family
- means you are eating foods closer to the way nature intended
- doesn't defy commonsense!

Not only that. You will feel better and have more energy – and you don't have to deprive or discipline yourself. A low GI diet is *easy*.

How do you do it?

Low GI eating fits with the first dietary guideline of countries all around the world: 'Eat a wide variety of foods.' There is a large range of low GI foods from which to choose. In fact, low GI foods can be found in four of the five food groups:

- wholegrains and pasta in the bread and cereal group
- milk and yoghurt among the dairy foods
- pulses (beans, peas and lentils) of all types in the meat and alternatives group
- virtually all fruits and vegetables

This is what makes it so easy to eat the low GI way every meal, every day.

> **Did you know?**
>
> The foods most strongly associated with high GI diets are white bread and refined cereals. High intakes of fruit and vegetables are associated with lower GI diets.

GETTING STARTED ON LOW GI EATING

To get started, you need to:

- *eat* a lot more fruit and vegetables, pulses (beans, peas and lentils) and wholegrain products such as barley and traditional oats
- *pay attention* to breads and breakfast cereals – these foods contribute most to the glycaemic load of a typical British diet
- *minimise* refined flour products and starches such as crumpets, crackers, biscuits, rolls and pastries, irrespective of their fat and sugar content

• *avoid* high GI snacks such as pretzels, corn chips, rice cakes and crackers

In Part 2 (page 33) you'll find step-by-step guidelines for making the switch to everyday low GI eating.

Three key habits to ensure a low GI diet

1. If you eat breakfast cereal, check out the GI of your favourite brand – you might get quite a surprise. Most of the popular big-name cereals have high GI values in the 70s and above.
2. Choose low GI bread. Check the tables in this book or look for an accredited low GI symbol on the pack-aged bread you buy. Ask for a grainy bread whenever buying sandwiches. Steer clear of sweet biscuits, cakes, scones, doughnuts and bread rolls made of refined flour (except sourdough) as much as you can.
3. Eat fruit for at least one of your daily snacks and have a low fat milk drink or low fat yoghurt for another.

Getting familiar with the GI of popular carbs

In the table on pages 17 and 18 you will find some common carbohydrate foods, listed according to their GI value. Take a look to see where your favourite carbs fit on the GI scale.

Where does your favourite food fit on the GI scale?

LOW GI <55	MEDIUM GI 56–69	HIGH GI >70
FRUIT		
apples	canned apricots	watermelon
oranges	cantaloupe	
pears	mango	
peaches		
banana		
For more low GI fruits see pages 107–129		
VEGETABLES		
sweetcorn	new potatoes	chips
sweet potato	beetroot	mashed potato
baked beans		baked potato
BREADS		
wholegrain bread	pitta bread	white bread
fruit bread	croissant	wholemeal bread
		doughnuts
CEREALS/GRAINS		
pasta	couscous	jasmine rice
noodles	basmati rice	cornflakes
porridge		
muesli		
bran cereal		
SUGARS		
pure floral honey	sugar	glucose
maple syrup		maltodextrins
DAIRY FOODS		
ice-cream		
yoghurt		
custard		
SNACKS		
nuts	crisps	
chocolate		

(cont.)

LOW GI <55	MEDIUM GI 56–69	HIGH GI >70
BEVERAGES		
milk	beer	
juice	cordial	
flavoured milk	soft drink	

Note: Some foods such as cheese, eggs, bacon, meat, lettuce, avocado and fish don't appear on this table – because they don't contain any carbs.

GL (GLYCAEMIC LOAD) VS GI

Don't restrict high GI fruit and vegetables, other than potatoes. Because most are not major sources of carbs, their GI is not that important.

Your blood glucose rises and falls when you eat a meal containing carbohydrate. How high it rises and how long it remains high is critically important to your health and depends on the quality of the carbohydrate (its GI value) as well as the quantity of carbohydrate in your meal. Researchers at Harvard University came up with a term that combines these two factors – glycaemic load (GL).

GL = GI/100 x carbs per serving

Some people think that GL should be used instead of GI when comparing foods because it reflects the glycaemic impact of both the quantity and quality of carbohydrate in a food. But more often than not, it's low GI rather than low GL that best predicts good health outcomes.

So what should you use? Our advice is to stick with the GI in all but a few instances. When you choose low GI carbs, your diet is invariably healthy with the appropriate quantity and quality of carbohydrate. Following the alternate low GL path could mean you're eating a decidedly unhealthy diet, low in carbs and full of the wrong sorts of fats and proteins.

You may be wondering what the fuss is all about. Well, some carb-rich foods such as pasta – which have a good fill-up factor – have a low GI but could have a high GL if the serving size is large. Portion size still counts. And while it's true that a handful of high GI foods, such as watermelon, have a low GL, we don't want you to restrict any fruit and vegetable other than potato.

There's no denying that it is easier to overeat certain foods. This is where low GI foods are star performers – the versions with the lowest GI values also have the best fill-up factor. If you listen to your true appetite, you are far less likely to overeat when you are choosing low GI foods.

To give you the easy picture of the glycaemic impact of foods, we have taken both the GI and the GL into account in our tables (see page 219).

> Don't get carried away with GL: it doesn't distinguish between foods that are **low carb or slow carb**.

Avoiding the post-lunch dip

Have you ever experienced what nutritionists describe as the 'post-lunch dip'? It's that sleepy feeling that hits you, typically mid-afternoon. Your high carb lunch and the subsequent surge in insulin levels sends your blood glucose plummeting, driving you out to seek a sweet fix and some caffeine. The trick to preventing this dip is lowering the glycaemic load of your lunch: eat less carbohydrate, choose lower GI carbs and add some protein (such as canned tuna, a couple of eggs, some cottage cheese or lean meat or chicken). And tuck into as many green, red and yellow vegetables as possible.

EAT LOW GI CARBS TO LOSE WEIGHT

There is no doubt that reducing portion sizes and eating fewer calories will lead to weight loss. Just how you do this is the name of the game. These days, we are eating less fat but getting fatter. Instead of eating fewer calories we are eating more, especially in the form of high GI refined starches and sugars.

Cutting out all carbs is not the answer (remember the carb deficit problem we mentioned on page 9). The real solution to both weight loss and weight maintenance is to be choosy about the type of carbs you eat. Here are some good reasons why.

How do high GI carbs make us fat?

- Eating high GI carbs causes a surge of glucose in the blood.
- Although the body needs glucose, it doesn't want it all in one hit, so it pumps out insulin to drive the glucose out of the blood and into the tissues.
- Insulin switches muscle cells from fat burning to carbo-hydrate (glucose) burning.
- Insulin also directs excess fuels to storage – glucose to glycogen and fats to fat storage.
- The action of insulin means blood glucose levels begin to decline rapidly.
- The brain detects falling blood glucose and sends out hunger signals.
- Low levels of fuel and high levels of insulin then trigger the release of stress hormones such as adrenalin to scour the body for more glucose. This translates to hunger,

light-headedness and feeling shaky. The only way to relieve the state of hunger is with another snack.

How can low GI carbs help?

If you feel hungry all the time, low GI foods can help you turn off the switch. Here's how and why . . .

- Low GI foods are rich in carbohydrate – an appetite suppressant far superior to fat.
- Many low GI foods are less processed, which means they require more chewing – helping to signal satiety to your brain.
- Low GI foods often come in the company of fibre so they swell and create a greater feeling of fullness in your stomach.
- Low GI foods are more slowly digested, which means they stay in your intestines longer, keeping you feeling satisfied.
- Being slowly digested, low GI foods trickle glucose into your blood stream slowly, helping to ward off hunger.
- Low GI foods help overcome the body's natural tendency to slow down fuel usage (your metabolic rate) while dieting.

The fill-up factor

Can you imagine feeling satisfied after eating just a fraction of your usual calories? Low GI foods help make this possible.

In the early days of GI research at the University of Sydney, we discovered a match between the GI of foods and how satisfying they were to eat. Our readers regularly tell us how easy they find low GI diets because they feel far less hungry. We now know this has a scientific basis – secretion of one of the most powerful satiety hormones (called GLP-1) is higher after consuming the low GI version of your usual bread, breakfast cereal or rice.

Test for yourself and feel the difference

You can experience one benefit of low GI carbs with this simple breakfast challenge. Try out each of the following breakfasts on consecutive mornings, one high GI and one low GI, and feel the difference yourself. By mid-morning you'll be thinking better, feeling better and have more insight into your natural hunger and satiety cues with Breakfast 1.

Breakfast 1 – a low GI option
50 grams (1¾ oz) natural muesli
with 125 ml (4 fl oz) cup low fat milk
and ½ a banana

Breakfast 2 – a high GI option
30 grams (1 oz) cornflakes
with 250 ml (9 fl oz) low fat milk
and a few strawberries

 ## Health tip:

Low GI foods alleviate hunger, making it easier to eat less. Studies show that, on average, kilojoule intake is 20 per cent greater after consumption of high GI meals than after low GI meals.

> ### The weight of the evidence
>
> Studies in adults lasting up to 12 months have consistently shown that people lost more body fat following a diet rich in low GI carbs compared with conventional diets.
>
> In 2004, a study was published in the prestigious medical journal The Lancet confirming that changing only the GI of the carbohydrate in a diet (keeping everything else exactly the same), leads to reduced body fat in animals.

The bottom line: 4 keys to long-term weight loss

1. Choose low GI carbs. Eat regularly and try to include low GI carbs at every meal. This will stave off hunger and strengthen your resolve against temptation.
2. Reduce your fat intake by cutting out the saturated fat in foods such as chocolate, biscuits and crisps.
3. Snack smarter, snack low GI and say 'no thanks' to high GI biscuits, crackers, sweets and soft drinks.
4. Think balance and moderation. Eat a little less. Do a little more.

Health tip:

There's no magic button. It's no secret, either. The evidence from people who have lost weight and maintained it over the long haul is that they:

- Wanted to change their diet to improve their health
- Were willing to lose weight slowly
- Made lasting changes to their diet and activity patterns

LOW GI CARBS CAN REDUCE YOUR RISK OF DIABETES

Did you realise that the higher the GI of your diet, the greater your risk of diabetes? Yes, you read it right. An Australian study of 31,000 people over 10 years found that those who had the highest GI diets were more likely to develop diabetes. In fact they found that eating white bread (not sugar!) was the food most strongly related to the development of diabetes.

Foods with a high GI are digested quickly and cause a rapid rise in blood glucose, and an outpouring of insulin (the hormone that removes glucose from the blood and stores it in cells). If you're eating high GI meals all the time you end up with chronically high insulin levels which could contribute to insulin resistance. This means the cells that normally respond to insulin become insensitive to it, so your body thinks it has to make even more insulin to do the job.

Often, type 2 diabetes is only diagnosed once the pancreas (which produces insulin) is absolutely worn out and cannot maintain sufficient insulin production to normalise blood glucose. Before you get to that point, eating a moderately high carbohydrate, low GI diet can actually improve the function of your pancreas and improved glycaemic control can prevent the onset of type 2 diabetes.

In case you still have your doubts . . .

- In US studies of thousands of people followed up over eight years, researchers found that those who ate a high GI diet were almost twice as likely to develop type 2 diabetes. Interestingly, the effect was most pronounced in those with low levels of physical activity, a known way of overcoming insulin resistance.

- In the US in the past 100 years, the prevalence of obesity and type 2 diabetes has increased directly in proportion to the consumption of refined carbohydrate.

Are you at risk of type 2 diabetes?

About 1.8 million people in Britain are known to have diabetes and another million have diabetes but don't know it, and all are at risk of heart disease and stroke. To find out if you are at risk of type 2 diabetes, answer the following questions.

❐ 1. Tick the box if you have a family history of any of the following:

- diabetes
- heart disease
- high blood pressure
- polycystic ovarian syndrome

❐ 2. Tick the box if you are:

- overweight
- over 40 and of European descent; or over 25 and of Indian, Middle Eastern, African or Afro-Caribbean heritage
- a woman who had diabetes in pregnancy
- a woman who has polycystic ovarian syndrome

If you have ticked either or both boxes above you are at risk of developing type 2 diabetes and should discuss screening tests for this condition with your doctor.

What are the key signs and symptoms of diabetes?

- increased thirst
- going to the lavatory all the time – especially at night
- extreme tiredness
- unexplained weight loss
- genital itching or regular episodes of thrush
- poor healing of wounds
- blurred vision

For more information go to **www.diabetes. org.uk**

Did you know?:

Some diet books demonise sugar and advocate strict avoidance, but a modest serving of 2 teaspoons of sugar actually has a GL of only 7.

> A meal with a high GI can result in glucose concentrations twice the level compared with the same amount of food with a low GI.

Low GI carbs – giving people with diabetes a new lease on life

When it comes to diabetes, following a low GI diet can be as effective at lowering your blood glucose as taking diabetes tablets. This is not an exaggeration! A scientific analysis of 14 different studies from around the world of people with diabetes showed that low GI diets improved glycaemic control significantly more than high GI or conventional diets. Improved glycaemic control can prevent the onset and progression of diabetes complications.

On a day-to-day basis, low GI foods can minimise the peaks and troughs in blood glucose that make life so difficult when you have diabetes. Since they are slowly digested and absorbed, low GI foods reduce insulin demand – lessening the strain on the struggling pancreas of a person with type 2 diabetes and potentially lowering insulin requirements for those with type 1 diabetes. Lower insulin levels have the follow-on benefit of reducing the risk of large blood vessel damage, lessening the likelihood of developing heart disease.

The bottom line: the optimum diet for people with diabetes

There isn't any one optimum diet for all people with diabetes. Whether you eat higher fat, low fat, high protein, high carb or whatever, certain characteristics are desirable. They are:

- Eating regular meals and choosing slowly digested carbs with a low GI.
- Including plenty of vegetables and fruits.
- Eating only small amounts of saturated fat.
- Including a moderate amount of sugar and sugary foods.
- Drinking only a moderate quantity of alcohol.
- Including a minimum amount of salt and salty foods.

LOW GI CARBS & A HEALTHY HEART

Eating a high GI diet isn't only related to diabetes. Heart disease is the single biggest killer of Britons and having high glucose levels after meals is a predictor of future heart disease. Sound far fetched? Here's how it happens . . .

A high level of glucose in the blood means:

- excess glucose moves into cells lining the arteries, causing inflammation, thickening and stiffening – the making of 'hardened arteries'
- highly reactive, charged particles called 'free radicals' are formed which destroy the machinery inside the cell, eventually causing the cell death
- glucose adheres to cholesterol in the blood which promotes the formation of fatty plaque and prevents the body from breaking down excess cholesterol
- higher levels of insulin raises blood pressure and blood fats, while suppressing 'good' (HDL) cholesterol levels

How's your shape?

Fat around the middle part of our body (abdominal fat) increases our risk of heart disease, high blood pressure and diabetes. In contrast, fat on the lower part of the body, such as hips and thighs, doesn't carry the same health risk. Your body shape can be described according to your distribution of body fat as either an 'apple' or a 'pear' shape. There are significant health benefits in reducing your waist measurement, particularly if you have an 'apple' shape.

For more information on heart disease go to **www. heartuk.org.uk**

Halve your risk of heart attack with a low GI diet

This might sound like an inflated newspaper headline – it isn't! The results of a Harvard University study of over 100 000 people over 10 years found that those who ate more high GI foods had nearly twice the risk of heart attack compared with those eating low GI diets. This was independent of other risk factors such as age, obesity and smoking, although, surprisingly, in those who were lean, high GI foods did not pose excess risk.

The bottom line: reduce your risk of heart disease

Along with exercise, a diet rich in slowly digested, low GI carbs will reduce your risk of heart disease in several ways. By lowering your blood glucose after meals and reducing high insulin levels, you'll have:

- healthier blood vessels that are more elastic, dilate more easily and aid blood flow

- improved blood flow and less inflammation
- more potential for weight loss and therefore less pressure on the heart
- better blood fats – more of the good cholesterol and less of the bad

LOW GI CARBS AND PCOS

Polycystic ovarian syndrome (PCOS) is thought to affect one in four women in developed countries. Characteristics of the syndrome can include irregular periods, infertility, heavy body hair growth, obstinate body fat, diabetes and cardiovascular disease. In many women it goes undiagnosed because the symptoms may be subtle, such as faint facial hair.

Insulin resistance – where the body resists the normal actions of the hormone insulin – is at the root of PCOS. In an effort to overcome insulin resistance the body secretes more insulin than normal. Among other effects, this leads to growth and multiplication of cells in the ovaries, causing hormonal imbalances.

The problem of insulin resistance

Elevations in blood glucose after eating high GI foods are followed by elevations in insulin. When insulin levels are chronically raised, the cells that usually respond to insulin become resistant to its signals. The body responds by secreting more insulin, a neverending vicious cycle that spells trouble on many fronts.

A low GI diet is invaluable in the management of insulin resistance because it will:

- result in lower blood glucose after meals and thereby
- *reduce the demand for insulin* which can

- help *appetite control* and improve *weight loss*
- normalise fertility hormones

Managing the symptoms of PCOS

> For more nformation on PCOS, go to **www.verity-pcos.org.uk** or **www.diagnose mefirst.com**

To manage PCOS symptoms effectively you need to take charge of your health by managing your weight (body fat), making the change to low GI eating and building more activity into your life. The benefits will include:

- improving PCOS symptoms
- achieving and maintaining healthy weight
- controlling blood glucose and insulin levels
- boosting fertility
- gaining control and quality of life

The bottom line: eating well if you have PCOS

If you have PCOS, eating well is not just about managing your weight. It can also improve your overall health and energy levels, and reduce your risk of developing diabetes or heart disease. It's essential to eat in a way that helps to control your insulin levels. This means eating small regular meals and snacks spread throughout the day and choosing low GI carbs. Your healthy eating plan should include:

- fresh vegetables and salads
- fresh fruit
- wholegrain breads and cereals
- low fat dairy foods or non-dairy alternatives such as soya
- fish, lean meat, skinless chicken, eggs, pulses (beans, peas and lentils) and soya products

- small amounts of healthy fats including nuts, seeds, avocados, olives, olive oil, rapeseed oil or peanut oil

LOW GI CARBS & ANTI-AGEING

Scientists are beginning to find connections between high blood glucose levels and diseases such as dementia. As we age, abnormal protein deposits form in parts of the brain and eventually interfere with normal mental functioning. High glucose levels accelerate this process. Indeed, the abnormal proteins are called advanced glycosylated endproducts (AGE for short!).

To get a feel for how this happens, think about the browning reactions that occur naturally during cooking – think of toasting, baking and grilling. When sugar is present, the reactions occur faster, sometimes leading to excess browning, i.e. burning!

The same reactions between sugars and proteins occur very slowly inside the body. Gradually the proteins become burdened by the presence of the freeloading sugar molecules and lose the ability to do their job. When that happens to a long-lived protein like the collagen in skin, the elasticity and natural glow of youthful skin fades. The result: wrinkles. We can't stop it entirely but we can slow it down.

PART 2

Everyday
low gi eating:
Making the switch

Don't diet. Focus on eating well and moving more. Enjoy food and make sure you choose a diet that will give you energy to burn. And remember, we all need to be active. Every day.

LOW GI EATING: FOR EVERYBODY, EVERY DAY, EVERY MEAL

We love hearing our readers' stories of how low GI eating has transformed their lives. Success stories like the woman with gestational diabetes who swapped high GI for low GI carbs and found she did not need to take insulin – their stories inspire us all.

These examples and hundreds more have helped us understand what works for people and what doesn't. And that's what this section is about. It covers the sorts of questions our readers and clients actually ask. The answers will show you how easy it is to make simple changes in your food choices that will have a big impact on your overall health – for life.

One of our most frequently received requests is 'just tell me what to eat!'. So, in this section, we focus on food and give you some simple guidelines about making the switch to everyday low GI eating. You'll find out how to:

- put together a balanced low GI meal
- how to eat low GI when socialising with friends and family and eating out
- what to buy and how to stock your larder

Exactly how you incorporate low GI eating into your life is up to you. Some people want to eat low GI foods all the time, others some of the time. That's OK. There's room for both approaches. And in reality that's how we eat, too.

LOW GI EATING – THE BASICS

First let's show you how easy it is to eat the low GI way. There's no specific order in which you have to do things, no strict week-by-week list of diet do's and don'ts, no counting, calculating or measuring. However, there are some basics – daily and weekly eating and activity habits essential to good health. After all, this is not a magic pill. It's an eating plan that will help you nourish your body, feel better and promote optimum health. So, to help you get started, here are the basics.

Every day you need to:

- Eat at least three meals – don't skip meals. Eat snacks too if you are hungry.
- Eat fruit at least twice – fresh, frozen, cooked, dried or juice.
- Eat vegetables at least twice – cooked, raw, salads, soups, juices and snacks.
- Eat a cereal at least once – such as bread, breakfast cereal, pasta, noodles, rice and other grains in a whole-grain or low GI form.
- Accumulate 60 minutes of physical activity (including incidental activity and planned exercise).

Health tip:

Make healthy eating a habit. Here are some tips.
- Make breakfast a priority.
- If it's healthy keep it handy.

- Don't buy food you want to avoid.
- Focus on the positive – think about what to eat, rather than what not to eat.
- Listen to your appetite – eat when you are hungry and stop when you are full (you don't have to leave a clean plate all the time).

Every week you need to:

- Eat beans, peas and/or lentils – at least twice. This includes baked beans, chickpeas, red kidney beans, butter beans, split peas and foods made from them such as hummous and dhal.
- Eat fish and seafood at least once, preferably twice – fresh, smoked, frozen or canned.
- Eat nuts regularly – just a tiny handful.

What to choose?

- ❏ Low GI breads – wholegrain, sourdough and other low GI breads
- ❏ Low GI breakfast cereals – muesli, porridge, rolled oats, etc.
- ❏ Low GI cereals – pasta, noodles, basmati rice, whole-grains etc.
- ❏ Lean meat and skinless chicken
- ❏ Low fat milk, yoghurt, or soya based, calcium-enriched alternatives
- ❏ Omega-3-enriched eggs
- ❏ Olive and rapeseed oils as your main cooking and salad oils

Three tips for making the switch

Here's how you can make it easier to develop and maintain your new low GI eating habits.

Start with something simple
Nothing inspires like success so attack the easiest changes first, such as eating one piece of fruit every day.

Do it gradually
Choose one aspect of your diet that you want to work on, for example, eating more vegetables, and make that your focus for at least six weeks. It can take at least this long for a new behaviour to become habit.

Don't expect 100 per cent success
A lapse in your eating habits is not failure. It's a natural part of developing new habits. Falling over is easy, but getting up and keeping going can take real effort. Believe in yourself. You can do it!

How does your daily diet rate?

Try our quick quiz.

1. I mostly eat reduced fat or semi-skimmed dairy foods. ❑ YES ❑ NO
2. I include at least 250 ml (9 fl oz) milk or 200 grams (7 oz) yoghurt or calcium-enriched soya alternative every day. ❑ YES ❑ NO
3. When I drink alcohol, I would mostly drink no more than two standard drinks per day. (Tick YES if you don't drink alcohol.) ❑ YES ❑ NO

4. I generally don't eat takeaway/fast food more than once a week. ❑ YES ❑ NO

5. I eat regular meals. ❑ YES ❑ NO

6. I eat skinless chicken. ❑ YES ❑ NO

7. I avoid adding salt to my food. ❑ YES ❑ NO

8. I include fish or some other seafood at least once a week. ❑ YES ❑ NO

9. I rarely eat packaged snacks such as crisps. ❑ YES ❑ NO

10. I would usually eat five or more different vegetables in a day. ❑ YES ❑ NO

11. I use an unsaturated margarine spread rather than butter. (Tick YES if you use neither.) ❑ YES ❑ NO

12. I use unsaturated oils such as olive, rapeseed, sunflower, sesame, macadamia and mustard seed for cooking and food preparation. ❑ YES ❑ NO

13. I eat at least one piece of fruit every day.

14. I limit fatty meats such as sausages, luncheon meat, salami, hamburger mince, lamb chops to less than once a week. ❑ YES ❑ NO

Score 1 point for each YES

What your score means.

12–14   Excellent. It looks like you have the balance right and your basic dietary habits are sound. Read on to make sure what you are eating is low GI.

9–11   It sounds like your dietary habits aren't bad but you have work to do in achieving the right balance and lowering the GI of your diet.

Less than 9   Oops! Room for a lot of improvement here
               – just to boost the basic nutritional quality
               of your diet. So, back to the basics (page
               35) and good luck.

THIS FOR THAT

Simply substituting high GI foods with low GI alternatives
will give your overall diet a lower GI and deliver the benefits
of a low GI diet. Here's how you can put slow carbs to work
in your day by cutting back consumption of high GI foods
and replacing them with alternatives that are just as tasty.

If you are currently eating this (high GI) food	Choose this (low GI) lternative instead
Biscuits	A slice of wholegrain bread or toast with jam, fruit spread or Nutella®
Breads such as soft white or wholemeal; smooth textured breads, rolls, scones	Dense breads with wholegrains, wholegrain and stoneground flour and sourdough; look for low GI labelling
Breakfast cereals – most commercial, processed cereals including cornflakes, rice bubbles, cereal bars	Traditional rolled oats, muesli and commercial low GI brands which have been glycaemic index tested – look for low GI labelling
Cakes and pastries	Raisin toast, fruit loaf and fruit buns are healthier baked options; yoghurts and low fat mousses also make great snacks or desserts

(cont.)

If you are currently eating this (high GI) food	Choose this (low GI) lternative instead
Crisps and other packet snacks such as pretzels, Hula Hoops Crackers	Fresh grapes or strawberries or dried fruit and nuts Crisp vegetable strips such as carrot, pepper or celery
Doughnuts and croissants	Try a skimmed milk cappuccino or smoothie instead
Chips	Leave them out! Have salad or extra vegetables instead. Corn on the cob or coleslaw are better takeaway options
Sweets	Chocolate is lower GI but high in fat. Healthier options are sultanas, dried apricots and other dried fruits
Muesli bars	Try a nut bar or dried fruit and nut mix
Potatoes	Prepare smaller amounts of potato and add some sweet potato or sweetcorn. Canned new potatoes are an easy and lower GI option. You can also try sweet potato, yam or baby new potatoes – or just replace with other low GI or no-GI vegetables
Rice, especially large serves of it in dishes such as risotto, nasi goreng, fried rice	Try basmati rice, Japanese Koshihikari (sushi) rice, pearled barley, cracked wheat (bulghur), quinoa, pasta or noodles
Soft drink and fruit juice drink	Use a diet variety if you drink these often. Fruit juice has a lower GI (but it is not a lower calorie option). Water is best

(cont.)

If you are currently eating this (high GI) food	Choose this (low GI) lternative instead
Sugar	Moderate the quantity. Consider pure floral honey, apple juice, fruit sugars (fructose) such as Fruisana® or Tate & Lyle Fruit Sugar and grape nectar as alternatives

LOW GI EATING GIVES YOU A HEALTHY BALANCE

Everyday low GI eating is easy. Although the glycaemic index itself has a scientific basis, you don't need to crunch numbers or do any sort of mental arithmetic to make sure you are eating a healthy low GI diet.

By following the low GI eating basics we described earlier (page 35) you'll find you are enjoying foods from all the food groups and reaping the benefits of 40-plus nutrients. You'll also be taking in the protective anti-oxidants and phytochemicals your body needs each day for long-term health and wellbeing.

FAQs about the GI

Are sugary foods all high GI?
No. This is one of the most widely perpetuated myths, even by so-called proponents of the GI – the sweeter it is the more it spikes your blood glucose. Long-held beliefs are hard to shift. In our food finder (page 101) you'll

discover many deliciously sweet low GI foods from ice-cream and chocolate milk to floral honey and fresh fruit.

Should I add up the GI each day?

No. In some of our early books we included sample menus and calculated an estimated GI for the day. As our understanding of the GI grew and we talked to our clients and heard from our readers, we realised how unnecessary and misleading this was. The GI value of a food can be altered by the way it is processed or cooked, so we don't believe it is possible to calculate a precise GI value for recipes or to predict the GI of a menu for the whole day. That's why we now prefer simply to categorise foods as low, medium or high GI in most circumstances. We have also found that many people who simply substitute low for high GI foods in their everyday meals and snacks reduce the overall GI of their diet, gain better blood glucose control and lose weight.

Should I avoid all high GI foods?

No. There is no need to eat only low GI foods. While you will benefit from eating low GI carbs at each meal, this doesn't have to be at the exclusion of all others. High GI foods such as potatoes and wholemeal bread make a valuable nutritional contribution to our diet and when eaten with protein foods or low GI carbs, the overall GI value of the meal will be medium.

What's the GI of meat, chicken, fish, eggs and cheese?

There is no point wondering about the GI of meat, eggs, fish and cheese – these foods don't have one. The same goes for most of the vegetable kingdom – foods such as broccoli, tomatoes, pumpkin and parsnips contain so little carbohydrate that their GI is either impossible to measure or irrelevant. But these foods are part of a healthy, balanced diet and we're asked about them all the time, so we have included them in our tables.

Should I be pedantic about GI values?

No. Whether a food's GI is 56 or 64 isn't biologically distinguishable. Normal day-to-day variation in the human body could obscure the difference in these values. Generally a variation of more than 10 could be considered different.

Does a food's GI value make it good or bad for you?

No. When choosing foods the glycaemic index is not intended to be used on its own. A food's GI value doesn't make it good or bad for you. The nutritional benefits of different foods are many and varied. Meat and fish are protein rich, wholegrains are rich in carbs, while fruit and vegetables are rich in vitamins, minerals and anti-oxidants. We suggest you base your food choices on the overall nutritional content, along with the amount of saturated fat, salt, fibre and, of course, the GI value. In the food finder we highlight some of the many important nutritional benefits of the top 100 low GI foods.

Avoid these common mistakes about food and eating

Giving food a low priority

People who give food a low priority often skip meals, grab food on the run, or become overhungry then overindulge to compensate. Usually all three and in this order! Some people take better care of their cars than their bodies. Remember, food is our fuel for a healthy life – we need it to live, breathe and go about our everyday tasks. So schedule choosing, preparing and eating healthy food into your day.

Not eating enough vegetables

Three vegetables on your dinner plate is not enough. You need to eat a variety of vegetables in different forms at different times of the day. When you follow our '1, 2, 3 ... putting it on the plate' plan (see page 47), you'll find it easy to enjoy fruit or vegetables at every meal.

Comparing your food intake with others

This is a pointless exercise. First, it's almost impossible to get an accurate picture of what other people really eat (they lie). Secondly, food requirements vary so much between people. Gender, size, activity and age all come into play along with a range of individual factors. Some lucky people just need to eat more than others.

Going on a restrictive diet

If you want to lose body fat and keep it off, restrictive dieting isn't the answer. This kind of dieting that has you obsessively counting calories and cutting out whole food groups is almost impossible to stick to in the long term and can set you on the dreaded 'yo yo' dieting cycle. Instead of trying to control every urge to sneak a morsel of chocolate or feeling guilty when you fall off the dieting wagon, give yourself a treat and enjoy a regular splurge. It's a more sensible approach to eating – and living.

The only way to lose weight and body fat permanently is to change your eating habits and include regular physical activity in your day. We know this can mean changing the habits of a lifetime. We know this is hard. That's why we suggest you make gradual changes, one step at a time, that fit in with your way of living and that you can maintain for life.

Filling the shopping trolley with 'fat-free' foods

Low fat or no fat is a recent trend in food manufacturing. But '99% fat free' doesn't mean calorie free; all too often much of it is high GI and will still cause weight gain if eaten to excess. Here's an example. Take a regular 100 ml/50 gram (3½ fl oz/1¾ oz) scoop of vanilla ice-cream:

- regular ice-cream (10% fat) = 375 kJ/90 Kcal (average)
- reduced fat ice-cream (6.5% fat) = 355 kJ/85 Kcal (average)
- low fat ice-cream (less than 4% fat) = 295 kJ/70 Kcal (average)

So, enjoy a scoop of low fat ice-cream, but say 'no thanks' to seconds.

Health tip:

Commit time to being more active. This is just as important as committing to three meals a day, or substituting low GI for high. In our modern lifestyle, exercise seldom just happens. Like anything else that we want to do, we have to plan it and allocate time for it. It's not 'optional'.

Food minus exercise = fat

SIMPLE STEPS TO DEVELOPING GOOD EATING HABITS

Listen to your appetite

Eat when you are hungry and put your knife and fork down when you are full (not stuffed). If you have a tendency to overeat, serve food in the kitchen and bring it to the table to remove the temptation of helping your-self to seconds and thirds at the table. Also, be aware that we all have 'hungry days', so it's quite normal to eat more on some days and less on others.

Watch for signs of non-hungry eating

It's also normal to reach for food when you are tired, bored or stressed. We call this 'non-hungry eating'. It isn't wrong, but it tends to contribute to overeating. If you are aware of it, you can do something about it – such as drink a glass of water or make yourself busy.

Think about what to eat, rather than what not to eat

Be positive. Make planning and preparing meals fun. Our food finder on page 101 is packed with hundreds of delicious foods, meal ideas and recipes you can enjoy every day.

Eat regularly

Remember the basics: three meals a day is a must. It's probably easier to stick to regular meal and snack times to start with, too. So make meals a time to relax and enjoy food whether you are on your own or with family or friends – you are more likely to feel satisfied if you do.

If it's healthy, keep it handy

Stock your cupboards and fridge with healthy low GI foods and snacks. Increase your chances of eating them by keeping them handy!

Keep occasional foods out of sight

Make overeating as hard as possible by putting occasional and treat foods well out of sight, preferably out of easy reach.

Health tip:

Low GI foods can form the basis of a healthy and flexible diet whoever you are and wherever you live.

1, 2, 3 . . . PUTTING IT ON THE PLATE

Main meals for most Britons consist of some sort of meat (or chicken or fish) with vegetables and potato (or rice or pasta). This is a good start and a little fine-tuning will ensure a healthy, balanced meal. All you need to do is adjust your proportions to match our 'plate'. Here are the three simple steps to put together a balanced low GI meal.

1 is for carb

It's an essential, although sometimes forgotten part of a balanced meal. What do you feel like? A grain like rice, barley or cracked wheat? Pasta, noodles or bean vermicelli? Or perhaps a high carb vegetable like sweetcorn, sweet potato or pulses such as beans, peas and lentils? Include at least one low GI carb per meal.

2 is for protein

Include some protein at each meal. It lowers the glycaemic load by replacing some of the carbohydrate – not all! It also helps satisfy the appetite.

3 is for fruit and vegetables

This is the part we often go without. If anything it should have the highest priority in a meal, but a meal based solely on fruit and low carb vegetables won't be sustaining for long. A plain salad sandwich is a recipe for hunger.

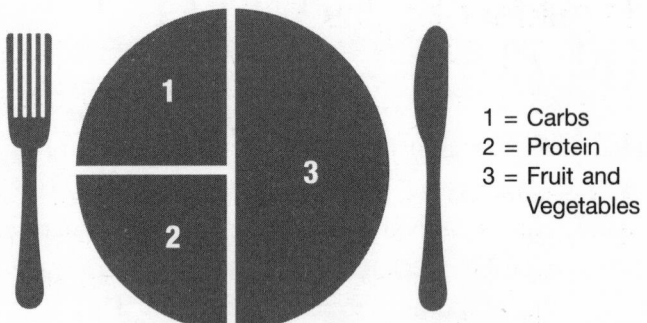

1 = Carbs
2 = Protein
3 = Fruit and Vegetables

The plate model is adaptable to any serving sizes.

- As long as you keep food to the proportions shown here, the meal will be balanced.
- As long as the types of food you choose fit within the guidelines for healthy eating, then you should have a healthy diet overall.

 ## Health tip:

Choose healthy foods that you like eating – put them together to make balanced, low GI meals.

BREAKFASTS THAT SUSTAIN YOU THROUGH THE MORNING

No doubt you know it's a good idea to eat breakfast if you want to keep healthy, but did you realise that your food choices may also be a critical factor? Firing up your engine with high GI crispy flakes or soft, light toast provides a short-lived fuel supply that will send you in search of a top-up within a few hours. If you want something to nourish your body and sustain you right through the morning, follow our breakfast basics.

Breakfast basics

Choose foods from each group – carbohydrate, protein and fruit and vegetables.

1. **Carbohydrate** – breakfast cereal, bread, baked beans
3. **Protein** – low fat milk, calcium-enriched soya milk, low fat yoghurt, eggs, tofu, lean ham or bacon, sardines or a little cheese
3. **Fruit and vegetables** – the choice is yours, fresh, frozen or canned fruit and vegetables, dried fruit, fruit or vegetable juice

> **Eating breakfast can improve:**
>
> - speed in short-term memory tests
> - alertness, which may help with memory and learning
> - mood, calmness and reduce feeling of stress
>
> Breakfast also helps schoolchildren do better in creativity tests.

Health tip:

A healthy breakfast including wholegrains and fruit is a great start in meeting your daily fibre intake.

Seven everyday low GI breakfasts

Kaye's Favourite Breakfast

1. **Carbohydrate**: natural muesli
2. **Protein**: skimmed milk, low fat natural yoghurt
3 **Fruit**: strawberries

Add a little skimmed milk to a big bowl of natural muesli to moisten, plus a generous dollop of low fat natural yoghurt. Top with a handful of chopped strawberries (or any other fruit).

Creamy Porridge

1. **Carbohydrate**: rolled oats
2. **Protein**: skimmed milk
3. **Fruit**: raisins, honey

Cook traditional rolled oats according to the packet instructions in skimmed milk to make a creamier porridge. Serve topped with a scattering of raisins and a drizzle of honey.

Fruit Toast with Ricotta and Pear

1. **Carbohydrate**: dense fruit and nut bread
2. **Protein**: reduced fat ricotta cheese
3. **Fruit**: pear

Spread thick slices of a dense fruit and nut bread with reduced fat ricotta cheese and top with sliced fresh pear (peeled if you prefer). Sprinkle with cinnamon sugar to serve.

Eggs with Mushrooms and Parsley

1. **Carbohydrate**: soya and linseed bread
2 **Protein**: eggs
3 **Vegetables**: mushrooms, parsley

Slice a generous handful of button mushrooms and cook in a little olive oil. When softened, add some fresh chopped parsley and season with salt and pepper if desired. Serve on toasted soya and linseed bread with poached or scrambled eggs. A grilled tomato alongside makes this breakfast extra tasty.

> **Did you know?**
>
> Highly processed breakfast cereals are some of the highest GI foods and cost a lot more than traditional cereal grains such as porridge.

Oats with Apple, Raisins and Almonds

1. **Carbohydrate**: rolled oats
2. **Protein**: skimmed milk
3. **Fruit and nuts**: apple, raisins, almonds

Soak traditional rolled oats in skimmed milk in the refrigerator overnight. Next morning add 1 grated Granny Smith apple, a small handful of raisins and a sprinkle of slivered almonds, stir and serve.

Smoothie 'On the Go'

1. **Carbohydrate**: processed bran cereal
2 **Protein**: semi-skimmed milk, low fat yoghurt
3. **Fruit**: banana, honey

Combine 1 banana, 1 tablespoon of bran cereal, 250 ml (9 fl oz) of low fat milk, 2 teaspoons of honey and 100 grams (31/2 oz) of low fat yoghurt in a blender. Blend until smooth and thick.

Lazy Weekend French Toast

1. Carbohydrate: sourdough bread
2. Protein: eggs, skimmed milk
3 Fruit: pear or apple

Beat together 2 eggs, 60 ml (2 fl oz) of skimmed milk and 1 teaspoon of pure vanilla extract. Dip 4 thick slices of sourdough bread in the egg mixture, then cook over medium heat in a lightly greased non-stick frypan for 2–3 minutes on each side until golden. Serve topped with pan-fried pear or apple slices and a sprinkling of cinnamon.

LIGHT & LOW, THE SMART CARB LUNCH

It is important to take a break and refuel properly at lunchtime. A healthy low GI lunch will help maintain energy levels and concentration throughout the afternoon and reduce the temptation to snack on something indulgent later in the day. It does not need to be a big meal. In fact, if you find yourself feeling sleepy in the afternoon, cut back on the carbs and boost the protein and light vegetables at lunchtime. (Of course a cup of coffee may help too!). Try these light meal suggestions for lunch – or for dinner if you prefer to eat your main meal at lunchtime.

Lunch and light meal basics

Choose a food or foods from each group – carbs, protein and fruit and vegetables.

1. Start with a low GI carb such as wholegrain or sourdough bread, pasta, noodles, sweetcorn or canned mixed beans.
2. Add some protein such as fresh or canned salmon or tuna, lean meat, sliced chicken, reduced fat cheese or egg.
3. Plus vegetables or salad to help fill you up. A large salad made with a variety of vegetables would be ideal. Round off the meal with fruit.

Seven everyday low GI lunches and light meals

Minestrone and Toast

1. Carbohydrate: beans, pasta, sweet potato, barley, rice, low GI bread
2. Protein: Parmesan, beans
3. Vegetables: tomato, carrots, onion, celery and other soup vegetables

When making minestrone yourself or buying it ready-made, choose a filling combination that includes pulses (beans, peas and lentils) and plenty of chopped vegetables. Serve topped with some freshly shaved Parmesan and enjoy with low GI toast or a crusty grainy roll.

Tasty soups for light meals and lunches

- lentil and spinach soup
- split pea and ham soup
- chicken and sweetcorn soup
- long or short soup with noodles and tofu
- bean soup
- tom yum soup
- pumpkin soup
- mushroom soup

Health tip:

Of all foods eaten by populations around the world, pulses (beans, peas and lentils) are associated with the longest lifespan. Aim to include them at least twice a week.

Pulses

Versatile, filling, nutritious beans, peas and lentils are low in calories and provide a valuable source of protein and carbs, which is why we include them as both a carb and protein food in our ingredient listing.

Snack Bar Sandwich

1. **Carbohydrate**: mixed grain, soya and linseed or seeded bread
2. **Protein**: canned salmon, tuna or hardboiled egg
3. **Vegetables**: tomato, sprouts, grated carrot, finely sliced onion rings, mixed salad greens

Try a smear of mayonnaise on the bread instead of margarine.

Lebanese Roll-ups

1. **Carbohydrate**: wholemeal flatbread, hummous
2. **Protein**: reduced fat cheese, hummous
3. **Vegetables**: tabbouleh, shredded lettuce

Spread flatbread with hummous, roll up around a filling of tabbouleh and shredded lettuce sprinkled with grated cheese and warm through in a sandwich press.

Mexican Bean Tortilla

1. **Carbohydrate**: Mexican beans (red kidney beans in a tomato and mild chilli sauce), corn tortilla
2. **Protein**: reduced fat cheese, red kidney beans
3 **Vegetables**: avocado, shredded lettuce, sliced tomato

Warm about 75 grams (2½ oz) of beans and serve in a corn tortilla with 2–3 avocado slices, lots of shredded lettuce, tomato slices and grated reduced fat cheese.

Simple Long Soup

1. Carbohydrate: vermicelli noodles, creamed sweetcorn
2. Protein: chicken stock, chicken, egg
3. Vegetables: carrot, shallots

Bring 500 ml (17 fl oz) of chicken stock to the boil, add a handful of dry vermicelli noodles and 1 finely diced carrot. Cook the noodles and carrot for 3–4 minutes then stir in 125 grams (4½ oz) of creamed sweetcorn, strips of cooked chicken (a great way to use leftovers) and chopped shallots. Heat through. Beat 1 egg and slowly pour it into the boiling soup in a thin stream, stirring quickly.

Frittata

1. Carbohydrate: sweet potato, sweetcorn kernels
2. Protein: egg, skimmed milk, lean ham, reduced fat cheese
3. Vegetables: courgette, red and green peppers, tomato, onion, mushroom, shallots and parsley

Stir-fry about 200 grams (7 oz) of chopped vegetables with 2 slices of chopped ham in a little oil until soft. Beat 2 eggs with 125 ml (4 fl oz) of skimmed milk and season with freshly ground black pepper and 1 tablespoon of chopped parsley. Pour the egg mixture over the vegetables and cook over a low heat (preferably covered) until set. Sprinkle a little grated cheese over the top and brown under a hot grill.

Salmon Salad with Chilli Dressing

1. Carbohydrate: sourdough or wholegrain bread
2. Protein: red salmon
3. Vegetables: cherry tomatoes, red onion, red and yellow peppers, mixed salad and baby spinach leaves

Combine 1 small can of red salmon (drained and flaked) with ½ punnet of cherry tomatoes, slices of red onion, red and yellow pepper strips and mixed salad and baby spinach leaves. Toss in a chilli dressing made from olive oil, lemon juice and minced chilli and serve with bread or a crusty roll.

TAKE TIME OVER ONE MAIN MEAL EVERY DAY

What to make for dinner is the perennial question. Most people know that eating well is important, but it can be hard to get motivated to cook at the end of a long day. You don't have to spend hours preparing. If your cupboards and refrigerator are stocked with the right foods, you should be able to put a meal together in under 30 minutes.

Involve everybody at mealtimes

When you can, involve everybody in the household in choosing and preparing meals. Even if you love cooking, it's fun having an offsider – someone to spin the lettuce, turn the meat, set the table, or simply chat to while you chop or stir, etc. It's also a great opportunity to find out about what's happening in other family members' lives! Lots of our readers say they hate cooking, but preparing and cooking meals is an integral part of healthy eating. Easy meals for family and friends can revolve around platters of foods on the table from which everyone can serve themselves. This avoids any complaints about being served foods they don't like.

If you live alone . . .

If you live alone, why not prepare food for two and put a meal away for another night? To avoid overeating on the night you cook, divide up all the food before you sit down to eat. Make use of partially prepared convenience foods such as chopped salads, filled pastas and frozen mixed vegetables to make meal preparation a little easier.

If you like using frozen meals, choose a low fat type and add your own cooked vegetables to bulk it out. Make a point of taking time over your meal and enjoy what you're eating. Don't gulp it down without thinking in front of the television – you can end up eating more than you should. The experts have even given this habit a name: 'mindless eating'.

Eating together as a family not only improves relationships but eating habits, too. In a recent study, researchers found that children who regularly ate dinner at home had:

- higher intakes of fruit and vegetables

- higher nutrient intakes

- lower intakes of soft drinks and fried food

- lower saturated fat intakes as a proportion of their total energy intake

Main meal basics

Choose a food or foods from each group – carbs, protein and fruit and vegetables.

1. **Start** with a low GI carb such as sweet potato, pasta, noodles, sweetcorn, beans, peas or lentils.
2. **Add** some protein such as lean meat or chicken, fish or seafood, eggs and pulses.
3. **Plus** plenty of vegetables and salad to help fill you up – remember our plate model (page 48). A large salad made with a variety of vegetables would be ideal. Round off the meal with fruit.

Alcohol

If you like to have a drink, that's OK – there might even be some health benefits. Both red and white wines contain powerful anti-oxidants, which may work to reduce heart disease risk. But go easy. While studies show some health benefits in those who drink one to two standard drinks a day, compared to none at all, there is a very steep increase in health risk from increased consumption. 100 ml/3½ fl oz (for women) to 200 ml/7 fl oz (for men) of wine per day is the maximum recommended by health authorities. Keep in mind that alcohol:

- is addictive
- can be fattening
- contributes to dehydration

Seven everyday low GI main meals

Peppered Steak with Sweet Potato Mash

1. **Carbohydrate**: sweet potato (allow 115 grams/4 oz per person)
2. **Protein**: fillet, rump or topside steak (allow 150 grams/ 5½ oz per person)
3. **Vegetables**: mushrooms, green beans, salad vegetables including tomato

Sprinkle steak with pepper seasoning and barbecue or pan-fry. Serve with steamed sweet potato mashed with skimmed milk, sliced mushrooms cooked in a little olive oil, steamed green beans and a crisp salad tossed in a vinaigrette dressing.

Lamb and Vegetables

1. **Carbohydrate**: canned or baby new potatoes (allow 2–3 per person), sweetcorn on the cob (allow 1 small cob per person)
2. **Protein**: trimmed lamb loin chops or cutlets (allow 200 grams/7 oz per person) or lean lamb fillet (allow 150 grams/5½ oz per person)
3. **Vegetables**: carrot, broccoli (allow 100 grams/3½ oz per person)

For extra flavour, coat the meat with a spice blend such as chermoula or garlic and rosemary and allow to 'dry marinate' for about 20 minutes. Barbecue or grill lamb (trim off the fat if you are cooking chops). Serve with steamed vegetables – baby new potatoes, corn cob, sliced carrots and broccoli florets – and your favourite condiments.

Thai-style Kebabs

1. **Carbohydrate**: basmati rice
2. **Protein**: chicken, beef, firm white-fleshed fish, or tofu (allow 500 grams/ 1 lb 2 oz for 4 kebabs)
3. **Vegetables**: courgette, onion, mushrooms (add extra vegetables such as red pepper if you like)

Prepare a marinade using the following ingredients: juice and grated rind of 2 limes, 1 teaspoon of crushed garlic, 1 tablespoon of grated ginger, 2 teaspoons of chopped chilli, 1 tablespoon of chopped lemongrass and 1 tablespoon of chopped coriander.

Marinate diced chicken, beef, firm fish or tofu, 2 courgettes sliced into rounds, 1 onion quartered and layers separated and 8 mushrooms, halved, or quartered if they are large, for at least 20 minutes, longer if you have the time. Thread the different ingredients alternately on skewers, brush with a little oil and barbecue or grill under a preheated grill for about 10 minutes, turning regularly and basting with the marinade. Serve with basmati rice and lime wedges.

Honey and Mustard Pork

1. **Carbohydrate**: baby new potatoes (allow 2–3 per person), or sweet potato (allow 115 grams /4 oz per person)
2. **Protein**: pork cutlets (allow 200 grams (7 oz) per person)
3. **Vegetables**: red pepper, broccoli

Prepare a marinade with the following: 1 tablespoon of olive oil, 1 tablespoon of seeded mustard, 2 teaspoons of honey, 2 tablespoons of lemon juice and freshly ground black pepper. Trim the fat off the pork cutlets, marinate for an hour then pan-fry for about 5 minutes on each side. Cut the peppers into strips lengthwise and stir-fry in the remaining marinade. Serve with steamed broccoli florets and potato or sweet potato, spooning the juices over the meat. Serve with additional mustard or apple sauce.

Spicy Fish with Rice and Vegetables

1. **Carbohydrate**: basmati rice
2. **Protein**: firm white fish fillets (allow 150 grams (5½ oz) per person)
3. **Vegetables**: frozen vegetable combination (peas, carrots, beans, sweetcorn, etc.)

Brush firm white fish fillets with your favourite curry paste blended with some lemon juice. Pan-fry and serve with basmati rice and steamed vegetables.

Spaghetti with Tomato Salsa and Feta

1. **Carbohydrate**: spaghetti (or your favourite pasta shapes)
2. **Protein**: feta cheese
3. **Vegetables**: tomato, onion, basil, olives, salad vegetables

To make enough salsa for 4 people, chop 4 tomatoes, ½ red onion, a handful of basil leaves and 75 grams (2½ oz) of pitted kalamata olives and combine in a bowl. Toss cooked spaghetti in a little olive oil and top with the tomato salsa and 150 grams (5½ oz) of crumbled feta. Serve with a crispy green salad.

Red Lentil and Vegetable Curry

1. Carbohydrate: split red lentils, basmati rice
2. Protein: lentils, yoghurt
3. Vegetables: onion, pumpkin, carrots, vegetable stock, spinach, coriander

Cook 1 finely chopped onion in a little oil in a large frying pan until soft and golden. Add 2 tablespoons of curry paste, 400 grams (14 oz) of diced pumpkin, 2 diced carrots and 125 grams (4½ oz) of split red lentils. Stir in 500 ml (17 fl oz) of vegetable stock and simmer, uncovered, until just cooked. Stir in the leaves from a bunch of spinach and simmer gently just until they wilt. Serve over steamed basmati rice with natural yoghurt, topped with finely chopped fresh coriander. Serves 4 people.

DESSERTS FOR
SWEET FINISHES

The idea of dessert puts a smile on everyone's face but so often we keep sweet treats for special occasions. Well, you don't need to worry with these recipe ideas – they are easy, everyday fare made with just a few ingredients in a matter of minutes. Finishing your meal with something sweet can help signal satiety/satisfaction to the brain's appetite centre, and stop you hunting around the kitchen afterwards. They're also a great source of fruit and calcium- and protein-rich dairy foods.

Seven everyday low GI desserts

Caramelised Apples

Cut 4 apples into quarters, remove the core and seeds and slice thinly. Cook in 1 tablespoon margarine for 4–5 minutes, or until golden. Reduce the heat and add 2 tablespoons brown sugar, stirring until it dissolves. Increase the heat and add 150 ml (5 fl oz) light evaporated milk and stir to combine and heat through. Serve the apples with the sauce and a dollop of low fat natural yoghurt.

Honey Banana Cups

Slice a large banana and halve 2 fresh passionfruit. Divide half a 200 gram (7 oz) pot of low fat honey-flavoured yoghurt between 2 small cups or glasses. Top with half the banana and one of the passionfruit. Top with the rest of the yoghurt and remaining banana, finishing with the passionfruit. Serve with a coconut macaroon alongside.

Health tip:

Low fat dairy products generally contain more calcium, phosphorus, potassium and magnesium than their full fat counterparts. So do your heart and your health a favour and eat lots of low fat dairy.

Strawberries with Honey Yoghurt

Toss 2 punnets of washed, hulled strawberries with 2 table-spoons of caster sugar in a frying pan for 5 minutes. Serve with low fat natural yoghurt combined with 1–2 table-spoons of honey, to taste.

Peaches with Cinnamon Ricotta

Beat 300 grams (10½ oz) of low fat ricotta cheese with 2 tablespoons of icing sugar, ½ teaspoon of cinnamon and ½ teaspoon of vanilla essence. Divide dollops of the mixture between 4 side plates and add a halved fresh peach (or any other fruit) and 2 almond wafers.

Banana Split

Cut 4 bananas in half lengthways and place in dessert bowls. Add 2 scoops of low fat ice-cream and top with the pulp of ½ passionfruit.

Summer Fruit Salsa

Dice a large mango, a handful of strawberries and a peeled orange into 1 cm (½ inch) pieces. Mix with fresh passion-fruit pulp and serve with low fat ice-cream or frozen yoghurt.

Fruit Toast

Toast thick slices of continental fruit loaf and spread with light cream cheese or ricotta sweetened with a teaspoonful of caster sugar and a few drops of vanilla essence. Top with fresh fruit: sliced banana, peach or strawberries, or whole fresh blueberries or raspberries. Sprinkle with icing sugar to serve.

> ### Sugar
>
> Many people pride themselves on not keeping sugar in their larder, yet have a bottle of fruit juice in the fridge. Sure, fruit juice does provide vitamin C and other phytonutrients but it also contains about five teaspoons of sugar per glass, the same as soft drink.
>
> Sugar can be a concentrated source of calories, with few nutrients, but no more so than a bottle of oil or alcoholic spirits or a block of butter. It isn't advisable to consume sugar to excess but you can use it in moderation without adversely affecting your health.

TIME FOR A SNACK

Most people feel like eating every three to four hours. Eating frequently can help you avoid becoming too hungry and lessen the chance of overeating when meal times come around. Depending on what you choose, snacks can also make a valuable contribution to your vitamin and mineral intake.

Quick snacks you can make anytime

- fresh fruit salad
- a handful of fresh or frozen grapes

- vegetable sticks with hummous or yoghurt-based dip: cut fresh celery, cucumber, carrots, red peppers and courgettes
- low fat natural yoghurt with fresh fruit
- a smoothie made with fruit and skimmed milk and yoghurt
- a scoop (just one!) of low fat ice-cream
- hummous with pitta bread
- a bowl of cereal with low fat milk
- a slice of fruit or raisin toast
- an apple muffin
- 2 oat biscuits with a slice of cheese and an apple
- wholewheat breakfast biscuits with milk (Note: eating sweetened cereals dry is hazardous for teeth – always add milk.)

> ### How to make pitta chips
>
> Open out Lebanese bread, spread lightly with bottled sweet chilli sauce and grill until just crisp.

Portable pack-and-go snacks

- a juicy orange
- a small banana
- a large peach or pear
- single-serve pear or peach snack pack in natural juice
- a handful of dried fruit and nut mix
- a handful of dried apricots, apple rings, sultanas or raisins
- a pot of low fat yoghurt or a dairy dessert
- low fat cheese or cheese sticks
- popcorn
- 4 squares (25–30 grams/about 1 oz) of chocolate (very occasionally for a treat)

Hot snacks for cold days

- corn on the cob
- a mug of vegetable soup with toast or crackers
- toasted sandwich on low GI bread

- small can of baked beans
- small serving of instant noodles with vegetables
- toasted fruit loaf lightly spread with margarine or low fat ricotta
- low GI toast fingers lightly spread with Nutella®, peanut butter, honey, fruit spread or Marmite®

Nibbles

- a small handful of unsalted, roasted nuts
- a small handful of dried fruit and nut mix
- carrot, celery and other vegetable sticks
- fruit platter – berries, orange segments, dried fruit, nuts, etc.
- marinated vegetable platter (use paper towels to soak up some of the oil before arranging the platter) with pitta bread

Drinks

- a small glass of fruit juice (150 ml/5 fl oz)
- low fat milk or calcium-enriched soya milk
- low fat flavoured milk
- warm flavoured milk drink (Milo®, Horlicks®, Ovaltine® etc.)
- a low fat smoothie
- café latte or cappuccino with semi-skimmed milk

 Health tip:

Make a delicious low fat milkshake by combining a cup of low fat milk with a tablespoon of skimmed milk powder, 2 tablespoons of low fat vanilla yoghurt and a tablespoon of ice-cream topping. Blend until frothy.

WHAT TO DRINK?

Water

It's calorie-free and cheap – surely two good reasons for drinking water. However, it isn't necessary to drink eight glasses a day. Food contributes at least one-third of our daily fluid requirement, so we need five to seven cups of fluid to make up the remainder. Aim to make at least two or three of these water.

Fruit juice

It's widely considered a healthy drink, but if your diet includes fruit and vegetables, fruit juice really isn't necessary. If you like to include it, one glass (150 ml/5 fl oz) a day is enough, and think of it as a (low fibre) serving of fruit.

Tea

Drinking a cup of tea often provides the opportunity to take time out and relax – there is a benefit in this. Tea has also been recognised recently as a valuable source of anti-oxidants which may protect against several forms of cancer, cardiovascular disease, kidney stones, bacterial infection and dental cavities. A maximum of two to three cups of tea a day is recommended.

Coffee

Did you know that 80 per cent of the world's population consumes caffeine daily? For most people, no more than two cups of coffee a day is recommended, but if you are pregnant, caffeine sensitive or have high blood pressure it is probably best to cut down to one cup per day. Both tea and coffee are a major source of anti-oxidants in the diet, simply because they are so widely and frequently consumed.

> Energy drinks available in the UK that have been GI tested so far are Gatorade®, Isostar® and Lucozade®, and all have a high GI. This means they are a rapidly available source of glucose and makes them better suited to fluid replacement after strenuous exercise. For the recreational couch potato they may be just adding extra calories.

Three tips for making the switch

1. Start with something easy.

2. Do it gradually.

3. Don't expect 100 per cent.

Milk

Milk is a valuable source of nutrients for adults and children but, being a liquid, it is easily overconsumed. Think of it as food in a liquid form. Recommended intakes vary for different ages, but for normal, healthy, non-pregnant adults, around 300–450 ml (10½–16 fl oz) of semi-skimmed milk a day is suitable.

LIVING EVERYDAY LOW GI EATING

Five typical menus

Wondering if you can really make this low GI diet work for you? Here's how some of our readers have changed to everyday low GI eating.

Barbara, 65, small eater

'When I gave up work to become a full-time home-maker I found I piled on the weight – and I wasn't happy about that at all! I keep myself busy looking after the house, my husband and my three young grandchildren several times a week. To get myself back into shape, I go for a brisk walk for at least 20 minutes, sometimes 40 minutes, in the morning, as often as I can. I've been eating low GI food for a year now and I'm used to it. That's just the way I (and my husband) eat now. I've lost 10 kilograms (22 lb) so far – down to 82 kilograms (12 stone 9 lb), but I'd like to lose a lot more!'

Breakfast

- small cranberry juice
- 30 grams (1 oz) Guardian® with 125 ml (4 fl oz) semi-skimmed milk
- white tea with 1 sugar

Mid-morning

- low fat yoghurt
- 1 fresh apricot

Lunch

- cheese and tomato sandwich on multigrain bread (with light margarine)
- white tea

Mid-afternoon

- 1 peach

Dinner

- grilled trout fillet
- 2 small jacket potatoes
- mixed salad
- low fat ice-cream in cone

After-dinner snack

- small bunch grapes
- 6 almonds

Harry, 55, medium eater

'I am on the road as a sales rep. I'd like to lose weight to look better – I actually need to lose about 20 kilograms (3 stone). Because my job is quite sedentary – I spend so much time sitting at a desk or behind the wheel of a car – I make the effort to walk for half an hour most weekday mornings. On the weekend I'll do a longer walk for an hour or so. So far I have lost 8 kilograms (18 lb). I eat out most lunchtimes and I'm now a three-meals-a-day person and I'll eat in between if I get hungry. It was a big change for me to start eating breakfast.'

Breakfast

- 2 slices multigrain toast spread with light margarine plus 2 slices of low fat processed cheese and half a tomato
- 1 banana

Mid-morning

- skinny cappuccino

Lunch

- 1 bowl miso soup
- teppanyaki chicken
- salad
- 200 grams (7 oz) cooked Japanese sushi rice

Dinner

- 200 grams (7 oz) cooked spaghetti
- 200 grams (7 oz) meat and tomato sauce
- 1 dessert bowl green salad
- 1 banana
- 1 fresh peach
- 100 grams (3½ oz) fat-free yoghurt
- glass of chardonnay

Fiona, 38, medium eater

'I have a more-than-fulltime, stressful job and work long hours. I have little time for planned exercise, so rely on 'incidental exercise' around the office or shopping, etc. I am not trying to lose weight – but I don't want to gain any! So I am careful with my diet and fussy about the food I eat. I take my lunch to work – it saves time and I know I am eating healthily!'

Breakfast

- small freshly squeezed orange juice
- 50 grams (1¾ oz) muesli with natural yoghurt
- a nectarine
- tea with low fat milk

Mid-morning

- nut bar
- tea with low fat milk

Lunch

- 2–3 slices grain bread, no butter
- mixed salad
- 100 gram (3½ oz) can tuna or salmon
- salad dressing
- grapes

Mid-afternoon

- white coffee
- low fat fruit yoghurt
- an apple

Dinner

- 150 grams (5½ oz) chicken strips
- 200 grams (7 oz) stir-fried noodles
- 400 grams (14 oz) stir-fried vegetables

After-dinner snack

- 2 scoops of low fat ice-cream or a choc-chip biscuit

David, 50, bigger eater

'I work fulltime as a warehouse manager, which I guess could be classified as 'light activity' – my job certainly gives me a good level of incidental activity. I socialise a fair bit and go square dancing twice a week. I have lost 10 kilograms (22 lb) and am now maintaining stable weight. I wouldn't really say I'm on a diet. We just eat well, we made a few changes to our bread and I eat more fruit than I used to.'

Breakfast

- 30 grams (1 oz) Special K® with 10 grams (⅓ oz) All-Bran® with 200 ml (7 fl oz) semi-skimmed milk
- ½ sliced banana

Mid-morning

- an apple and a banana

Lunch

- 4 slices grainy bread
- low fat cheese and ham
- pickles, tomato, lettuce
- diet drink

Mid-afternoon

- 3–4 oatmeal cookies or home-made muesli slice
- white coffee

Dinner

- lean steak
- 2 new potatoes, plus a chunk of sweet potato
- mini corn cob
- broccoli, carrot, pumpkin, beans

Dessert

- canned fruit and 125 ml (4 fl oz) low fat custard

> **Did you know?**
>
> An 85-gram (3 oz) packet of instant noodles supplies as many calories as five slices of bread. Low GI they may be, but low calorie they definitely are not.

Vicki, 29, medium eater

'I am a vegetarian but I do eat dairy foods. I work full-time in an office. I catch a train to work so I accumulate about 30 minutes of walking each day. On the weekends I do lots of outdoors things – go to the beach, swim, walks. Although I don't need to watch my weight, I am aware that I need to get plenty of iron from my diet. Eating low GI foods, I just feel better and have more energy to do things. It's the ideal way of eating to me!'

Breakfast

- 30 grams (1 oz) Ultra-Bran Soy and Linseed cereal with 2 tablespoons low fat plain yoghurt, skimmed milk and a small handful of raisins
- skim latte (decaf!)

Mid-morning

- 1 nectarine
- herbal tea

Lunch

- Avocado sushi roll, tofu sushi roll

Mid-afternoon

- 1 apple and a small handful of cashews
- tea with milk

Dinner

- 2 tortillas with red kidney bean and lentil chilli sauce with light sour cream, grated cheese and lettuce
- green side salad with vinaigrette

CLUED IN ON EATING OUT?

Quite often it's the high-calorie (kilojoule) foods you unknowingly choose from the menu that tip your healthy eating plans out of balance. If you eat out more than once a week, it's worth thinking about what you're actually eating. Check out your knowledge with this quick quiz.

Which of these has the lowest fat content?

a) combination Chinese meal with fried rice/lemon chicken/sweet and sour pork
b) lasagne with meat
c) Japanese bento box including beef with rice, sushi and salad
d) fish and chips, including battered fish

Which is the lowest calorie option when you catch up for coffee?

a) skimmed-milk hot chocolate
b) cappuccino
c) skimmed-milk latte

Which drink is less fattening?

a) Bacardi Breezer
b) Corona beer
c) glass of wine

Which is the healthiest fast-food snack?

a) 2 slices of super-supreme pizza
b) roast chicken Subway® sub with cheese
c) chicken burger

Which light meal is a low GI choice?

a) grilled chicken, avocado, pepper and cheese toasted
   Turkish bread sandwich
b) wedges with sour cream and sweet chilli sauce
c) fettuccine Napolitana

Which makes the healthiest café snack?

a) chunky raisin toast and butter
b) low fat banana smoothie
c) carrot cake

The secrets revealed

Which of these has the lowest fat content?

The meat lasagne is the lowest fat option here with an average serving containing only 16 grams of fat. Next is the Japanese Bento Box at 33 grams; fish and chips at 35; and a massive 40 grams in the Chinese meal.

Which is the lowest calorie option when you catch up for coffee?

The skimmed milk latte is the winner here in terms of calories (335 kJ/80 Kcal, 0.5 grams fat) and has the added bonus of extra calcium. Although the hot chocolate is made with skimmed milk it has twice the calories (670 kJ/160 Kcal) and eight times the fat. The cappuccino is in between at 375 kJ/90 Kcal and 5 grams of fat.

Which drink is less fattening?

Depending on your knowledge of alcoholic beverages, you might have guessed that the glass of wine is least fattening, containing the lowest number of calories. It's closely followed by the beer at 545 kJ/130 Kcal and the 'alcopop' Bacardi Breezer tops the list at 880 kJ/210 Kcal per serve. That's as much as three slices of bread!

Which is the healthiest fast-food snack?

Subway® fast food can be a lower calorie snack, depending on your toppings, but it whacks a pretty high glycaemic load on your plate with even the standard 'sub' which contains 44 grams of carbohydrate, and bread which is probably high GI (it hasn't been tested). None of the other options here are any better in the GI stakes and are all higher in calories.

Which light meal is a low GI choice?

Pasta has a low GI, so the fettuccine is the best option. Potato and refined flour in the other choices make them high GI. All of these options will have a high GL because of their large carbohydrate content, so team the pasta with salad and pass on the garlic bread!

Which makes the healthiest café snack?

Sustaining, nutritious and delicious – how could you go past a banana smoothie for a premium low GI snack? The raisin toast also has a low GI, but is best with the butter served separately so you control the amount.

MAKING THE RIGHT CHOICES WHEN EATING OUT

Fast-food outlets

Burgers and French fries are a bad idea – quickly eaten, high in saturated fat and rapidly absorbed high GI carbs that fill you with calories that don't last long. Some fast-food chains are introducing healthier choices but read the fine print. Look out for lean protein, low GI carbs, good fats and lots of vegetables.

You can choose:

- **marinated and barbecued chicken**, rather than fried
- **salads** such as coleslaw or garden salad; eat the salad first
- **corn on the cob** as a healthy side order
- **individual menu items** rather than meal deals, and never upsize

Lunch bars

Steer clear of places displaying lots of deep-fried fare and head towards fresh food bars offering fruit and vegetables. Tubs of garden or Greek salad finished with fruit and yoghurt make a healthy, low GI choice.

With sandwiches and melts, choose the fillings carefully. Including cheese can make the fat exceed 20 grams (¾ oz) per sandwich (that's as much as chips!).

Make sure you include some vegetables or salad in or alongside the sandwich.

You can choose:

- **mixed grain** bread rather than white
- **salad** fillings for sandwiches or as a side order instead of chips

- **pasta** dishes with both vegetables and meat
- **Lebanese kebabs** with tabbouleh and hummous
- **grilled fish** rather than fried
- **vegetarian pizza**
- **gourmet wraps**

In cafés

Whether it's a quick snack or a main meal, catching up with a friend for coffee doesn't have to tip your diet off balance. Pass on breads, but if you really must, something like a dense Italian bread is better than a garlic or herb bread.

Whatever you order, specify: 'no French fries – extra salad instead' so temptation does not confront you. If you want something sweet try a skimmed iced chocolate or a single little biscuit or slice.

You can choose:

- **semi-skimmed** or **skimmed milk coffee** rather than full cream milk
- **sourdough** or **wholegrain bread** instead of white or wholemeal
- **bruschetta** with tomatoes, onions, olive oil and basil on a dense Italian bread rather than buttery herb or garlic bread
- **salad** as a main or side order, with the dressing served separately so you control the amount
- **char-grilled steak** or **chicken breast** rather than fried or crumbed
- **vegetable-topped pizza** – such as pepper, onion, mushroom, artichoke, aubergine
- **lean meat pizza** – such as ham, fresh seafood or sliced chicken breast
- **pasta** with sauces such as marinara; Bolognese; Napolitana; arrabiata (tomato with olives, roasted pepper

and chilli); and piccolo (aubergine, roasted pepper and artichoke)

- **seafood** such as marinated calamari, grilled with chilli and lemon or steamed mussels with a tomato sauce
- **water, mineral water** or **freshly squeezed fruit and vegetable** juices rather than soft drinks

Asian meals

Asian meals including Chinese, Thai, Indian and Japanese offer a great variety of foods, making it possible to select a healthy meal with some careful choices.

Keeping in line with the 1, 2, 3 steps to a balanced meal, seek out a low GI carb such as basmati rice, dhal, sushi or noodles. Chinese and Thai rice will traditionally be jasmine and although high GI, a small serve of steamed rice is better for you than fried rice or noodles.

Next add some protein – marinated tofu, stir-fried seafood, Tandoori chicken, fish tikka or a braised dish with vegetables. Be cautious with pork and duck, for which fattier cuts are often used; and avoid Thai curries and dishes made with coconut milk because it's high in saturated fat.

And don't forget, the third dish to order is stir-fried vegetables!

You can choose:

- **steamed dumplings, dim sum** or **fresh spring rolls** rather than fried entrees
- **clear soups** to fill you up, rather than high fat laksa
- **noodles** in soups rather than fried in dishes such as pad Thai
- **noodle and vegetable stir-fries** – if you ask for extra vegetables you may find that the one dish feeds two
- **seafood** braised in a sauce with vegetables
- **tofu (bean curd), chicken, beef, lamb** or **pork fillet** braised with nuts, vegetables, black bean or other sauces

- **salads** such as Thai salads
- **smaller serves of rice**
- **vegetable dishes** such as stir-fried vegetables, vegetable curry, dhal, channa (a delicious chickpea curry) and side orders such as pickles, cucumber and yoghurt, tomato and onion
- **Japanese dishes** such as sushi, teriyaki, sashimi, salmon steak or tuna, teppanyaki (which is char-grilled) in preference to tempura, which is deep-fried

Airlines and airports

Airports are notoriously bad places to eat – fast-food chains, a limited range, pre-made sandwiches, sad-looking cakes, a lack of fresh fruit and vegetables – and it's expensive!

In airline lounges you will do better, although, again, the range is limited. Fresh fruit is always on offer and usually some sort of vegetables either as salad or soup. The bread is usually the super-high GI white French type and with crackers as the only other option, you would do better to rely on fruit, fruit juices, yoghurt or a skimmed milk coffee for your carbs.

In-flight, unless you have the privilege of a sky chef, meals are fairly standard fare, including a salad and fruit if you're lucky. Many airlines offer special diets with advance bookings and although there's no guarantee it meets your nutritional criteria, it may give you healthier choices compared to what everyone else is having.

Travelling domestic economy these days, it's probably best to eat before you leave, take your own snacks with you and decline the in-flight snack (you really will be better off without that mini chocolate bar, biscuit, cake or muffin, and on some airlines you have to pay for it).

You can choose to eat:

- **fresh fruit, soup** and **salad items** in airline lounges rather than white bread, cheese, cakes and salami
- **small meals** in-flight, rather than eating everything put in front of you
- **water** to drink, wherever you are
- **dried fruit, nut bars, bananas** or **apples** that you have taken along yourself

WHAT TO PUT IN THE SHOPPING TROLLEY

The perfect place to get started on healthy low GI eating is the supermarket, whether you are pushing a trolley up and down the aisles, or shopping online. This is where we make those hurried or impulsive decisions that have a big impact. If you see chocolate on sale, do you stock up or keep walking? One little decision – what a big impact.

Make a list

Spend a little time each day, or weekly if it suits, planning what to eat when. It makes life simpler. Meal planning is just writing down what you intend to eat for the main meals of the week, then checking your fridge and pantry for ingredients available and noting what you need to purchase. We've included more ideas on meal planning in the menu section on pages 49–64. So study the GI tables, look at the meal ideas in this book and browse through some recipes with a notepad handy.

The shopping list on pages 87–90 is just to get you started. Bear in mind that it doesn't contain all low GI foods, and individual choices will be dictated by your tastes and budget. Make a photocopy and take it with you to the shops if you like, or just use it for ideas. For more tips on what to pop in the trolley and stock in your pantry, check out Part 3: The Top 100 Low GI Food Finder.

WHY IT'S IMPORTANT TO READ THE LABEL

Often we're asked questions like: 'What should I look for on the label?' and 'Can I believe what it says?'

Reading the fine print

Remember, the GI alone doesn't identify a healthy food. If you like to keep some numbers in your head when you're shopping, then the following details are for you. Keep in mind that they are a general guide and shouldn't be used definitively to exclude or include foods in your diet.

Health tip:

Remember, if you don't buy it, you can't eat it.

Energy – This is a measure of how many kilojoules (kJ) or calories (Kcal) we get from a food. For a healthy diet we need to eat more foods with a low energy density and combine them with smaller amounts of higher energy foods. To assess the energy density of a packaged food, look at the kJ or Kcal per 100 grams. A low energy density is less than 500 kJ per 100 grams or 120 Kcals per 100 grams.

Fat – Seek low saturated fat content, ideally less than 20 per cent of the total fat. For example, if the total fat content is 10 grams, you want saturated fat to be less than 2 grams. A food can be labelled as being low fat only if it contains less than 1.5 grams of saturated fat per 100 grams/100 ml and the saturated fat provides less than 10 per cent of the total energy of the product.

Carbohydrate – This is the starch plus any naturally occurring and added sugars in the food. There's no need to look at the sugar figure separately since it's the total carbohydrate that affects your blood glucose level. You could use the total carbohydrate figure if you were monitoring your carbohydrate intake and to calculate the GL of the serving. The GL = grams of total carbohydrate x GI/100.

Sample Nutritional Information

Typical values per 100 grams

Energy	245kJ/58 Kcal
Protein	4.6 g
Carbohydrate	7.2 g
of which sugars	6.5 g
Fat	1.2 g
of which saturates	0.2 g
Fibre	0.2 g
Sodium	0.1 g

For more information on food labelling go to **www.eatwell.gov. uk/foodlabels**

Can I believe what it says?

Consumers are increasingly interested in what is in the food they eat. That's where the Food Standards Agency (FSA) comes in. This independent food safety watchdog was set up by an act of parliament to provide consumers and government with advice and information on nutrition and diet, and on food safety from farm to fork. It also protects consumers through effective monitoring and enforcement of regulations. For more information visit: www.food.gov.uk or www.eatwell.gov.uk

Fibre – Most of us don't eat enough fibre in our diet (the average intake for adults in the UK is around 12 grams a day – 6 grams short of the recommended 18 grams a day). So seek out foods that are high in fibre. Foods and food products that contain 6 grams of fibre per 100 grams (or 100 ml) may be labelled as being a 'high fibre' food.

Sodium – This is a measure of the nasty part of salt in our food. Our bodies need some salt but many people consume much more salt than the 6 grams a day they need. Canned, convenience and ready-to-eat foods in particular tend to be high in sodium. When shopping, check the nutrition label for the sodium content. If a food contains between 0.1 grams and 0.5 grams of sodium per 100 grams, this could be considered a moderate amount. A small amount would be less than 0.1 grams of sodium per 100 grams of the food. Sometimes sodium is listed in milligrams (mg). There are 1000 mg in 1 gram, so 600 mg = 0.6 grams and 1200 mg = 1.2 grams. For more information on sodium and salt go to www.salt.gov.uk

Health tip:

Seventy-five per cent of most people's salt intake comes from the supermarket (in processed foods and ready-to-eat meals) and from takeaways. What can you do to cut down?

- Check the labels for sodium content.
- Never add salt to your food.
- Minimise the frequency with which you eat salty foods.

How do you know if it's low, medium or high GI?

When it comes to the supermarket shelves, it's getting easier to identify foods that have been GI tested by the use of special GI symbols. Unfortunately, however, not all claims are reliable. Why? Well, the GI rating of a food must be tested physiologically and only a few centres around the world currently provide such a testing service. In fact the GI is defined by its internationally standardised method of testing in human subjects (we call this in vivo testing). You may hear about in vitro (test tube) methods, but these are simple short cuts, which may be useful for food manufacturers developing new products, but may not reflect the true GI of a food.

The GI Symbol Program

This international symbol is a guarantee that the product meets the Sydney University GI Research Service (SUGiRS) program's strict nutritional criteria. Whether high, medium or low GI, you can be assured that these foods are healthier choices within their food group. A number of leading food manufacturers in Australia have had their products GI tested by SUGiRS, an international program established by the University of Sydney, Diabetes Australia and the Juvenile Diabetes Research Foundation.

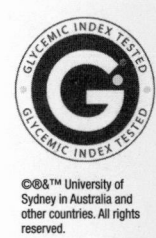

Some supermarket chains in the UK are glycaemic index testing products and labelling them 'Low GI' or 'Medium GI'.

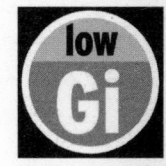

Sainsbury's

Sainsbury's launched low and medium GI labelling progressively across a range of products that meet strict nutritional criteria and that were tested by the Hammersmith Food Research Unit at Hammersmith Hospital.

Tesco

Tesco launched GI labelling across a range of products that were tested by Oxford Brookes University. Products are labelled 'Low Gi' or 'Medium Gi'.

EVERYDAY LOW GI SHOPPING

Having the staples on hand

Our shopping list will help you stock the larder and refrigerator with the staples you require to turn out a meal in minutes. It includes everything you'll need for the low GI meal ideas in the food finder.

To make your own shopping list, use the same headings. They will take you to the appropriate aisles of the supermarket or to the shops you usually favour.

We've included convenience foods such as canned beans, bagged salads, bottled sauces and pastes, canned fruits and chopped vegetables (fresh and frozen) in the list. There's no need to feel guilty about using these items. Remember, this book is about making eating a healthy, low GI diet as easy as possible and although some convenience items such as frozen vegetables or canned beans may be a little more expensive, the time savings and health benefits can outweigh the costs.

If you want to know more about some of the foods on the shopping list, check the food finder in Part 3. We have included lots of meal ideas and even some recipes in this section.

 ## Health tip:

We need to eat foods with fibre for bowel health and to keep regular. In fact we need about 18 grams of fibre a day (most of us fall short of that – about 6 grams short). It's easy to increase your intake. Just make sure your shopping list includes high fibre breakfast cereals and porridge oats, wholegrain or granary breads, fresh fruit and vegetables and canned (or dried) beans, peas and lentils. You'll find plenty of ideas for using these low GI high fibre foods in our Top 100 Food Finder.

The bakery

Fruit loaf
Low GI bread
   Granary or wholegrain
   Sourdough

English-style muffins
Pitta bread

The refrigerated cabinet

Milk
   Semi-skimmed
   Skimmed
   Low fat flavoured
Margarine
Cheese
   Reduced fat grated
   cheese
   Parmesan cheese
   Reduced fat ricotta
   or cottage cheese
   Reduced fat cheese
   slices
Yoghurt
   Low fat plain/natural
   Low fat fruit or vanilla
   flavoured
   Low fat drinking
   yoghurt

Soya alternatives
   Low fat calcium-enriched
   soya milk
   Soya yoghurt
Dairy desserts
   Crème fraîche desserts
   Custard
Fruit juice
   Apple juice
   Orange juice
   Grapefruit juice
   Cranberry juice
Fresh noodles
Fresh pasta
   Ravioli
   Tortellini
Tofu
Sushi
Dips such as hummous

Your everyday checkout choice

To cut back the fat, choose:

- lean cuts of meat and skinless chicken

- low fat dairy and soya milk products

- vegetable oils and cooking sprays

- 'lite' spreads and dressings

- tomato and pepper sauces and salsas to serve with pasta

Health tip:

If they have been stored and cooked carefully, frozen vegetables can provide similar levels of nutrients to those of fresh vegetables, sometimes even more.

The freezer

Ice-cream
  Reduced or low fat
  vanilla or flavoured
  Frozen yoghurt
Frozen fruit desserts
or gelato
Frozen vegetables
  Peas

Beans
Corn
Spinach
Mixed vegetables
Stir-fry mix
Broccoli
Cauliflower

Your everyday checkout choice

To fill up with fibre choose a cereal containing at least 9 grams of fibre per 100 grams.

Fresh fruit and vegetables

Basics
  Sweet potato
  Yam
  Sweetcorn
  Lemons or limes
  Onions
  Carrots
  Garlic
  Ginger
  Chillies
Leafy green and other
seasonal vegetables
  Spinach or silverbeet
  Cabbage
  Broccoli
  Cauliflower
  Asparagus
  Asian greens such
  as bok choi
  Leeks
  Fennel
  Mangetout

Beans and peas
Courgette or marrow
Brussel sprouts
Aubergine
Mushrooms
Salad vegetables, depending
on season
  Lettuce (choose a variety)
  Rocket
  Tomato
  Cucumber
  Pepper
  Spring onions
  Celery
  Bagged mixed salad
  greens
  Sprouts – mung bean,
  mangetout, alfalfa etc.
  Avocado
  Fresh herbs, depending
  on season
  Parsley

Your everyday checkout choice

To bone up on calcium choose low fat dairy products.

Basil
Mint
Chives
Coriander
Fresh fruit, depending
on season
  Apples
  Oranges

Pears
Grapes
Grapefruit
Peaches
Apricots
Strawberries and other
berries
Mango

General groceries

Eggs
Beverages
  Tea
  Coffee
  Flavoured milk
  powders such as
  Milo®, Horlicks®
  or Ovaltine®
Herbs, spices, condiments
and sauces
  Tube or jar of minced
  ginger, garlic, chilli
  Mustard
  Creamed horseradish
  Tomato sauce
  Asian sauces
  Soy sauce
  Bottled pasta sauce
  Jar of curry paste
Deli items or pre-packed jars
  Sundried tomatoes
  Olives
Spreads
  Pure floral honey
  Apricot jam

Nutella®
Peanut butter
Marmite®
Oils and vinegars
  Rapeseed or olive oil
  cooking spray
  Olive oil
  Rapeseed or vegetable oil
  Balsamic vinegar
  White wine vinegar
Breakfast cereals
  Traditional rolled oats
  Natural muesli
  Low GI packaged
  breakfast cereal
Cereals and wholegrains
  Pasta
  Noodles, rice, buckwheat
  Rice – basmati or
  Japanese sushi rice
  such as Koshihikari
  Couscous
  Bulghur/cracked wheat
  Pearl barley
  Oat biscuits

Did you know?

Highly processed breakfast cereals have high GI values, not because they're high in sugar but because they're high in refined starch.

Your everyday checkout choice

To increase iron intake choose lean red meat.

Dried pulses
  Beans – keep a variety
  in the cupboard
  including cannellini,
  borlotti, lima, kidney,
  soya, pinto etc.
  Chickpeas
  Lentils
  Split peas
Canned foods, including
pulses
  Baked beans
  Mexi-beans
  Chickpeas
  Lentils
  Beans – keep a variety
  in the cupboard
  including cannellini,
  butter, borlotti, lima,
  kidney, soya, pinto etc
  Four bean mix
  Corn kernels

Tomatoes, whole, crushed
  and tomato paste
Tomato soup
Tuna packed in
  spring water or oil
Salmon packed in
  water
Sardines
Canned fruit and single
serve pots
  Pears
  Peaches
  Mixed fruit salad
Dried fruit and nuts
  Apricots
  Sultanas
  Raisins
  Prunes
  Apple rings
  Unsalted natural
  almonds, walnuts,
  cashews, etc.

Butcher/meat department

Lean ham
Lean beef for grills,
barbecues and casseroles
Lean lamb fillets
Lean pork fillets
Lean minced beef

Chicken
  Skinless chicken breast
  or drumsticks
Fish
  Any type of fresh fish

Health tip:

Low iron levels can cause tiredness, physical weakness and increased sensitivity to cold. Lean red meat is a rich and highly bio-available source of iron, so aim to include it in your diet at least three times a week.

READY . . . SET . . . GO – MOVE IT & LOSE IT!

> Remember, all you have to do is accumulate 60 minutes of physical activity every day.

When we explained the basics of everyday low GI eating at the beginning of this section, we mentioned that one of the golden rules is to accumulate 60 minutes of physical activity every day, including incidental activity and planned exercise. This will help you control your weight for a whole host of reasons. To make a real difference to your health and energy levels, exercise has to be regular and some of it needs to be aerobic. But every little bit counts – and, best of all, any extra exercise you do is a step in the right direction.

Though some people can make a serious commitment to 30-plus minutes of planned exercise three or four times a week, most of us have a long list of excuses. We're too busy, too tired, too rushed, too stressed, too hot, too cold to go to the gym or take a walk or do a regular exercise routine. But there's good news. Research tells us that the calories we burn in our everyday activities are important too, and that any amount of movement is better than none at all.

Changing the habits of a lifetime isn't easy. We know how hard it can be to find time to fit everything into a day, especially if you are working and have a family. That's why we suggest you move it and lose it with our '1, 2, 3 one step at a time, in your own time' approach.

1. *Start* with extra incidental activity.
2. *Add* time to move more.
3. *Plus* planned exercise – it's worth it.

1. Start with extra incidental activity

> Think of extra incidental activity as an opportunity, not an inconvenience.

Incidental activity is the exercise we accumulate each day as part of our normal routines – putting out the rubbish, making the bed, doing chores, walking to the bus stop, popping out for a coffee and walking up a flight of stairs. If you make a conscious effort to increase the amount of this kind of activity in your day, it will eventually become second nature.

With just a little extra effort, here's how you can build more incidental physical activity into your life. You've probably heard these ideas before, so read this list as a timely reminder. It would be great if you could use just one of these ideas regularly.

- Use the stairs instead of taking the lift. Walk up them as quickly as you can. Try taking them two at a time – to strengthen your legs.
- Don't stand still on the escalator – walk up and down.
- Take the long way around whenever you can – popping down to the corner shop, getting a drink from the office water cooler, going to the bathroom.
- Make the time to walk your children to or from school.
- Catch up with a friend by meeting for a walk, rather than talking on the phone or over coffee.
- Get off your chair and talk to your colleagues rather than sending endless emails.
- Walk the dog instead of hitting tennis balls for him or her to chase and retrieve.
- Get rid of the leaf blower and rake the leaves or sweep the courtyard the old-fashioned way.

- Park the car at the opposite end of the carpark and walk to the cash machine, post office or dry cleaners.
- Walk to a restaurant (or park a good distance from it) to force yourself to take a walk after dinner.

Think of extra incidental activity as an opportunity not an inconvenience. The following table shows how 'spending' five minutes here and there every day can add up to potential fat 'savings' in the long term.

Take 5 minutes everyday to:	Potential savings in kilos of fat*	
	in 1 year	in 5 years
Take the stairs instead of the lift	3.7	18.5
Vacuum the living room	0.7	3.5
Walk 150 metres from the car to the office	0.7	3.5
Carry the groceries 150 metres to the car	0.9	4.5

* Figures based on a 70 kg (11 stone) person

2. Add time to move more

Exercise is more likely to be achieved when scheduled into your day, just like any other appointment. So think about your day, make a note in your diary and prioritise exercise. To reap the benefits, exercise doesn't have to be intense: exercise of moderate duration and intensity – including walking – is associated with reduced risk of disease. While brisk walking is best, even slow walkers benefit!

For most of us, walking fits the bill perfectly. It keeps us fit, it's cheap and convenient, it gets us out and about, and

If you do regular exercise you:

- will tend to have lower blood pressure
- will feel more energetic
- are less likely to have a heart attack or develop diabetes
- will reduce your insulin requirements if you have diabetes
- will find it easier to stop smoking
- will be better able to control your weight
- can increase levels of 'good' HDL cholesterol
- will sleep better

If you do regular exercise you:

- will have stronger bones and muscles

- are less likely to develop colon cancer

- will feel happier, more confident and relaxed

- can ease depression

it becomes even more important as we grow older. You can walk alone, or with friends. In fact, talking while you walk can have important emotional benefits: Not only do our bodies produce calming hormones while we walk, but the talk itself can be great therapy – and good for relationships in general. But don't hesitate to walk alone if you prefer, or with your dog – your pet will love you all the more for it. And you'll be able to take some time to think and relax.

How often? Try to walk every day. Ideally you should accumulate 30 minutes or more on most days of the week. The good news is, you can do it in two 15-minute sessions or six 5-minute sessions. It doesn't matter.

How hard? You should be able to talk comfortably while you walk. Find a level that suits you. If you feel sore at first, don't worry; your body will adapt and the soreness will decrease. Stretching for 2 minutes before and after your walk will help minimise aches and pains.

Getting started Before beginning a walking (or any exercise) program, see your doctor if you have:

- been inactive for some time
- a history of heart disease or chest pains
- diabetes
- high blood pressure

Or if you:

- smoke
- weigh more than you should

 ## Health tip

For more information, step out and check out these walking programs:
www.whi.org.uk
www.ramblers.org.uk
www.healthierweight.co.uk
www.foodfitness.org.uk
www.everydaysport.com

How many steps will make a difference?

Go out and buy a cheap pedometer (step counter). Research has shown that every day we need to take about:

- ❏ 7500 steps to maintain weight
- ❏ 10 000 steps to lose weight
- ❏ 12 500 steps to prevent weight regain

For most of us this means taking a walk on top of our incidental activity. In the normal course of a day – just living and working – it is virtually impossible (unless you deliver the mail or walk other people's dogs for a living!) to achieve that 10 000 steps a day. The following table gives you an idea of how many steps are equivalent to 15 minutes of certain activities.

15 minutes of activity	Equivalent number of steps
Moderate sexual activity	500
Watering the garden	600
Vigorous sexual activity	750
Clearing and washing the dishes	900
Standing cooking at the barbecue	950
Standing while playing with kids	1100
Carpentry – general workshop	1200
Playing golf at the driving range	1200
Food shopping with a trolley	1400
General house cleaning	1400
Sweeping and raking	1600
Digging the garden	2000
Mowing the lawn with a hand mower	2350
Moving furniture	2350
Carrying bricks or using heavy tools	3150

To achieve:

- 4000 steps you need about 30 minutes of moderately paced walking

- 7500 steps you need about 45 minutes of moderately paced walking

- 10 000 steps you need about 60 minutes of briskly paced walking

3. Plus planned exercise – it's worth it

> To help you achieve your walking goal, clip a pedometer to your waistband or belt in the morning and start counting. Of course the pedometer only counts steps and not any other activities.

Exercise and activity speed up your metabolic rate (increasing the amount of energy you use) which helps you to balance your food intake and control your weight. Exercise and activity also make your muscles more sensitive to insulin and increase the amount of fat you burn.

A healthy low GI diet has the same effect. Low GI foods reduce the amount of insulin you need, which makes fat easier to burn and harder to store. Since body fat is what you want to get rid of when you lose weight, exercise or activity in combination with a low GI diet makes a lot of sense.

Best of all, the effect of exercise doesn't end when you stop moving. People who exercise have higher metabolic rates and their bodies burn more calories per minute even when they are asleep!

If you are ready to improve your fitness, making a commitment to a planned exercise programme including aerobic, resistance and flexibility/stretching exercises will give you the best results. Variety is also important.

Planned exercise doesn't mean having to sweat it out in a gym. The key is to find some activities you enjoy – and do them regularly. Just 30 minutes of moderate exercise each day can improve your health, reducing your risk of heart disease and type 2 diabetes. If you prefer you can break this into two 15-minute sessions or three 10-minute sessions. You'll still see the benefits. Remember, every little bit counts.

What about personal trainers?

Working with a personal trainer can be a great way to improve your health and fitness and work towards your goals. A good trainer will design an exercise programme tailored to your needs and fitness level as well as providing motivation and support. Many personal trainers now provide services for a reasonable rate and you can choose to use a health club or train at home or outdoors. If cost is an issue, you could train with a small group of three or four others with similar fitness levels, or you could just have a few sessions initially. If you can, try to budget for at least 10 sessions. This will help you achieve your goals and increase your confidence with the new exercises.

How to find a good personal trainer

Many trainers are attached to health clubs, but if you don't belong to one or you would prefer to train at home or outdoors, look in your local newspaper or search online for someone in your area. Ask to see their qualifications – they should have at least Level 3 in Instructing Physical Exercise & Exercise. Go to *www.exerciseregister.org* for more information. A good trainer should offer you at least one complimentary session to 'try before you buy'.

What to expect when you see a personal trainer

In your first session, a good personal trainer will ask you about your current lifestyle, your goals and expectations and any health or medical problems. He or she will then work out a programme to help you reach your goals and work closely with you to implement the plan, supervising each of your exercise sessions to make sure you are performing the exercises correctly and pushing you to the next level. He or she will also help to motivate you when the going gets tough.

Health tip:

Did you know that the benefits of exercise don't stop when you stop? People who exercise have higher metabolic rates and their bodies burn more calories per minute – even when they are sound asleep!

Before starting . . .

If you have any concerns about your health, or any illnesses such as diabetes or heart problems or an injury, discuss your activity plan with your GP first.

Here are some ideas to get you started

- aerobics
- aqua-robics
- cycling
- dancing
- exercise balls
- exercise bikes
- exercise classes
- exercise DVDs and videos
- golf
- health clubs and gyms
- paddling, rowing and kayaking
- Pilates
- spin classes
- surfing and bodysurfing
- swimming
- table tennis
- tai chi
- team sports
- tennis, squash and other racket sports
- treadmills
- weight training
- yoga

PART 3

The Top 100
low gi food finder

Everyone can benefit from the low GI approach to eating. It is the way nature intended us to eat – slow-burning, nutritious foods that satisfy our hunger.

- Fruit & vegetables (page 104)

- Breads & cereals (page 142)

- Pulses including beans, peas & lentils (page 181)

- Nuts (page 197)

- Fish & seafood (page 201)

- Lean meat, chicken & eggs (page 204)

- Low fat dairy foods & calcium-enriched soya products (page 206)

To pick the top 100 low GI foods for healthy eating and to give you plenty of choice, we pushed our shopping trolley up and down the supermarket aisles. We have listed the foods in this section A to Z within the appropriate food group to make meal planning and shopping easier.

We are often asked about foods such as lean red meat, chicken, eggs, fish and seafood – foods that don't have a GI because they don't contain carbs. As a result we have also included brief sections on these protein-rich foods because they are an important part of a healthy diet.

The food groups

When planning meals, choose foods from all the groups to make sure you gain the benefits of the 40+ essential nutrients along with the protective anti-oxidants and phytochemicals your body needs each day for long-term health and wellbeing.

We have also included a few 'borderline' low–medium GI foods as they are great additions to your diet.

Which brand?

Low GI eating often means making a move back to staple foods – pulses, whole cereal grains, vegetables and fruit – which naturally have a low GI, so it doesn't matter what brand you buy.

Knowing which brand to buy is important, however, when it comes to choosing carb-rich processed foods such as breads and breakfast cereals whose GI values can range from low to high.

To find the GI of your favourite brands you can:

- Look for a low GI symbol on foods.
- Check the nutritional label – some manufacturers include the GI.
- Visit **www.glycemicindex.com** to search a reliable database of GI values.
- Check the GI tables on page 219.

If you can't find the GI of your favourite breakfast cereal or bread, contact the manufacturer and suggest they have the food tested by an accredited laboratory.

GI values

A low GI value is 55 or less

A medium value is 56–69

A high GI value is 70 or more

Are you eating enough fibre?

Many low GI foods are good sources of dietary fibre, which is a terrific bonus since we need about 18 grams of fibre a day for bowel health and to keep regular. Filling, high fibre foods can also help you maintain a healthy weight by reducing hunger pangs.

Dietary fibre comes from plant foods – it is found in the outer bran layers of grains (corn, oats, wheat and rice and in foods containing these grains), fruit and vegetables and nuts and pulses (dried beans, peas and lentils). There are two types – soluble and insoluble – and there is a difference.

A word on processed food

Try to avoid highly processed foods as much as possible. Think of it this way: you should do the processing, not the food company!

- *Soluble fibres* are the gel, gum and often jelly-like components of apples, oats and pulses (beans, peas and lentils). By slowing down the time it takes for food to pass through the stomach and small intestine, soluble fibre can lower the glycaemic response to food.
- *Insoluble fibres* are dry and bran-like and commonly thought of as roughage. All cereal grains and products made from them that retain the outer coat of the grain are sources of insoluble fibre, e.g. wholemeal bread and

All-Bran®, but not all foods containing insoluble fibre are low GI. Insoluble fibres will only lower the GI of a food when they exist in their original, intact form, for example in whole grains of wheat. Here they act as a physical barrier, delaying access of digestive enzymes and water to the starch within the cereal grain.

FRUIT & VEGETABLES

When it comes to fruit and vegetables think colour, think variety, think protective anti-oxidants, and give these foods a starring role in your meals and snacks.

Fruit and vegetables play a central role in a low GI diet. While we all remember being told to eat our greens, we believe that it's important to eat seven or more serves of fruit and vegetables every day for long-term health and wellbeing. The greater the variety, the better.

Green

- artichokes, Asian greens, asparagus, avocados, bok choi, broccoli, broccolini, Brussel sprouts, cabbage and Chinese cabbage, celery, chard, chicory, courgettes, cress, cucumber, endive, green beans, green peppers, leafy greens, leeks, lettuce, marrow, mesclun, okra, peas (including mangetouts and sugar snap peas), rocket, silverbeet, spinach, spring onions, watercress
- green apples, figs, green grapes, honeydew melons, kiwi fruit, limes, green pears

Red/pink

- red peppers, radishes, red onions, tomatoes, yams
- red apples, blood oranges, cherries, cranberries, red grapes, pink/red grapefruit, guavas, plums, pomegranates, raspberries, rhubarb, strawberries, tamarillo, watermelon

White/cream

- bamboo shoots, cauliflower, celeriac, daikon, fennel, garlic, Jerusalem artichoke, kohlrabi, mushrooms, onions, parsnips, potatoes (white-fleshed), shallots, swedes, taro, turnips, white onions
- bananas, lychees, nectarines, white peaches

Orange/yellow

- butternut squash, carrots, yellow/orange peppers, pumpkin, marrow, sweetcorn, sweet potato, winter squash, yellow beets, yellow tomatoes
- yellow apples, apricots, cantaloupe, custard apple, gooseberries, grapefruit, lemons, mandarins, mangoes, nectarines, oranges, papaya (pawpaw) peaches, persimmons, pineapple, tangerines

Blue/purple

- aubergine, beetroot, purple asparagus, radicchio lettuce, red cabbage
- blackberries, blackcurrants, blueberries, boysenberries, purple figs, purple grapes, plums, raisins

Wash first

Wash all fruit and vegetables before you eat or cook them. If you are going to eat the skins, use a scrubbing brush on vegetables such as potatoes and carrots. For leafy vegetables such as cabbages and lettuce, remove the outer leaves first, then wash leaves individually and dry in a salad spinner.

Why are fruit and vegetables so important?

A high fruit and vegetable intake has been consistently linked with better health. It could be because they are packed with anti-oxidants – nature's personal bodyguards – which protect body cells from damage caused by pollutants and the natural ageing process.

Some key anti-oxidants

Beta-carotene – the plant form of vitamin A, used to maintain healthy skin and eyes. A diet rich in beta-carotene may even reduce damage caused by UV rays. Apricots, peaches, mangoes, carrots, broccoli and sweet potato are particularly rich in beta-carotene.

Vitamin C – nature's water-soluble anti-oxidant found in virtually all fruits and vegetables. Some of the richest sources are cantaloupes, guavas, oranges, peppers and kiwi fruit. Vitamin C is used to make collagen, the protein that gives our skin strength and elasticity.

Anthocyanins – the purple and red pigments in aubergine, blackberries, blueberries and peppers also function as anti-oxidants, minimising the damage to cell membranes that occurs with ageing.

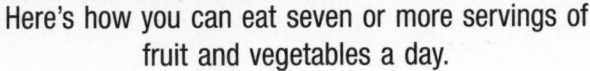

> **Here's how you can eat seven or more servings of fruit and vegetables a day.**
>
> ❑ Top muesli or *breakfast* cereal with sliced fruit.
> ❑ Sip a small juice for a *morning snack*.
> ❑ Enjoy a vegetable soup or salad for lunch.
> ❑ Boost your brainpower *mid-afternoon* with a snack such as a handful of grapes or crispbread topped with ricotta and tomato slices.
> ❑ Brighten your *dinner* plate with a variety of vegetables such as sweet potato, green beans and red and yellow peppers plus a big salad.
> ❑ Finish your meal with a fruity *dessert* or a fruit platter.

FRUIT

People who eat three of four serves of fruit a day, particularly apples and oranges, have the lowest overall GI and the best blood glucose control.

Naturally sweet and filling, fruit is widely available, inexpensive, portable and easy to eat – just like other snack foods, but without the added fat and sugar. So, buy the best you can and enjoy a lifetime of benefits.

The sugars in fruits and berries have provided energy in the human diet for millions of years. It shouldn't come as too much of a surprise, therefore, to learn that these sugars have low GI values. Fructose, in particular – a sugar that occurs naturally in all fruits and in floral honey – has the lowest GI of all. Fruit is also a good source of soluble and insoluble fibres which can slow digestion and provide a low GI. And as a general rule, the more acidic a fruit is, the lower its GI value.

Temperate climate fruits – apples, pears, citrus (oranges, grapefruit) and stone fruits (peaches, plums, apricots) – all have low GI values.

Tropical fruits – cantaloupe, pineapple, papaya (pawpaw),

banana and watermelon tend to have higher GI values, but their glycaemic load (GL) is low because they are low in carbohydrate. So keep them in the fruit bowl and enjoy them every day if you wish as they are excellent sources of anti-oxidants.

How much?

One serving is equivalent to:

- 1 medium piece of fresh fruit such as an apple, banana, mango, orange, peach or pear (about 115 grams/4 oz)
- 2 small pieces of fresh fruit such as apricots, kiwi fruit or plums (about 60 grams/2¼ each)
- 115 grams (4 oz) of fresh diced or canned fruit pieces including grapes and chopped berries and strawberries
- 4–5 dried apricot halves, apple rings, figs or prunes (about 30 grams/1 oz)
- 1½ tablespoons sultanas (about 30 grams/1 oz)
- 150 ml (5 fl oz) fruit juice, homemade or unsweetened, 100 per cent juice

How much a day?

- Smaller eaters: 2 serves
- Medium eaters: 3 serves
- Bigger eaters: 4 serves

Serving suggestions

1. Fruit is nature's takeaway food. Carry fresh fruit or a small container of fruit pieces or dried fruit to snack on.
2. Top your breakfast cereal with fresh fruit such as berries and sliced bananas or add diced fruit to low fat yoghurt snacks.
3. Whip up smoothies with fresh fruit, juice and low fat yoghurt or make fresh fruit ice-cubes with juice or simply freeze some fruit!

4. Toss fresh fruit slices (apples, citrus segments, straw-berries, pears) or whole grapes into crispy green salads. Add a few nuts and serve with a light oil and vinegar or citrus dressing.

5. Prepare a fruit platter (including grapes, strawberries, slices of melon, apple or pear, orange segments, etc.) for dessert or to nibble on while watching television; or keep a bowl of your favourite fruit within reach.

6. It's more likely to tempt you if it's right in front of you, so store fruit or vegetable pieces (such as diced melon or carrot sticks) in a clear container in the refrigerator.

7. Sliced pear, apple, banana or pineapple make great toasted sandwich fillings.

8. Serve fresh fruit salsa with meat, chicken or fish, or use as a salad dressing or dip.

9. Make fruit compotes for desserts or toppings for low fat ice-cream, pancakes and waffles.

10. Try apple or pear slices with some cheese and whole-grain crackers or top grainy toast with thinly sliced peaches, strawberries, apples or pears and a dollop of ricotta or cottage cheese.

Thirst-quencher

Eating fruit regularly is a great way to keep hydrated: some fruits such as watermelon contain up to 90 per cent water. If you're not well hydrated, all your body functions, from joint lubrication and muscle contraction through to digestion and mental performance can be compromised.

APPLES

GI 38

Apples are the ultimate portable snack. It's said that the Roman legions munched them as they marched, the *Mayflower* Pilgrims packed them when they set sail for America, and Captain Phillip stocked up before heading for Botany Bay. Just one fresh apple will give you about one-third of your vitamin C needs for the day and by stimulating saliva it can also help prevent dental decay. Apples are a good source of dietary fibre, particularly pectin, which promotes a healthy balance of bacteria in the intestine. On top of this, apples, particularly the skins, are packed with anti-oxidants.

Simply wash, dry and enjoy as a snack, skin and all

(some people even eat the core), or eat one for a sweet finish to meals. Cooking apples is likely to raise the GI *slightly*.

Serving suggestions

- Add coarsely grated apple to your muesli or favourite low GI breakfast cereal, or to muffin mixes when baking.
- Bake or microwave whole apples for a warm and filling dessert, or core and stuff with dried fruit, a little honey and a sprinkle of cinnamon, then bake.
- Add apple slices to sandwiches and salads or serve apple slices with fruit and cheese platters.
- Slice into segments and use to make stewed apple with cloves, open apple tarts or apple crumbles with a crunchy toasted muesli topping.

APPLE RINGS, DRIED
GI 29

A rich source of fibre, dried apple rings are great for lunch boxes, and a tasty ingredient to chop and add to muesli and other breakfast cereals, fruit and nut mixes, health bars and fruit slices and desserts. Drying concentrates the calories, so count about 10 rings as a serving.

Serving suggestions

- Make a compote by microwaving or simmering dried apple with other fruits and a cinnamon quill in just enough water to cover.
- Soak dried apple in boiling water for about 30 minutes and use in desserts or baking or to make an apple sauce for serving with meat.

APPLE JUICE
GI 40 (unsweetened)

Apple juice is a good source of vitamin C and potassium. The fibre, however, is lost during processing, along with many of the other nutrients in apple skin. When buying juice, look for unsweetened, 100 per cent juice. To make your own, quarter and core two apples and cut into pieces that will fit into the food tube of your juicer, process and enjoy a small glass of juice (150 ml/5 fl oz) as a snack or to finish a meal. Add sticks of celery, carrot or a little fresh ginger for variety.

Serving suggestions

- Sip on a long apple spritzer made with 125 ml (4 fl oz) of juice plus plenty of crushed ice, soda water and fresh mint leaves.
- Make apple juice ice-cubes to cool down on hot days.
- Start the day with muesli moistened with apple juice rather than low fat milk.
- Use apple juice to sweeten breakfast cereal and other foods.

> For maximum health benefits, be choosy about the juice you buy. Look for brands with no added sugar and juices that are pressed whole including the skins, pips and cores.

APRICOTS
GI 57

For fragrance and flavour, fresh apricots are almost irresistible. This sweet 'borderline' low–medium GI fruit is delicious as a snack or to finish a meal. Like all orange–yellow fruits and vegetables, they are rich in beta-carotene and a good source of vitamin C, fibre and potassium.

Cooking apricots draws out their flavour, so they are delicious stewed. If they are not quite ready for eating when you buy them, they should ripen in a day or two at room temperature in your fruit bowl (or in a paper bag away from heat and light). To eat your fill of apricots year round, choose canned or dried apricots. Canned apricots have a medium GI (64). Or, for a delicious topping on grainy toast, use apricot fruit spread (GI 56) in moderation.

Serving suggestions

- Grill apricot halves (stones removed) and serve with custard, ice-cream or yoghurt.

- Halve fresh apricots, remove the stones, stuff with a teaspoon of ricotta and top with chopped nuts.
- Gently poach whole or halved apricots in fruit juice with cloves or a cinnamon quill.

APRICOTS, DRIED
GI 30

Dried apricots can be so more-ish it's often hard to stick to just a handful – five or six halves is the equivalent of a serve. However, if you do overindulge, remind yourself of their health benefits: they are high in fibre, a rich source of beta-carotene and provide reasonable amounts of calcium, iron and potassium.

Dried apricots are a delicious snack food whether you are on the run or desk-bound. They also bring a natural sweetness to many recipes: soaked and pureéd for desserts, added whole to casseroles, or chopped and mixed with couscous or rice as a main meal accompaniment.

Serving suggestions

- Simmer dried apricots in a little water, white wine or fruit juice to soften and plump up and serve on their own or with a dollop of low fat yoghurt or ice-cream.
- Add chopped apricots and other dried fruits to home-made muesli.
- Dice and add dried apricots to the mix when baking fruit slices and cookies.
- Make a Moroccan-flavoured casserole with diced lamb or chicken, onions, dried apricots and spices such as paprika and cumin.

BANANAS
GI 52

Bananas are one of the world's most popular fruits. Eat this versatile fruit raw or cooked; whole, sliced or mashed; or as a snack or part of a dessert, fruit salad or meal. They are also a nutritional goldmine: high in fibre, folate and vitamin C and rich in potassium, which is why sportspeople consume them in great numbers after intense exercise to replace nutrients and help maintain peak performance.

Unlike most other fruit, bananas contain both sugars and starch. The less ripe the banana, the lower its GI – ripening causes the starch to turn to sugars and the GI increases. The starch in raw bananas is resistant to digestion and reaches the large intestine intact, where it is fermented by the resident microflora. The products of fermentation are believed to be important for large intestine health and may reduce the risk of bowel cancer. Cooking bananas increases the GI because it gelatinises the starch so that it becomes easily digested.

> Did you know that if you place bananas in a mixed fruit bowl they'll help other fruit ripen?
>
> To prevent a peeled banana from going brown, brush it with a little lemon juice.

Serving suggestions
- If the bananas in your fruit bowl are looking over-ripe, freeze them in their skins, then peel and add to the blender. They make the most delicious ice-cream alternative for creamy thickshakes and smoothies.
- Enjoy banana custard or ice-cream made with semi-skimmed milk or soya drink.
- Add mashed banana to the mixing bowl for muffins and fruit breads.
- Gently fry banana slices in a little margarine and brown sugar and serve with pancakes or a dollop of low fat yoghurt – or both.
- Bake or steam green bananas (about 30 minutes) and serve as a vegetable accompaniment with barbecued meats.

CRANBERRY JUICE
GI 52 (unsweetened)
Cranberries have earned a reputation for promoting urinary tract health and research is now confirming this. Whole cranberries are an excellent source of iron, vitamin C and fibre

and are packed with anti-oxidant power. Cranberry juice is a healthy option but, like all juices, drink it in moderation. Remember, drinking a large glass can mean you are taking on board more energy (calories) than you intended – or need. As an alternative, try a cranberry spritzer with ice and soda.

Berries – enjoy them by the bowlful

Apart from strawberries (GI 40), most berries have so little carbohydrate it's difficult to test their GI. Their low carbohydrate content means their glycaemic load (GL) will be low, so enjoy them by the bowlful. They are a good source of vitamin C and fibre and some berries also supply small amounts of folate and essential minerals such as potassium, iron, calcium, magnesium and phosphorus.

Berries are best eaten as soon as possible after purchase. If you need to keep them for a day or two, here's how to minimise mould. Take them out of the punnet and store in the refrigerator on a couple of layers of paper towel and cover loosely with plastic wrap.

Serving suggestions

❑ Combine your favourite berries with a little caster sugar and a tablespoon or two of balsamic vinegar or a little white wine or orange juice. Let the flavours develop for 30 minutes or so at room temperature then serve.
❑ Top gelato, low fat ice-cream or yoghurt with a spoon or two of berries for a snack or dessert.
❑ Make berry smoothies with semi-skimmed milk, soya milk or yoghurt for breakfast or a meal in a glass when you are on the run.
❑ Purée berries for coulis, salsas, sauces, sorbets and ice-creams.
❑ Serve berries for breakfast with muesli or your favourite low GI cereal and a dollop of low fat vanilla or honey yoghurt.

See also Strawberries (page 127).

Serving suggestions

- Blend a tangy cranberry cooler by combining 250 ml (9 fl oz) of cranberry juice with ½ banana, a tub of low fat yoghurt, 100 g (3½ oz) fresh or frozen raspberries and a handful of crushed ice
- Whip up a creamy cranberry-banana flip for two. Blend 1 small banana with ½ pot vanilla low fat yoghurt, 250 ml (9 fl oz) of cranberry juice and 125 ml (4 fl oz) skimmed milk. Add more yoghurt if you like it when the straw stands up straight!

Citrus fruit – nutritional powerpacks

Citrus fruit – oranges, mandarins, lemons, grapefruit and limes – have among the highest levels of anti-oxidants of all fruit. They are also rich in folate, fibre, vitamin C and vitamin A. We know that oranges and grapefruit have a low GI, while the juice of lemons and limes provides acidity that slows gastric emptying and lowers the overall GI of a meal. Try a fresh squeeze of lemon or lime on vegetables with a twist of black pepper just before serving, or toss salad in a dressing made with oil, lemon juice and salt and pepper to taste.

See Grapefruit (page 118); Oranges (page 122).

CUSTARD APPLES
GI 54

Although you may not find custard apples in your local supermarket every day, the range of exotic and tropical fruits available is on the increase to satisfy consumer demand. In fact, with online shopping options, exotic fruit such as custard apples, which are also grown in Spain, can be delivered to your door. Creamy custard apples, originally from South America, taste like a tropical fruit

Dried fruit – concentrated flavour

Drying is the oldest known method of preserving fruit. It often happens naturally on the tree or vine and animals love the results too. It intensifies the flavour and sweetness and at the same time effectively concentrates the nutrients and retains the fibre. If you are watching your weight, keep in mind that the calorie content of dried fruit is higher than for fresh fruit.

salad and are virtually a complete low GI food source on their own, providing some protein, carbohydrate and fibre along with many essential vitamins and minerals, including vitamin C, potassium and magnesium.

If you haven't tried this fruit before, choose one that's just soft to touch (like an avocado) without splits or bruises. A few black spots on the skin don't matter. Ripe fruit will yield to gentle pressure and can be kept in the crisper section of the refrigerator for up to two days – but be aware that the skin will blacken. If unripe, store fruit at room temperature until ripe. To eat, simply cut in half or twist open and eat the creamy flesh straight away with a teaspoon discarding the black seeds, or scoop out the flesh and add to salads. The flesh discolours rapidly, so brush it with a little lemon or lime juice if you aren't eating it immediately. Add puréed custard apple to yoghurt or to desserts such as cake, sorbets, parfait and ice-cream for a taste of the tropics. Cooking alters the flavour, so stir segments into savoury dishes or curries just before serving to heat through.

Serving suggestions

- Power your day with an energy breakfast of muesli moistened with fresh orange juice and topped with scoops of custard apple.
- For a meal on the run, sip a custard apple smoothie made with low fat yoghurt and semi-skimmed milk with a little honey to sweeten.
- Sleep soundly after a custard apple egg nog made with low fat milk and honey to taste.

Dried dates update

Dates are one of the oldest cultivated fruits and a staple food throughout the Middle East. Rich in carbohydrate, dried dates are a good source of fibre, minerals such as iron, potassium and magnesium and vitamins B6, niacin and folate. Unlike most fruits they contain almost no vitamin C. It would appear that the GI value of dried dates could vary significantly depending on the variety (and there are approximately 600 varieties).

When dried dates were first tested their GI value was 103. This high value was puzzling and was rechecked a number of times. It may be that the amount of carbohydrate per serve on the packaging label was incorrect. A team in the Faculty of Medicine and Health Sciences at the United Arab Emirates University tested the khalas variety of dates in 2004 and found that the average GI value was 39.

Dried dates are a delicious snack or addition to stuffings, pilafs, muffins and winter warming desserts. Like all dried fruits, a little goes a long way.

GRAPEFRUIT
GI 25

Just half a grapefruit contains about 35 mg of vitamin C, which is almost your recommended daily intake. This is one of the lowest GI fruits and provides some fibre too. Choose fruit that feels 'heavy' for its size – this tends to indicate a thinner skin and plenty of juice. Store in your fruit bowl as they are juicier eaten at room temperature.

Serving suggestions

- Start your day with zest with juicy grapefruit's refreshing tang. Halve a grapefruit, loosen the segments and eat as is, or sweeten with a little sugar or a drizzle of pure floral honey.
- Toss segments in salads with smoked salmon and avocado; prawn and avocado; or Belgian endive, radicchio, beetroot and avocado; or simply add to Asian greens and a citrus dressing.
- Combine with chopped pepper, finely chopped onion and a little chilli for a tangy salsa to accompany barbecued meats.
- Enjoy as part of a winter fruit salad with sweeter ingredients such as oranges and raisins and a drizzle of honey.

GRAPEFRUIT JUICE
GI 48 (commercial)

Cool and refreshing as a snack or after a workout, one small glass of grapefruit juice is rich in vitamin C. The grapefruit juice you buy in the supermarket has a much higher GI than the whole fruit, possibly because manufacturers reduce its acidity to produce a juice with wide consumer appeal. If you squeeze your own grapefruit for juice, however, the GI will be similar to that of whole fruit.

Serving suggestions

- Combine with soda or mineral water for a cool, tangy spritzer.
- Add juice to desserts such as sorbets and mousses.

GRAPES
GI 46 (green)

Grapes are a perfect low GI finger food fruit – grab a small bunch and enjoy as a no-mess, no-fuss snack or with a fruit or cheese platter to finish a meal. They are a good source of vitamin C, provide some fibre and red-skinned grapes contain protective anti-oxidants called antho-cyanins. They have one of the highest sugar contents of all temperate fruits, which is one reason why they make such a good starter for alcoholic drinks – more sugar means more alcohol. The first wine (recorded in Mesopotamia and Egypt around 3000 BC) was probably made by accident by allowing a container of grapes to ferment naturally.

Choose bunches with plump, undamaged fruit (avoid split, sticky or withered grapes) and don't be shy about asking if you can taste-test for flavour.

Serving suggestions

- Top cereal with low fat vanilla yoghurt and a handful of fresh grapes to start the day.
- Put a bowl of grapes on the table after dinner.
- Add red and green grapes to fruit salads and side salads.
- Cool off with frozen fruit skewers – grapes, strawber-ries, banana slices and melon or pineapple chunks make a colourful combination.

HONEY

It could be said that we are all born with 'a sweet tooth'. We don't know why, but it may have something to do with the brain's dependence on glucose as its sole source of fuel. Our hunter–gatherer ancestors relished honey and all sorts of other sources of concentrated sugars such as maple syrup, dried fruits and honey ants and went to great trouble to obtain them. So, if you like to sweeten your food with honey or use it as a spread, you are following a long tradition!

The colour and flavour of honey differs depending on the nectar source (the flowers) visited by the honey bees. We now know from our testing in Australia that the GI of honey can vary too, depending on where the bees have been buzzing. We found that in Australia the lower GI honeys are what are called pure floral honeys (average GI 55) from the blossoms of particular eucalyptus nectar sources rather than the mass market blended honeys from a variety of nectar sources (GI more than 70).

Supermarkets do stock pure floral honeys including Tasmanian Leatherwood Honey (Sainsbury's) and Manuka honey but as yet, we don't know their GI. However, there's no need to go without honey, as a modest serving of 2 teaspoons of even a high GI blended honey, actually has a GL of only 5.

JAM

GI 55 (average)

A dollop (1–2 teaspoons) of jam or fruit spread on grainy bread or toast contains fewer calories than lightly spreading it with butter or margarine. So enjoy a little jam on your bread or toast and give fat the flick.

- Strawberry jam GI 51
- Apricot fruit spread GI 56

KIWI FRUIT
GI 53

The furry kiwi fruit provides plenty of vitamin C – just one will meet your daily requirements. They are also rich in fibre, a good source of both vitamin E and potassium and a moderate source of iron. They are renowned as a meat tenderiser thanks to the enzyme actinidin – simply rub cut or mashed fruit over the meat and leave for about 30–40 minutes before barbecuing or grilling.

The best way to eat them is simply to cut them in half and scoop out the flesh. Alternatively peel and slice or dice and add to fruit and green salads, and fruit and cheese platters, or purée and serve with low fat yoghurt, ice-cream, gelato and sorbets.

Serving suggestions

- Toss kiwi fruit slices with watercress and avocado chunks in a light citrus dressing.
- Bring colour and variety to a cheese platter with slices of kiwi fruit, small bunches of purple–red grapes, dried apricot halves and walnuts.

MANGOES
GI 51

Mangoes are one of the few tropical fruits that squeeze into the low GI range. They are also a rich source of vitamin C (one provides your recommended daily intake) and beta-carotene, and a useful source of fibre and potassium.

This versatile fruit is delicious fresh, sliced and puréed in desserts, or combined with fish, meat, poultry along with flavours such as lime juice, chilli and coriander for main meals. You can even eat them green in Asian-style salads and pickles, although you need to choose the right variety of mango. Ask your greengrocer to recommend a green eating mango or visit an Asian produce store.

Serving suggestions

- Stir-fry strips of duck or chicken breast and make a warm salad tossed with golden mango slices, bean sprouts, chopped onion, chilli, fresh mint leaves and a tangy Thai dressing.
- Combine diced mango with chopped red onion, tomatoes, red pepper and coriander and a dash of lime juice to serve as a salsa with seafood.
- Try chopped fresh mango with a scoop of low fat chocolate ice-cream and an almond wafer for a delicious and easy dessert.

ORANGES
GI 42

One orange is something of a personal protection powerhouse, providing you with your whole day's vitamin C requirement. Oranges are rich in anti-oxidants and are good sources of folate and potassium. Much of their sugar is sucrose, a 'double' sugar made up of glucose and fructose. When digested, only the glucose molecules have an impact on your blood glucose levels. This, plus the high acid content, account for the low GI.

Serving suggestions

- Peel and enjoy the juicy segments with breakfast cereal, as a snack, or as an after-dinner palate cleanser.
- Chop into fruit salads, toss into salads, add to soups or casseroles or to couscous.
- Slice and add to fruit punch.
- Carrot and orange make a great couple – enjoy this perfect partnership in soup, salad or juice.
- Oranges make delicious desserts – jellies, sorbets, souffles, crepes, ice-cream
- Try a citrus salad with orange and grapefruit segments, a can of chickpeas, cherry tomatoes and peppery rocket tossed in an oil and lemon juice dressing.

ORANGE JUICE

GI 50 (unsweetened)

Freshly squeezed juice has most of the health benefits of a whole orange, but lacks the fibre unless you throw in the pulp. Its GI will be similar to that of whole fruit. If you are buying oranges specifically for juicing, choose ones that are firm and heavy for their size.

The juices you buy from the supermarket tend to have a slightly higher GI than the whole fruit because they contain equal amounts of fructose, glucose and sucrose. During processing much of the original sucrose is partially split or 'hydrolysed' to glucose and fructose. When shopping look for unsweetened, 100 per cent juice.

Use orange juice to moisten breakfast cereal as a change from milk, or add to meat dishes, couscous or spinach salads to help increase iron absorption. And remember, it's all too easy to overdo your juice intake – a serve is just 150 ml (5 fl oz).

Serving suggestions

- Add juice to fruit punches, fruit salad, milk shakes and egg nog.
- Use orange juice's zesty flavour in marinades, sauces and dressings.
- Freeze juice to make summer treats such as ice-lollies and ice pops.

PAPAYA/PAWPAW

GI 56

You can be forgiven for being confused about whether to call this large, oval-shaped tropical fruit papaya or pawpaw, or even whether it's the same fruit, as the names are used interchangeably even by the experts. Native to the Americas, the tropical papaya (*Carica papaya*) is a completely different fruit from Asimina triloba – the true

> **The true pawpaw**
>
> The true pawpaw or papaw (*Asimina triloba*) is a North American native from the same family as custard apples. It has creamy-yellow, sweet flesh with a custard-like texture and looks rather like a fat, brown banana.

pawpaw (see sidebar). Papayas range in colour from a deep orange to a pale green, and in size from looking rather like a small football to an overgrown pear, depending on the variety. Whichever you buy, however, it will be rich in vitamins A and C, a moderate source of fibre and will have a low–medium GI.

Like many tropical fruits, a ripe papaya is best raw. Simply cut it in half lengthways, scoop out the seeds, peel away the skin, cut the flesh into slices or wedges and enjoy. The green or unripe fruit can be cooked as a vegetable or cut into strips or grated and added to Asian-style salads. The shiny black–grey seeds are usually thrown away, but they are also edible (they have a peppery flavour) – crush them and add to dressings or sprinkle over salads.

Serving suggestions

- Serve papaya slices for breakfast sprinkled with lemon or lime juice for a fresh-tasting start to the day, or dice papaya and add to tropical fruit salads with mangoes, kiwi fruit, passionfruit and berries.
- Purée ripe papaya and use as a sauce or topping or to flavour sorbets and ice creams (but not jellies – fresh papaya will not set in gelatine desserts).
- Serve seafood or chicken with a coriander and papaya salsa.
- Purée ripe papaya and add to marinades (it contains papain, a protein-splitting enzyme which can be used as a meat tenderiser) or just rub a little juice over meat and leave for about 20 minutes before cooking.

PEACHES
GI 42

It's nice to know that something as juicy and delicious as a ripe, fresh peach is so healthy. Peaches are good sources of vitamin C, potassium and fibre.

For eating, look for bruise-free peaches with a fragrant aroma that give a little to touch. For cooking, freestone peaches (ask your greengrocer if unsure) are probably the better choice. The easiest way to peel a peach is to dip it in boiling water, then in cold water. The peel should slide off easily. To prevent discolouration if you are not eating the cut fruit immediately, brush with a little lemon or lime juice.

Canned peaches have many of the nutritional benefits of fresh fruit (with a little less vitamin C) along with a low GI and the convenience of being available year round. Try single serving cans or pots as a snack.

Serving suggestions

- Top grainy toast with ricotta and thinly sliced fresh peaches for an easy breakfast or a tasty snack.
- Halve, stone and poach peaches in champagne, white wine or fruit juice with or without the skin and serve with low fat yoghurt or ice-cream.
- Sip on a fruity whip of puréed peaches or nectarines blended with ice and orange juice.
- Sprinkle fresh peach halves with a little cinnamon and lightly grill.

PEARS
GI 38

Juicy, sweet pears are one of the world's most loved fruits – they've even been immortalised in poetry, paintings and a Christmas carol! They are renowned as a non-allergenic food, thus a favourite when introducing babies to solid foods. An excellent source of fibre and rich in vitamin C and potassium, fresh pears have a low GI because most of their sugar is fructose. Canned pears in 'natural juice' also have a low GI (44) because the fructose remains in high concentration during processing. Single-serve pots and cans are also available. Again, look for those in natural juice.

Although they are often hard when you buy them, pears will ripen at room temperature in a few days. Pack a pear for lunch or to snack on during the day – there's no need to peel as the skin is a good source of fibre.

Serving suggestions

- Dip pear slices in lemon juice and serve with cheese and walnuts.
- Toss in salads – try pear, avocado, rocket or radicchio and walnuts.
- Poach or bake pears in a light citrus syrup or red wine with a touch of cardamom.
- Try topping a bowl of porridge with grilled pear slices and a drizzle of honey or some brown sugar.

PLUMS
GI 39

Plum pudding, plum jam, Chinese plum sauce – this fruit is popular the world over. It's also a good source fibre and provides small quantities of vitamins and minerals. Fresh plums have a low GI and it's likely that canned plums in natural juice will also have a low GI. However they have not been tested yet.

Choose plump, undamaged fruit (no splits, bruises or signs of decay) with a slight whitish bloom and enjoy fresh as a snack or to finish a meal.

Serving suggestions

- Halve, remove stone and add to fruit salads and compotes or serve with cheese or fruit platters.
- Purée for making sauces and delicious sorbets and ice-cream – or plum soup.
- Top stewed plums with a sprinkle of toasted muesli and a dollop of yoghurt for a breakfast with a difference.
- Poach plums in red or white wine with a stick of cinnamon and serve hot or cold.

PRUNES
GI 29

Prunes have a reputation for keeping us regular, but there's more to this tasty dried fruit than that. They are a concentrated source of many nutrients including beta-carotene, B vitamins, potassium and phosphorus. Prunes are also a useful source of iron for vegetarians. Their sugar content, naturally occurring acids and fibre make them a great low GI food for snacks on their own or as part of a fruit and nut mix.

You can buy prunes with stones or pitted – but check for the occasional stone as the processing is not always perfect. Soften or 'plump' by simmering or soaking and enjoy in desserts, or add to lamb, pork, chicken and game dishes for a Moroccan flavour.

Serving suggestions

- Combine prunes with an equal amount of water in a small pan and gently simmer for about 5–10 minutes. Add a slice of lemon or some spices for extra flavour.
- To soften in the microwave, pour fruit juice or water over prunes, cover and cook.
- To soften overnight, place prunes in a heatproof bowl and just cover with boiling water. When cool, cover and store in the refrigerator.

STRAWBERRIES
GI 40

It's no wonder deliciously versatile strawberries are the world's most popular berry fruit. You can eat them fresh, add them to fruit salads and smoothies, use them in a delicious dessert, decorate cakes with them, or make them into jams, fruit spreads and sauces.

Fresh strawberries are rich in vitamin C, potassium, folate, fibre and protective anti-oxidants. Because the average serve has very little impact on blood glucose levels, people with diabetes can eat them freely. So reap the health benefits as you enjoy them by the bowlful, but hold the cream! A word of warning: don't eat too many in a single day. They can have diuretic and laxative effects if you overdo it.

If you aren't eating them immediately, spread the berries out in a single layer on paper towel on a plate and lightly cover with plastic wrap. Remove any damaged or mouldy ones first.

Serving suggestions

- For a perfect parfait, take a tall glass and arrange layers of sliced strawberries, whole blueberries and dollops of low fat vanilla yogurt. Mango slices are delicious with this combination, too.
- Blend strawberries for a bright and refreshing coulis to serve with low fat ice-cream or poached pears. Freeze for fruity ice-cubes.
- Add strawberries to smoothies and shakes with low fat yoghurt or ice-cream.
- Serve whole with fruit and cheese platters or dip in chocolate for a sweet treat with coffee at the end of a meal.
- Quarter fresh strawberries and soak in balsamic vinegar with a little sugar.
- Add to green salads with baby spinach, small cubes of mozzarella and a light balsamic dressing.
- Enjoy a dollop of strawberry jam (GI 51) on grainy fresh bread or toast in moderation.

SULTANAS
GI 56

For a quick and easy low GI snack it's hard to go past sultanas. They are a good source of fibre and also provide some potassium and vitamin E. They are juicier, softer and sweeter than their cousins the currant and raisin, which may account for their popularity in breakfast cereals, muesli and mixes with nuts and apricots. They also make a versatile cooking ingredient – add to all sorts of dishes from casseroles and compotes to couscous, cakes, cookies and crumbles.

Serving suggestions

- A mini-box of sultanas is ideal for school lunch boxes.
- Spread grainy bread with a little peanut butter and make a salad sandwich with grated carrot, cucumber slices, sultanas and shredded lettuce.
- Sweeten breakfast cereal and yoghurt with a spoonful of sultanas.
- Simmer sultanas in apple or orange juice with peeled and grated ginger to make a tasty compote for breakfast or dessert.
- Add sultanas to your favourite bread and butter pudding recipe along with chopped dates.

VEGETABLES

Think of vegetables as 'free' foods – they are full of fibre, essential nutrients and protective anti-oxidants that will fill you up without adding extra calories. And most are so low in carbohydrate that they will have no measurable effect on your blood glucose levels.

Pile your plate high with leafy green and salad vegetables and eat your way to long-term health and vitality.

Leafy green and salad vegetables, for example, have so little carbohydrate that we can't test their GI. Even in generous serving sizes they will have no effect on your blood glucose levels.

Higher carbohydrate vegetables include sweetcorn, potato, sweet potato, taro and yam, so you need to watch the portion sizes with these. Most varieties of potato tested to date have a high GI, so if you are a big potato eater, try to replace some with low GI alternatives such as sweetcorn, sweet potato, yam or pulses. Vegetables such as pumpkin, carrots, peas and beetroot contain some carbohydrate, but a normal serving size contains so little that it won't raise your blood glucose levels significantly.

How much?

One serving is equivalent to:

- About 80 grams (2¾ oz) cooked vegetables (other than potato, sweetcorn and sweet potato)
- 1 dessert bowl of raw salad vegetables
- 250 ml (9 fl oz) vegetable soup (without cream!)
- 250 ml (9 fl oz) pure vegetable juice

How much a day?

Even the smallest eater should aim to eat five or more servings of vegetables every day, including fresh and frozen vegetables, vegetable juices and soups. This is a minimum of 400 grams (14 oz) of cooked vegetables or 4 dessert bowls of salad.

Starchy vegetables – how much a day?

Starchy vegetables such as sweet potato, potato and sweetcorn are higher in carbohydrate so their GI and serve size is more relevant. One serving is equivalent to:

- 1 medium (115 grams/4 oz) potato (a touch smaller than a tennis ball)
- 100 grams (3½ oz) mashed potato
- 115 grams (4 oz) sweet potato
- 100 grams (3½ oz) corn kernels
- ½ cob sweetcorn
- 1 large (about 150 grams/5½ oz) parsnip

In addition to the five or more serves of other fresh or frozen vegetables:

- Smaller eaters: 1 serve
- Medium eaters: 3 serves
- Bigger eaters: 4 serves

Serving suggestions

1. Pile vegetables on your favourite sandwiches. Try sliced peppers, cucumber, onion, tomatoes, broccoli, courgettes, spinach and mushrooms. Or include salad ingredients or chopped up leftover vegetables in a pitta pocket, sandwich or tortilla wrap. Top grainy toast with leftover vegies.
2. Add vegetables to stir-fried meat, chicken, prawns, fish or tofu dishes.
3. Make a meal of stuffed vegetables – peppers, tomato, aubergine and onion all make great 'containers'.
4. Use herbs and spices for flavour and serve two or three portions of different vegetables such as broccoli, carrots and cauliflower or even a ratatouille of mixed vegetables including tomatoes, peppers, aubergine and onions.
5. Throw some vegetables under the grill or on the barbecue with meat. Try courgettes, corn, peppers, mushrooms, aubergine, onion or thick slices of parboiled sweet potato. (Use vegetable oil spray or a little olive oil on a cold grill to prevent sticking.)
6. Make homemade vegetable soups. Try combinations like onion, carrot, celery and tomato in a chicken or vegetable stock. Purée if you prefer a creamy texture.
7. Try a vegetarian main dish at least once a week such as creamy vegetarian lasagne with ricotta, onions, mushrooms, tomatoes, lentils and spinach.
8. Add grated carrot and courgettes to breads and muffins, or grated carrot and onion to rissoles and burgers.

Salad for starters

Enjoy a mixed salad (lettuce, tomato, cucumber, celery, peppers) tossed in an oil and vinegar dressing before moving on to your main course.
A recent study reported that eating a salad like this for starters helps to fill you up and you will eat less overall.

9. For quick munching, keep celery, peppers, baby carrots, cucumbers, broccoli or cauliflower florets and cherry tomatoes on hand. Dip them in hummous, low fat aubergine or tuna dips or a homemade tomato salsa.
10. Buy a vegetable cookbook packed with recipes you can't wait to try out and buy and try vegetables you haven't cooked before.

Storage and cooking tips

Vegetables are best fresh, so shop two or three times a week if you can and use them within two to three days.

Ethylene gas produced by ageing fruit and vegetables leads to their deterioration. You can minimise the effect of ethylene by storing vegetables in the fridge in long life bags, which are available in the food wrap section of supermarkets, or you can use special cartridges (available in some supermarkets) designed to absorb ethylene. Fruits give off more ethylene than vegetables, but vegetables are more sensitive to its effects so if you have two crispers, keep fruit in one and vegetables in the other.

Wash green leafy vegetables well to remove any soil or grit, then rinse before cooking. They are best steamed or cooked with a minimum of water. Tear salad leaves into small pieces and dry them thoroughly before adding to the salad bowl – the water will dilute the dressing. Salad spinners are great for this purpose, or simply use a clean tea towel.

To make sure you gain the benefit of all those essential nutrients when cooking:

- leave the skins on whenever you can, or peel very finely
- avoid soaking vegetables in water
- use a steamer or microwave for best results
- cook vegetables in big chunks rather than coarsely chopped
- reduce the amount of water you use, cover the pan and

cook quickly and as close to serving time as possible; never add bicarbonate of soda to the cooking water
- cook vegetables until they're softened but still firm to bite

Takeaway tips

When you are ordering takeaway food opt for choices that include vegetables, such as:

- regular hamburger with salad
- pizza piled with vegetable toppings – mushrooms, tomatoes, peppers, spinach, artichoke
- salad with sandwiches, wraps or rolls
- pasta with a tomato-based sauce and plenty of vegetables
- stuffed potato with Mexican-style beans, tomato salsa and cheese
- sweetcorn on the cob
- vegetarian nachos
- salad as a side order or a main course (hold the fries!)
- meat and vegetable fajitas
- corn tortilla with beans and salsa

CARROTS
GI 41

'Eating your carrots will help you see in the dark' – sound familiar? Carrots are rich in beta-carotene, a plant form of vitamin A or retinol, which we need to maintain normal vision. A deficiency in vitamin A produces night blindness (an inability to see in dim light). Carrots also provide some vitamin C and fibre, so add them when you're cooking soups, salads, stir-fries, stews, casseroles, cakes and puddings.

Because they make a deliciously crunchy raw snack, it's worthwhile being fussy when shopping and choose firm, bright orange carrots. Avoid the ones with cracks, soft patches or discoloured skin if you can. Grate and add to salads and sandwiches, cut into sticks for dips or snacks, or boil, steam or bake (whole or sliced) and serve with main meals.

Salad on the side

A side salad tossed in an oil and vinegar dressing with your meal, especially a high GI meal, will help to keep blood glucose levels under control.

Serving suggestions

- Enjoy a freshly grated carrot salad with a bunch of chopped chives and a dressing of oil and lemon juice.
- For a Middle Eastern flavour toss cooked carrot slices in a little oil and lemon juice with roasted cumin seeds crushed in a mortar and pestle.
- Make a creamy, puréed carrot soup with leeks, a potato, and a good quality chicken stock served with a dollop of low fat yoghurt.
- Peel and juice a couple of carrots or add other vegetables or fruit such as celery, apple and orange to start your day with a good healthy glow.

Keep a look out for cassava

Although you may never have seen this starchy tuber in your local supermarket, you may well use one of its best known by-products, tapioca (GI 70), when thickening sauces or making puddings. Cassava (GI 46), also called yuca, manioc and mandioca, is a high carbohydrate staple for millions of people around the world. It looks rather like an elongated potato (about 30 centimetres long) with coarse brown skin and white, fibrous flesh. The roots are usually peeled and boiled, baked or fried. They are also dried and processed into granules, pastes, flours – and even alcohol. The young leaves can be eaten as a vegetable, while the larger, older leaves are sometimes used for wrapping food before cooking.

CORN
See Sweetcorn, page 136.

PEAS, GREEN
GI 48

There's nothing like the aroma of shelling and eating fresh, green peas straight from the pod. Today, most of us buy them in frozen packs – the manufacturer has done the hard work. Green peas are actually a legume, but we have included them here as most of us think of them as a green vegetable. They are rich in fibre and vitamin C and higher in protein than most vegetables. Although a good source of thiamin, niacin, phosphorus and iron when fresh, cooking will reduce the nutrient levels. Frozen peas have about 60 per cent more beta-carotene than fresh peas that have been exposed to light during their trip to market.

If you do buy peas in the pod, you'll need about 350 grams (12 oz) of pods to fill a cup with shelled peas. And tempting as it is to pick up a pack of 'freshly' shelled peas from your greengrocer or supermarket, only do so if you know they really have been freshly shelled and you plan to use them immediately.

Boil, steam or microwave peas for about 4–5 minutes (remember, cooking destroys the nutrients) or add to rice dishes such as risottos, pasta dishes, omelettes, soups and stews (at the last minute), or combine with mashed potato or sweet potato.

Peas with edible pods such as mangetouts and sugar snaps (immature pods) only need the minimum of cooking time, too, and are delicious in stir-fries, or steamed or cooked in the microwave for a side dish.

Serving suggestions

- Whip up an omelette with onion, a little ham or lean bacon and fresh peas.
- If you feel like comfort food, purée or mash cooked peas with chicken stock and a little margarine.

- Add blanched mangetouts or sugar snaps to salads or serve with vegetable platters and dips.

See also Split Peas (page 194).

Have you heard about prickly pear?

The fleshy pads or 'paddles' (nopales) of the prickly pear cactus (nopal) with the spines removed are a traditional ingredient in Mexican cuisine. They are a good source of calcium and vitamin C and contain beta-carotene and iron. They have a small amount of carbohydrate and an amazingly low GI – 7. Sometimes called 'edible cactus', nopales are usually sold in Mexico and the US 'despined' although you'd probably have to trim the eyes with a vegetable peeler to remove any remaining 'prickers'. They can be diced for salads; steamed quickly as an accompaniment (the texture should be crunchy); added to soups, salsas, stews, stir-fries, fillings for scrambled eggs or tortillas; or stirred into Mexican-style recipes with chilli, tomatoes and corn.

SWEETCORN
GI 48 (on the cob)

Sweetcorn is actually the seed of a type of grass that grew in the Americas for thousands of years before Christopher Columbus arrived on the scene. It is rich in vitamin C and a good source of fibre, folate and beta-carotene. It also has higher amounts of protein and vitamin B than most other vegetables because it's actually a cereal grain. Canned and frozen kernels have a similar GI to corn on the cob.

Corn is often used as a base for gluten-free products. However, many products made from corn don't have a low GI at all – cornflakes (GI 77), popcorn (GI 72), cornmeal

(GI 68) and corn pasta (GI 87). Corn chips do (GI 42), but they are also very high in salt and fat.

For the sweetest flavour, buy corn on the cob with the fresh green husk intact, because the natural sugar in the kernels starts converting into starch the moment the husk is removed. To avoid disappointment, stay away from cobs with dry yellow husks and small shrinking kernels.

Boil, steam or microwave briefly, or bake or barbecue and serve piping hot topped with the merest hint of margarine or butter. Toss whole baby corn into stir-fries or cut kernels off the cob (slicing as close to the cob as possible) and add to soups and stews, fritters and frittata, chowders and crepes, salsa and salads. You can substitute canned kernels in recipes calling for fresh, but remember that the flavour won't be quite as sweet.

Serving suggestions

- Spice up barbecue meats with a tangy corn salsa made from diced tomato, red and green peppers, onion, chopped chilli (to taste), fresh coriander and a lime dressing.
- Barbecue cobs by pulling back the husk, removing the silk and then pulling the husk back over the kernels to cover before cooking. When barbecuing, the experts recommend plunging the whole cobs into iced water for an hour before cooking to help the corn cook slowly and evenly.
- Make a sweetcorn frittata with chopped onion, lean bacon, eggs, semi-skimmed milk and parsley and top with a sprinkle of reduced fat tasty cheese.
- Add the finishing touch to a warm salad of roast sweet potato, red onion, red pepper, baby aubergine and baby spinach with small corn cob chunks.

What about potatoes?

Boiled, mashed, baked or fried, everybody loves potatoes. However, we now know that the GI value of potatoes can vary significantly depending on variety and cooking method (GI 56 to 89) – according to University of Toronto researchers reporting in the Journal of the American Dietetic Association in 2005. Their study found that precooking and reheating potatoes or consuming cold cooked potatoes (such as potato salad) reduces the glycaemic response. The highest GI values were found in potatoes that were freshly cooked and in instant mashed potatoes.

In our testing so far in Australia, the only potatoes to make the moderate GI range are tiny, new canned ones (GI 65). The lower GI of these potatoes may be due to differences in the structure of the starch. As potatoes age, the degree of branching of their amylopectin starch increases significantly, becoming more readily gelatinised and digested, thus producing a higher GI. New potatoes are also smaller and there seems to be a correlation between size and GI – the smaller the potato the lower the GI.

Although GI values for potatoes available in UK supermarkets haven't been published yet, there's no need to say 'no' to potatoes altogether just because they may have a high GI. They are fat free (when you don't fry them), nutrient rich and filling. Not every food you eat has to have a low GI. So enjoy them, but in moderation. Try steaming small new potatoes (with their skin for added nutrients), or bake a jacket potato and add a tasty topping based on beans, chickpeas or corn kernels. Add variety to meals and occasionally replace potatoes with sweetcorn, sweet potato or yams, or serve pasta, noodles, basmati rice or pulses.

SWEET POTATO
GI 44

Sweet potatoes aren't a 'potato' at all, they are the roots of a vine from the sprawling morning glory family, and a staple food in many parts of the world. There are several varieties: orange fleshed with red skin (kumara); red-purple skinned with yellow flesh; and white skinned with yellow skin and flesh. All are rich in nutrients including beta-carotene, vitamin C and fibre plus vitamin E, thiamin and folate. A versatile vegetable with a low GI, they make a great substitute for potatoes and, like pumpkin, you can use them in sweet dishes, too. A big advantage over potatoes is that the skin does not develop green patches (which makes them inedible) when exposed to light.

They are as easy to prepare and cook as potatoes – peel or simply scrub the skins and steam, boil, bake or microwave. Try mashing peeled sweet potatoes with a little mustard oil or wrapping small chunks in foil and cooking them on the barbecue. Sliced or cut into chunks, they make a tasty addition to soups, stews, stir-fries and salads (roasted first); cooked and puréed you can add them to scone or cake mixes.

Serving suggestions

- Tuck into a winter-warming shepherd's pie with a sweet potato mash topping.
- Make a spicy stir-fry with onions, ginger, garlic, sweet potato slices, peas and water chestnuts.
- Create casseroles and stews by adding a variety of vegetables including sweet potatoes, tomatoes, onions and carrots to chicken or lean meat.
- Make a creamy soup with sweet potatoes and Granny Smith apples flavoured with cumin and cinnamon and topped with a dollop of low fat plain yoghurt.

> ### Have you heard about taro?
>
> Taro, sometimes called 'elephant ear', is an important food throughout the Pacific Islands. It's a good source of vitamin C and fibre and, like other traditional staples such as sweet potato and yam, it is slowly digested, which is probably why it offered protection against diabetes to at-risk populations such as Pacific Islanders, Maoris and Australian Aborigines. The increased incidence of diabetes in these groups today is linked to increased consumption of modern quickly digested starches.
>
> If you haven't tried taro before, look for firm, hairy tubers with no wrinkling of the skin. Wear rubber gloves when peeling as the juices occasionally cause a skin irritation. Taro flesh is similar to sweet potato in flavour and you can use it the same way – steamed, boiled or cut into wedges and baked.

TOMATOES

As with most vegetables you can tuck into tomatoes without thinking about their GI. They are so low in carbohydrate that they have no measurable effect on your blood glucose levels, but they do provide plenty of fibre, vitamins, minerals and health-giving lycopene, an anti-cancer anti-oxidant.

Products made with tomatoes such as tomato juice and tomato soup are more concentrated and can be a useful source of carbohydrate for light meals and snacks.

CANNED TOMATO SOUP
GI 38

While canned tomato soup is a quick and easy meal with a slice or two of grainy toast, it is also great for quick casseroles and sauces – try it as a bolognese sauce base. Many brands contain large amounts of sodium, so look for salt-reduced ones. A serving is 250 ml (9 fl oz).

COMMERCIAL TOMATO JUICE
GI 38

On the rocks or straight from the can you can feel good about drinking tomato juice (no sugar and minimal sodium added). A thirst-quenching glass provides vitamins A and C, potassium and folic acid. A serving is 150 ml (5 fl oz).

Serving suggestions

- Add beans to your favourite homemade tomato soup recipe and top with finely chopped fresh herbs for a satisfying meal.
- Oven-roast tomatoes and serve with pasta shapes or stir a fresh tomato sauce through spaghetti for a meal in minutes.

YAM
GI 37

Like sweet potato and taro, yams are high in fibre, nutrient dense and a good source of vitamin C and potassium. They have long been a staple food in Asia, throughout the Pacific Islands and in New Zealand. In Australia the Aborigines ate many species of yam; and when they led their traditional 'bush tucker' lifestyle they were protected from diabetes.

Use yams in your cooking in the same way you would use sweet potatoes, although yams tend to have an 'earthier' flavour. Wash and peel before baking, steaming, boiling or microwaving to serve as an accompaniment or add to salads, soups and stews.

Serving suggestions

- Purée yam cooked with leeks and chicken stock to make a creamy soup and flavour with fresh herbs such as dill or chives.

Vegetable juices

Watch the sodium content in commercial vegetable juices – look for brands with low- or reduced-sodium labels. Or make your own!

- Toss cooked bite-sized chunks of yam with mesclun, onion slices, peppers and chives in a light oil and vinegar dressing for a satisfying salad.
- Steam and mash yam chunks with skimmed milk and a teaspoon or two of margarine and season with salt and a few twists of freshly ground black pepper to taste.
- Bake a gratin at 180°C (350°F, Gas mark 4) with overlapping yam slices moistened with chicken stock, sprinkled with a teaspoon of dried sage topped with grated cheddar cheese and freshly grated nutmeg.

BREADS & CEREALS

High in fibre, rich in nutrients, bulky and filling, wholegrain cereal foods serve us well.

Did you know that the type of bread and cereal you eat affects the overall GI of your diet the most? Why? Well, cereal grains such as rice, wheat, oats, barley and rye and products made from them such as bread, pasta and breakfast cereals are the most concentrated sources of carbohydrate in our diet.

These days, supermarket shelves are packed with products based on quickly digested, high GI flours and grains. Breakfast cereals are a good example. Once, a bowl of slowly digested porridge made with traditional rolled oats gave most of us the energy to keep going from breakfast through to lunchtime. Nowadays we are more likely to fill that breakfast bowl with high GI crunchy flakes that will spike our blood glucose and insulin levels and leave us needing a mid-morning snack to keep going.

A simple swap is all it takes to reduce the GI of your diet. To get started, replace some of those high GI breads and breakfast cereals with low GI carbs that will trickle fuel into your engine. Here's how on the opposite page.

How much?

One serving is equivalent to:

- 1 medium slice bread (sandwich thickness) or ½ English-style muffin
- 30 grams (1 oz) breakfast cereal, rolled oats or muesli
- 100 grams (3½ oz) cooked rice or other small grains such as bulghur or couscous; or cooked pasta or noodles

How much a day?

- Small eaters: 4 servings
- Medium eaters: 6 servings
- Bigger eaters: 8 servings

Switch from this high GI food	To this low GI alternative
Bread – wholemeal or white	Bread and bread rolls containing visible grainy bits, multigrain, 100 per cent wholegrain stoneground, whole wheat, sourdough, sourdough rye, pumpernickel, soya and linseed and fruit breads.
Processed breakfast cereal such as cornflakes and rice bubbles	Rolled oats (not instant), and oat-based cereal such as muesli or a fibre-based cereal such as All-Bran®
Plain biscuits and crackers; wafers, rice cakes	Biscuits made with dried fruit, wholegrains and oats such as oatcakes, or make your own 'crisp' breads with baked or toasted thin slices of low GI breads.
Cakes and muffins,	Add fruit, oats and wholegrains to the mix. Look for recipes on wholegrain cereal packets. Go halves in a slice of fruit and nut cake or fruit and muesli muffin in a café.
Rice	Choose low GI varieties (basmati or Koshihikari sushi rice) or try buckwheat noodles or barley instead – you can even make a barley risotto.

Serving suggestions

1. Start the day with porridge or muesli, fruit and a dollop of low fat yoghurt.
2. Top grainy toast with creamed sweetcorn, grilled mushrooms or baked beans for something savoury; or ricotta and slices of peaches or apples for a fruity flavour.
3. When buying lunch, choose a grainy or low GI bread or roll for sandwiches.
4. Pack pitta pockets with a bean or chickpea salad, tomato and onion slices and lots of fresh basil or coriander.
5. Serve noodles, pasta, low GI rice, bulghur or quinoa with main meals instead of potato.
6. Add barley, pasta or a low GI rice to soups, stews and casseroles for a filling one-dish wonder.
7. Add bulghur or oats to homemade burger patties or rissoles and serve with a wholemeal bun.
8. Develop a taste for wholegrain bread (try toasting it to begin with), and commit to eating it as your main bread choice.
9. Develop a repertoire of low GI snacks – raisin toast or fruit loaf with a dollop of ricotta; pitta crisps dunked in hummous or salsa.
10. Get hold of a natural wholefoods cookbook, stock your pantry with wholegrain staples and try a new recipe each week.

What about gluten?

People with coeliac disease have a permanent intolerance of gluten, a type of protein in wheat, rye, barley, millet, triticale and oats. Even eating tiny amounts can cause a problem. There are a number of gluten-free products on the market, but with their refined corn or rice starch content many have intermediate or high GI values. If you are on a gluten-free diet and need to reduce the overall GI of your diet, opt for basmati rice or Koshihikari sushi rice, pastas made from soya, noodles made from rice or mung beans and pulses in any form.

Check the tables (page 219) or go to www.glycemicindex.com to find the latest GI values. Or contact manufacturers for information on the GI of their products.

BREAD

Brown or white, wholemeal or multigrain, sourdough or soya and linseed, sliced or in loaves or rolls, bread is truly a staple food – it's inexpensive, low in fat and a useful source of protein, carbohydrate and fibre along with essential vitamins and minerals. In Britain it represents at least 40 per cent of our cereal intake. Most breads sold today have a high GI because they are made from quickly digested refined flours – white or wholemeal. Choose a low GI bread and you are on your way to reducing the overall GI of your diet. Here's how.

Look for really grainy breads, granary, 100 per cent stoneground wholemeal or wholewheat, sourdough, or breads made from chickpea or other pulse-based flours such as soya, or with added soyabeans. Look for these breads in the bread or bakery section of your supermarket, in specialty bakeries or delis, and in health, natural and organic food stores. Check out the ingredient list on the packet. Good choices will list grains such as barley, rye, triticale, oats or oat bran and kibbled wheat; or seeds such as sunflower or linseed; and pulses such as soyabeans. If you want a general rule of thumb: the coarser textured, denser and less processed a bread is, the lower its GI is likely to be.

Don't over-spread yourself

Breads, bread rolls and pocket breads are not fattening in themselves. It's what goes on (or in) them that can pile on the calories. A smear of margarine is all you need – or none at all. For a change, try Nutella®, peanut butter, almond or cashew butter, or avocado. Or you can opt for low fat alternatives like ricotta or cottage cheese or a fresh fruit spread.

Baking your own fruit loaf

As yet we don't have a homemade wholegrain bread recipe with a low GI (although not for the lack of trying). It is very difficult to predict the GI of baked goods that include flour. However, we know that fruit loaves have a lower GI because some of the flour is replaced with dried fruit. This delicious homemade fruit loaf recipe is from *The Low GI Diet Cookbook* (Hodder Mobius). Enjoy it for breakfast, in a bread and butter pudding or toasted as a snack. The loaf is also packed with the fibre needed for a healthy digestive system – 1 slice contains about 4 grams fibre.

To make the fruit loaf put 50 grams (1¾ oz) All-Bran® cereal in a bowl, pour over 300 ml (10½ fl oz) skimmed milk and soak for 30 minutes. Preheat the oven to 180° C (350°F/Gas mark 4).

Sift 225 grams (8 oz) wholemeal self-raising flour and 1 teaspoon baking powder into a bowl and stir in the bran cereal mixture, together with any bran left in the sieve. Stir in 90 grams (3 oz) sultanas, 50 grams (1¾ oz) dried apricots (cut into small dice), 50 grams (1¾ oz) pitted prunes (cut into small dice), 75 grams (2½ oz) dark muscovado or dark brown sugar and 4 tablespoons pure floral honey, and mix well. Spoon the mixture into a non-stick 900 gram (2 lb) loaf tin (or brush the tin with oil to prevent sticking) and level the top. Bake for 1–1¼ hours, or until the loaf is cooked and golden brown on top. Allow the loaf to cool a little in the tin before turning it out onto a wire rack to cool completely.

CHAPATTI

GI 27 (made with besan flour)

Chapatti is an unleavened bread eaten every day by millions of people throughout India and Sri Lanka, and found on the menu in Indian restaurants worldwide. When made with besan flour, chapatti has a low GI. Besan flour is made from ground, dried chickpeas and is also used to make roti and other Indian breads. It's a heavy-textured flour with a distinctive nutty flavour and you can often find it in health food shops, Asian produce stores and the Asian foods section of supermarkets. Nutrient rich thanks to its pulse origins, besan is an excellent source of protein and the minerals potassium, calcium and magnesium.

Chapatti is also made from barley flour and from atta, a wheat flour with a higher GI (63) due to the nature of the starch – so if you are ordering chapattis in a restaurant, ask about the ingredients. If you are making them yourself, use a recipe that specifies besan or gram flour. One chapatti could be equivalent to as much as 3 bread serves, depending on size.

Serving suggestions

- Serve a curry with chapattis instead of basmati rice, or to mop up a delicious dhal.
- Use chapattis to wrap a curry mixture made from lean mince meat browned with your favourite curry paste, a chopped onion and a can of brown lentils or chickpeas. Heat through and stir in a couple of tablespoons of low fat natural yoghurt and freshly chopped mint. Spoon onto one side of the chapatti, roll up and serve while still warm.

FRUIT LOAF

GI range 44–54

There are several types of fruit loaves or breads which include raisins, sultanas, dried apricots or apple, figs and sometimes nuts and seeds. The dried fruit content means they can be a useful source of iron, protein, fibre, thiamin, niacin, riboflavin and magnesium. Generally, the heavier, dense fruity breads will have a lower GI. Enjoy fresh or toasted for breakfast or as a snack.

Serving suggestions

- Snack on toasted fruit loaf with a dollop of ricotta.
- Add flavour to a bread and butter pudding by making it with slices of fruit loaf – great comfort food or for filling hollow legs. Spread 8 slices of fruit loaf with a tablespoon of margarine. Cut into triangles and place in layers in a round casserole dish. Whisk 3 eggs with 500 ml (17 fl oz) of semi-skimmed milk or soya milk and 2 tablespoons of sugar or honey and pour over the bread layers. Stand the casserole dish in a baking pan filled with enough water to come halfway up the sides of the dish. Bake in a moderate oven (180°C/350°F, Gas mark 4) for 40 minutes or until browned on top.

PITTA BREAD

GI 57

Top it, stuff it, wrap it, cut it into wedges and dip it, or split it open and bake it to make 'crisps' – pitta is the ultimate meal-in-a-bread to have around for all occasions. With all the health benefits of ordinary bread, this traditional Middle Eastern flat two-layered bread splits open horizontally, making the perfect pocket for your favourite fillings.

Serving suggestions

- Wrap up with hummous, shredded lettuce, felafel, tabbouleh and a tangy tomato salsa; or avocado, mushrooms, bean salad, shredded lettuce and pepper strips; or tuna, borlotti beans, onion rings, cucumber, feta and a drizzle of oil and vinegar.
- Use pitta bread as an instant pizza base – top with tomato paste, mushrooms, peppers, finely sliced onion, olives and a sprinkle of Parmesan cheese.
- For breakfast, toast and top with fresh light ricotta and a dollop of blackberry all-fruit preserves.
- Serve dips such as hummous and babaghanoush with pitta crisps – simply cut the pitta bread into triangles, open out the 'halves' and spray with a little olive oil, sprinkle over paprika for extra flavour and bake at 180°C (350°F/Gas mark 4) for about 5 minutes, or until crisp.

PUMPERNICKEL
GI 50
This traditional rye bread from Germany can be something of an acquired taste. It's a very good source of fibre and thanks to its high proportion of whole cereal grains, has a low GI value. Also known as rye kernel bread, pumpernickel contains 80–90 per cent whole and cracked rye kernels.

Pumpernickel (no one is quite sure of the origins of the name) has a strong flavour and is dark, dense and compact – not 'airy' like some breads. It is usually sold thinly sliced and vacuum packed for long shelf life. You can crumble it to use in stuffings and for making desserts, but it is most popular as an appetiser.

Serving suggestions

- For an appetiser, top pumpernickel with tangy cheese and apple or pear slivers, spicy sausage and salsa, or smoked salmon, horseradish cream and dill.

Keep them cool

If you plan to make salad sandwiches ahead of time or pack them for your lunch, be sure to include a cold pack. If you're taking your sandwiches on a picnic, park the cooler in the shade. Foods most susceptible to bacteria growth are meats, poultry, eggs and mayonnaise, so be sure they are not left at room temperature for more than an hour.

- For breakfast, toast pumpernickel, spread lightly with margarine and accompany with a hot chocolate drink made with semi-skimmed milk.

SOURDOUGH
GI 54

Crusty, chewy white sourdough's characteristic flavour comes from the slow fermentation process, which produces a build-up of organic acids. It's about the best low GI bread substitute for people who absolutely insist they can only eat white bread. Use for sandwiches and toast (with sweet or savoury spreads and toppings) or serve with main meals, soups and salads.

Serving suggestions

Make bruschetta for a quick and easy light meal or snack. Simply brush slices of crusty sourdough with a little olive oil then lightly grill or bake on both sides and top with:

- fresh tomato and basil salsa with a dash of balsamic vinegar
- char-grilled red and yellow peppers with roasted artichoke hearts
- char-grilled aubergine with semi-dried tomatoes
- mushrooms sautéed with garlic, lemon juice and parsley
- tuna, rocket and capers

SOURDOUGH RYE
GI 54

Sourdough rye is made with rye instead of wheat flour. Slices of chewy, low GI sourdough rye piled with tasty hot or cold fillings make great sandwiches for workdays, picnics or travel. This bread's compact structure keeps the sandwich with all its fillings intact, while the slightly sour flavour combines well with a wide range of meat, poultry, fish and salad fillings.

Serving suggestions

Try these sandwich fillings:

- salad (the works) with rare roast beef and horseradish, or smoked ham and grainy mustard
- smoked turkey with cranberry, avocado and sprouts
- egg salad with fresh chopped chives and crispy cos lettuce
- chicken breast with watercress, apple slices and walnuts
- tuna melt – flaked tuna, finely sliced onion rings and a slice of gruyère cheese
- BLT – lean grilled bacon, lettuce and tomato slices

SOYA AND LINSEED BREAD

GI range 36–57

These moist breads with good keeping qualities are made by adding kibbled soya beans or soya flour and linseeds to bread dough. These phytoestrogen-rich ingredients have been shown to help relieve the symptoms of menopause. They are also rich in omega-3 fatty acids (the good essential oils). Unless you are on a very low fat diet, don't be deterred from enjoying soya and linseed breads as their fat content is unsaturated and they are a good source of fibre.

Serving suggestions

- Club sandwiches; open-faced sandwiches with cold meats and salad and toasted or grilled sandwiches for light meals and lunches.
- For a satisfying salad in a sandwich, skim two slices of soya and linseed bread with a little avocado and fill with a slice of lean ham, tomato, rocket, grated carrot, beetroot, spring onions and sprouts.
- To make a cheesy melt, spread a slice of soya and linseed bread with wholegrain mustard. Add chopped sun-dried tomatoes, grilled eggplant and a slice of mozzarella cheese. Melt the cheese under the grill, top with salad greens and another slice of soya and linseed, slice diagonally and serve.

STONEGROUND 100% WHOLEMEAL OR WHOLEWHEAT BREADS
GI 53

'Stoneground 100% wholewheat bread' means that the flour has been milled from the entire wheat berry – the germ, endosperm and the bran – and the milling process slowly grinds the grain with a burrstone instead of high speed metal rollers to distribute the germ oil more evenly. As a result, virtually none of the nutrient-rich ingredients are lost in the processing, making this bread a rich source of several B vitamins, iron, zinc and dietary fibre. If you can't find stoneground breads in the bakery section of your supermarket, try specialist bakeries or health, natural or organic food stores.

Serving suggestions

- Fill toasted sandwiches with tomato and a slice of cheese or banana, light cream cheese and honey.
- Top toast with a slice of lean ham, spinach, a perfectly poached egg and a drizzle of oil and vinegar.

TORTILLA
Corn tortilla GI 52
Wheat tortilla GI 30

Tortillas are a flat (unleavened) bread traditionally made from corn (maize) flour. A staple of Mexican cuisine, they are quite different from the Spanish tortilla, which is a type of omelette. And when made in the traditional Mexican way, whether from corn or wheat flour, they have a low GI.

Almost any kind of food that does not contain too much liquid – beans, corn or chicken, chilli or salsa – can be placed on or wrapped in the versatile tortilla for a complete meal. Make the most of them with your favourite recipes for burritos, enchiladas, fajitas and quesadillas (but hold the creamy dips) or use as rolls, wraps or scoops. Corn tortillas are also a good alternative to bread if you are gluten intolerant.

Serving suggestion

- To make bean and corn burritos, preheat the oven to 180°C (350°F/Gas mark 4). Combine a 400 gram (14 oz) can of corn kernels, drained, a 400 gram (14 oz) can of red kidney beans, rinsed and drained, 2 large ripe tomatoes, chopped, 2 shallots, finely sliced and 75 g (2½ oz) prepared taco sauce in a bowl. Wrap four 15 cm (6-inch) white corn tortillas in foil and warm in the oven for 5 minutes. To assemble, spread shredded lettuce over a warmed tortilla, and top with the bean mixture and a little grated reduced fat cheese. Fold the bottom of the tortilla over the filling, and roll up to enclose. Serve immediately. Makes 4.

WHOLEGRAIN BREAD
GI range 43–54
Wholegrain breads such as 'multigrain' or 'granary' breads contain lots of 'grainy bits' in the bread (not just on top for decoration). They tend to have a slightly grainy, chewy texture and provide a good source of fibre, vitamins, minerals and phytoestrogens, although this will depend on the flour mix. These are usually made from wholemeal or white flour (or a combination of the two) with kibbled and wholegrains added to the dough.

Choose breads with whole or kibbled grains such as barley, rye, triticale (a wheat and rye hybrid), oats, soya, cracked wheat and seeds such as sunflower seeds or linseeds.

Serving suggestions

- Make your own 'submarines' with wholegrain rolls or muffins
- Top a vegetable gratin with grainy breadcrumbs
- Enjoy a beef or chickpea burger on a grainy bun

BREAKFAST CEREALS

Whether you like waking up to a crisp, crunchy cereal, a warming bowl of porridge or a chewy, nutty muesli, a good breakfast can set you up for the day. Given the solid evidence that people who eat breakfast are calmer, happier and more sociable, the number of people skipping breakfast is an alarming trend. Studies regularly show that eating breakfast improves mood, mental alertness, concentration and memory. Nutritionists also know that having breakfast helps people lose weight, can lower cholesterol levels and helps stabilise blood glucose levels.

ALL-BRAN®
GI 30
With its malty taste, Kellogg's All-Bran® is a good source of B vitamins and excellent source of insoluble fibre. Made from coarsely milled wheat bran, it's among the most fibre-rich of all breakfast cereals on the market. It is also low in sodium and a good source of potassium.

Health tip:

Skipping breakfast is not a good way to cut back your food intake, and it can leave you feeling fatigued, dehydrated and without energy for the day's decisions. Breakfast-skippers tend to make up for the missed food by eating more snacks during the day, and more food overall.

Serving suggestions

- Top a bowl of All-Bran® with banana slices or canned pear slices and serve with low fat milk.
- Sprinkle a few tablespoons over low fat yoghurt as a fibre booster.
- Blend yourself a honey banana smoothie – a cup of low fat milk, a small banana, honey to taste and 15 grams (½ oz) of All-Bran® (or more if you like).
- Add 30 grams (1 oz) of All-Bran® to muffin mixes, banana and other fruit or vegetable breads, biscuits and slices when baking.

BRAN
GI 19 (extruded rice bran)
GI 55 (unprocessed oat bran, average)
You can buy unprocessed oat bran in the cereal section of supermarkets and in health, natural and organic food stores. Its carbohydrate content is lower than that of oats, and it is higher in fibre, particularly soluble fibre. Bran is a soft, bland product useful as an addition to breakfast cereals and as a partial substitution for flour in baked goods to help boost fibre and lower the GI. You can also add a tablespoon or two to meatball and burger mixes, use it in making muesli or add to porridge for extra fibre.

Serving suggestion
Enjoy one of these low GI Cherry Oat Crunchies made with fruit, nuts, oats and bran flakes. Just two delicious biscuits will give you 2 grams of fibre.

Preheat the oven to 180°C (350°F/Gas mark 4). Lightly spray two baking trays with olive oil. Put 55 grams (2 oz) soft brown sugar, 90 grams (3 oz) pure floral honey, 125 grams (4½ oz) reduced fat margarine or butter, 2 eggs, ½ teaspoon of bicarbonate of soda and 2 teaspoons of vanilla essence in a large mixing bowl. Beat using electric beaters on medium speed for 2 minutes. Fold in 150 grams (5½ oz) wholemeal flour, 200 grams (7 oz) rolled oats, 20 fresh cherries (pitted and roughly chopped), 60 grams (2 oz) roughly chopped walnuts and 80 grams (2½ oz) bran flakes cereal, crushed. Mix thoroughly. Drop spoonfuls of the mixture onto the prepared baking trays, spacing them about 5 cm (2 inches) apart. Bake for 15 minutes, or until light brown. Leave for 5 minutes before lifting off the tray and placing on a wire rack to cool. Store in an airtight container. Makes around 42.

MUESLI
GI 49 (natural muesli made with rolled oats, dried fruit, nuts and seeds)

Muesli originated as a Swiss health food, developed by Dr Max Bircher-Brenner who was a passionate advocate of the benefits of a vegetarian, especially raw, diet. It currently rates as one of the few relatively unprocessed breakfast cereals on the market. A good source of thiamin, riboflavin and niacin, its low GI value is the result of the slower digestion of raw oats. Oats also contain fibre that increases the viscosity of the contents of the small intestine, thereby slowing down enzyme attack. This same fibre has also been shown to reduce blood cholesterol levels.

There are essentially three basic types of muesli: toasted, natural (untoasted) and moist (Swiss or Bircher) muesli, but the list of possible ingredients is endless and generally includes:

- cereals: rolled oats, flakes of barley or rice, plus a processed bran cereal if you need to boost the fibre
- nuts: chopped almonds, walnuts, macadamias or hazelnuts
- seeds: sesame seeds, sunflower seeds, linseeds, pumpkin seeds
- dried fruit: sultanas, raisins, chopped dried apricots or figs, pears, bananas, apple rings, cranberries

- spices: cinnamon and other spices are sometimes added for extra flavour

Any muesli will fuel your day, but check the information label when buying toasted muesli as it can contain extra fat and sugar.

Serving suggestion

Try our low GI simple Swiss muesli:

Combine 100 grams (3½ oz) of traditional rolled oats, 125 ml (4 fl oz) of semi-skimmed milk and 2 tablespoons of sultanas in a bowl; cover and refrigerate overnight. Next morning add 100 grams (3½ oz) of low fat vanilla yoghurt, 2 tablespoons of slivered almonds and ½ an apple (grated). Mix well, adjusting the flavour with a little lemon juice if you wish. Serve with your favourite berries – such as strawberries or blueberries. Serves 2.

> Look for breakfast cereals with a 'low GI' label that have been tested by an accredited laboratory such as Sainsbury's Taste the Difference Scottish Jumbo Oats.

PORRIDGE

GI 42 (traditional rolled oats)

The first farmers back in Neolithic times knew that the best way to cook any grain was to make a 'porridge' – all they had to do was crack the grain, add water and cook the mixture in a pot on the edge of the fire. The basic recipe hasn't changed much over the years. The classic porridge we associate with Scotland was made from stone-ground oats simmered in milk or water until cooked, and served with salt or sugar and milk.

For a high-energy breakfast it's hard to go past porridge made with traditional oats – a good source of soluble fibre, B vitamins, vitamin E, iron and zinc. The GI value for porridge has been tested on a number of occasions and the published values range from 42 (for rolled oats made with water) to 82 (for instant oats).

Traditional rolled oats are hulled, steamed and flattened, which makes them a 100 per cent wholegrain cereal. The additional flaking to produce quick cooking or 'instant' oats not only speeds up cooking time, it increases the rate of digestion and the GI. This is why traditional rolled oats are preferred over instant in the low GI diet.

Porridge gourmets advocate steel-cut oats – the wholegrains are simply chopped into chunks. These oats are hard to find but worth the hunt if you like a chewier porridge – and it has a GI value of 51.

Follow the instructions on the packet (or use your favourite recipe) to make porridge. A fairly standard rule is one part rolled oats to four parts water. Cooking oats in milk (preferably semi-skimmed or skimmed) not only produces a creamy dish but supplies you with calcium and reduces the overall GI.

Serving suggestions

Don't skimp on the finishing touches for perfect porridge. Choose toppings such as:

- fresh fruit slices in season
- mixed berries
- unsweetened canned plums
- a teaspoon or two of maple syrup
- a tablespoon or two of dried fruit such as sultanas or chopped apricots

NOODLES

Noodles have long been a staple food in China, Japan, Korea and most of South-east Asia. Today, their meals-in-minutes value has made them popular worldwide – they are a great stand-by for quick meals. They are also a good source of carbohydrate, provide some protein, B vitamins and minerals and will help to keep blood glucose levels on an even keel.

Noodles are made from flour, water and sometimes egg which is mixed into a dough, rolled out to the appropriate thickness and cut into long ribbons, strips and strings – long noodles symbolise long life. Their dense texture and shape whether they are made from wheat flour, buckwheat, mung beans, soyabeans, rice or sweet potatoes contribute to their low to intermediate GI values (33 to 62). Choose lower GI noodles for everyday use.

You can buy noodles fresh, dried or boiled (wet). Fresh and boiled noodles will be in the refrigerator cabinets in your supermarket or Asian grocery store. Use them as soon as possible after purchase or store in the refrigerator for a day or two.

Dried noodles are handy to have in the larder for quick and easy meals in minutes. They will keep for several months, provided you haven't opened the packet.

Egg noodles are made from wheat flour and eggs. They are readily available dried, and you can find fresh egg noodles in the refrigerator section of the supermarket or Asian grocery store. Hokkien noodles are 'wet' egg noodles and will be in the refrigerator section too. Instant noodles are usually precooked and dehydrated egg noodles. Check the label as they are sometimes fried.

Served with fish, chicken, tofu or lean meat and plenty of vegetables, a soup, salad or stir-fry based on noodles gives you a healthy balance of carbs, fats and proteins plus some fibre and essential vitamins and minerals. Enjoy them hot or cold in soups, salads and stir-fries. If they are served crisp, it means that they have been deep-fried.

To cook, follow the instructions on the packet as times vary depending on types and thickness. Some noodles only need swirling under running warm water to separate, or soaking in hot (but not boiling) water to soften before you serve them or add to stir-fries. Others need to be boiled. Like pasta, they are usually best just tender, almost *al dente*, so keep an eye on the clock.

As it's all too easy to slurp, gulp, twirl and overeat noodles, keep those portion sizes moderate. While they are a low GI choice themselves, eating a huge amount will have a marked effect on your blood glucose. Instead of piling your plate with noodles, serve plenty of vegetables – a cup of noodles combined with lots of mixed vegetables can turn into three cups of a noodle-based meal and fit into any adult's daily diet.

Remember when planning meals that the sauces you serve with noodles and how you cook them can provide a lot more calories than the noodles themselves.

BUCKWHEAT NOODLES
GI 46 (soba noodles)

Japan's soba noodles are rather like spaghetti in both colour and texture. They are usually made from a combination of buckwheat and wheat flour and are a better source of protein and fibre than rice noodles. You can buy them fresh or dried, but fresh is better if available. Serve soba hot or cold. One of the classic soba recipes is zaru soba, in which boiled soba noodles are eaten cold with a soy dipping sauce.

Serving suggestions

- For a satisfying pork and noodle soup, season a pork fillet with freshly ground Szechuan pepper then sear on all sides in a little vegetable oil, to get a crust. Cook about 200 grams (7 oz) of buckwheat noodles following the instructions on the packet then drain and add to 2 cups of simmering chicken stock. Stir in a seeded and sliced dried red chilli, 100 grams (3½ oz) of thinly sliced shiitake mushrooms and 2 teaspoons of mushroom soy sauce. Add the thinly sliced pork, a handful of coriander leaves, heat through and serve.
- Make a buckwheat noodle salad by tossing 400 grams (14 oz) of cooked noodles in a dressing made with

about 1 tablespoon of light soy sauce, 2 tablespoons of white wine vinegar, 1 teaspoon of sesame oil, 2 teaspoons of rice wine, ½ teaspoon of finely chopped ginger, 1 clove of crushed garlic and a pinch of chilli (or to taste). Top with finely chopped spring onions and serve. If you like, add thinly sliced pieces of fresh bean curd, too.

CELLOPHANE NOODLES
GI 33

Cellophane noodles, also known as Lungkow bean thread noodles or green bean vermicelli, are fine, translucent threads made from mung bean flour, which is why they have the lowest GI value of noodles tested to date. When soaked they become shiny and slippery and are sometimes called slippery noodles or glass noodles. They are often used in soups, salads and stir-fries. They can also be deep fried. To soften simply soak them in hot (not boiling) water for a couple of minutes before adding them to the dish.

Serving suggestions

* Make a spiced seafood salad using seafood mix from the fish shop (including calamari, crab meat and prawns) with cellophane noodles, chopped Asian greens, mangetouts and a chilli lime dressing.
* Use leftover chicken to whip up a salad with noodles, blanched mangetouts, blanched green beans, rocket and a light sesame and hoi sin dressing.

INSTANT NOODLES
GI 46

Asian-style dried noodles are very popular as a quick meal or snack. They are a high-carbohydrate convenience food but they also contain a substantial amount of fat – over 35 per cent of their calories in fact. The flavour sachets supplied tend to be based on salt and flavour enhancers, including monosodium glutamate. Keep them for occasional use and add fresh or frozen chopped vegetables when preparing. These noodles can also be added to soups and stir-fries.

Serving suggestions

- For a meal in minutes, make a quick Thai noodle curry. Stir-fry sliced onion, red pepper, baby corn, broccoli florets and mangetouts in a large pan or wok. Add a tablespoon of Thai red curry paste. Prepare instant Asian noodles according to the instructions on the packet. Add to the vegetables with enough stock to make a sauce. Stir in a tablespoon of light coconut milk, heat through and serve.
- Make up a single-serve packet of quick-cook noodles with half the flavour sachet. Add a couple of tablespoons each of frozen peas and corn kernels and then microwave to heat through.

RICE NOODLES
GI 40 (fresh)
Made from ground or pounded rice flour, rice noodles are available fresh and dried. Run hot water through fresh rice noodles to loosen them then drain and combine with other ingredients. Dried rice noodles are rather brittle and need to be soaked for 10 to 15 minutes before adding to soups, salads and stir-fries.

Serving suggestions

- Enjoy rice noodles in broth served with a little lean meat, chicken or tofu and vegetables including chopped Asian greens, bean sprouts, mint leaves and some finely sliced chilli.
- Make up some fresh rice paper rolls: mix together

softened chopped rice vermicelli with grated carrot, fresh bean sprouts, chopped roasted peanuts (unsalted), chopped fresh mint and coriander or parsley and a dressing of sesame oil and lime juice with minced garlic, chilli and a pinch of sugar. Roll up spoonfuls of the mixture in softened rice paper rounds and serve alongside sweet chilli sauce for dipping.

WHEAT FLOUR NOODLES

GI 62 (udon noodles)
Japanese udon noodles are white and usually firmer and thicker than soba noodles. They are available dried, ready boiled and fresh. Cook them according to the instructions on the packet as times will vary depending on the type. Enjoy them hot in soup or cold with dipping sauces and salads.

Serving suggestions

- Combine cooked udon noodles with seared tuna and cucumber slices and toss in a tangy dressing made with soy sauce, lime juice, sesame oil and a dash of wasabi.
- Serve cooked udon noodles cold with a dipping sauce made from soy sauce, mirin and Japanese dashi soup stock and other accompaniments such as sesame seeds, grated fresh ginger, dried seaweed, chopped green onion and wasabi.

PASTA

It's said that pasta (Italian for 'dough') comes in more shapes and sizes than there are days of the year. Whatever the shape, it's perfect for quick meals and scores well nutritionally as a good source of protein, B vitamins and fibre. Pasta in any shape or form has a relatively low GI (30 to 60) –

Al dente

Cooked *al dente*, pasta does not cause sugar spikes when you eat *moderate* portions. *Al dente* ('firm to the bite') is the best way to eat pasta – it's not meant to be soft. It should be slightly firm and offer some resistance when you are chewing it. Its GI is lower, too – overcooking boosts the GI. Although most manufacturers specify a cooking time on the packet, don't take their word for it. Start testing about 2–3 minutes before the indicated cooking time is up.

great news for pasta lovers, but portion size is important. Keep it moderate.

Initially we thought that pasta's low GI was due to its main ingredient, semolina (durum or hard wheat flour). Scientists have now shown, however, that even pasta made with plain wheat flour has a low GI and the reason for the slow digestion is the physical entrapment of ungelatinised starch granules in a spongelike network of protein (gluten) molecules in the pasta dough. Pasta and noodles are unique in this regard. Adding egg to the dough lowers the GI further by increasing the protein content.

As a general rule, commercial dried pasta is made from durum wheat semolina and no eggs; commercial fresh pasta is made with durum wheat semolina and eggs. Homemade pasta tends to be made with plain wheat flour and eggs. There is also some evidence that thicker types of pasta tend to have a lower GI than thinner types perhaps due to their dense consistency and because they cook more slowly (and are less likely to be overcooked).

A number of pasta shapes and types have been tested. Note that canned spaghetti in tomato sauce and packet mix macaroni cheese are not low GI – they have medium to high GI values.

Watch that glucose load. While pasta is a low GI choice, eating too much will have a marked effect on your blood glucose. That's because if you eat too large a portion of even a low GI food the glucose load becomes too large. So, instead of piling your plate with pasta, fill it with vegetables – a cup of cooked pasta combined with plenty of mixed vegetables can turn into three cups of a pasta-based meal and fit easily into any adult's daily diet.

A moderate portion of pasta served with vegetables or tomato sauce or accompaniments such as olive oil, fish and lean meat, plenty of vegetables and small amounts of cheese provides a healthy balance of carbs, fats and proteins.

Pasta salads are ideal for people with busy lives. You can make them in minutes, or prepare beforehand and keep in the fridge until serving time.

Gluten free

These versatile products can be served with sauces, vegetables and used as the basis for salads. Gluten-free pastas based on rice and corn (maize) have moderate to high GI values.

CAPPELLINI
GI 45

This is the thinnest form of pasta (cappellini literally means 'fine hairs') and is made from semolina. Angel-hair pasta is similar in shape, but its dough is made with eggs. Because cappellini is so thin, it is all too easy to overcook it. For a perfect *al dente* product, the optimal cooking time is around 4 minutes. Cappellini comes fresh or dried and is best served with light, smooth or spicy sauces such as tomato, marinara or pesto.

Serving suggestion

A basic marinara sauce is essentially tomatoes and garlic to which seafood (most often these days) is added. To make a basic marinara, cook 2 cloves of crushed garlic and a finely sliced onion in a little olive oil until soft and golden. Add chopped fresh herbs such as parsley and basil (about 4 tablespoons), 2 x 400 gram (14 oz) cans of Italian tomatoes, a splash of white wine, a pinch of sugar and salt and freshly ground black pepper to taste. Simmer uncovered until the sauce is thick, rich and red – about half an hour. Add 250 grams (9 oz) of green prawns (shelled and deveined) towards the end of the cooking time. Cook until the prawns lose their translucency – just a few minutes depending on the size. Makes about 3 cups of sauce.

FETTUCCINE

GI 40

This is the familiar flat, long, ribbon-shaped pasta usually about ½ cm (¼ in) wide. Fettuccine is the term that Romans use for 'noodles'. It's made from semolina and other ingredients such as spinach, squid ink, tomato paste and even cocoa. Available fresh and dried, it's best with tomato- or cheese-based sauces.

Serving suggestions

- Toss cooked fettuccine in a tablespoon of pesto with diced tomatoes and top with a little grated Parmesan cheese. Try using a sundried tomato pesto as an alternative and topping with some pitted black olives.
- Fettuccine is delicious with seafood. While the pasta is cooking, combine a little finely chopped garlic, chopped red chillies and flat leaf parsley in a bowl (adjust the quantity to suit your tastebuds). Pan-fry about four scallops per person in a little olive oil for 2–3 minutes, then add the garlic mixture and heat through. Stir in the drained pasta and serve topped with more freshly chopped parsley.

LINGUINE

GI 46 (thick)

GI 52 (thin)

With its flat shape, linguine is great with many kinds of pasta sauces – pesto and clam or seafood sauces are ideal. It's available fresh and dried and in a variety of flavours including spinach and wholemeal.

Serving suggestions

- Toss *al dente* linguine with peppery baby rocket (stems removed), halved or quartered baby tomatoes, canned tuna and a little oil and lemon juice. Season with salt and freshly ground black pepper and serve warm topped with a little freshly grated Parmesan.

- Red pesto is a piquant coating sauce for all kinds of pasta shapes and ribbons. Combine the following ingredients in a food processor and blend: 15 grams (½ oz) of drained anchovy fillets, a clove of crushed garlic, a tablespoon of toasted pine nuts, a tablespoon of dried breadcrumbs (from grainy bread), a 180 gram (6½ oz) can of red pimiento (drained) or a small jar of roasted peppers, 1 large peeled and seeded tomato, 2 teaspoons of capers, 1 teaspoon of dried oregano and 1 tablespoon of chopped fresh parsley. Add 2 tablespoons of red wine and blend. Slowly add about ½ cup of olive oil and blend in bursts until the sauce has the consistency of pesto. Makes about 1 cup.

MACARONI
GI 47

These short, hollow pasta tubes of 'macaroni cheese' fame combine well with tomato- or other vegetable-based sauces. They are often used in baked dishes, soups and salads.

Serving suggestions

To make macaroni cheese, preheat the oven to 180°C (350°F, Gas mark 4) then cook 400 grams of macaroni following the instructions on the packet. Combine a 250 gram (14 oz) tub of ricotta with 300 ml (10½ fl oz) of semi-skimmed milk, 2 beaten eggs, 2 teaspoons of smooth Dijon mustard, 1 teaspoon of Tabasco sauce (or to taste) and freshly ground black pepper in a food processor and blend. Combine the cooked macaroni with 200 grams (7 oz) of shredded low fat tasty cheddar cheese and 2 handfuls of baby spinach leaves in a bowl. Stir in the ricotta mixture then spoon into a baking dish. Top with grated Parmesan cheese, grainy breadcrumbs and a little paprika and bake for 20–25 minutes. Serve with a crispy green salad. Serves 4.

PASTINA
GI 38 (star shaped)
Small pasta or 'pastina' comes in many shapes: stars, orzo, acini di pepe, and many more. But just like the larger pasta shapes, pastina is made from durum wheat semolina. It is used in vegetable, chicken and beef soups to provide some bulk and added calories to the soup. Children particularly love the shapes of these smaller pastas.

Serving suggestion
Cook 100 grams (3½ oz) of pastina according to the packet instructions and drain. Heat 6 cups of chicken stock and add the cooked pasta plus 2 cups of cooked shredded chicken fillet. Season with salt and freshly ground black pepper and serve with a little grated Parmesan cheese and chopped flat leaf parsley.

RAVIOLI
GI 39 (meat-filled)
Ravioli are small, square pasta 'pillows' with fillings such as meat, cheese and spinach, mushroom, pumpkin and tofu. Buy them fresh, frozen or vacuum packed and serve with a sauce that brings out the flavour of the fillings.

Serving suggestions

- A homemade tomato and basil sauce with a sprinkle of Parmesan cheese is a classic ravioli dish. What makes it even better is that by adding a large salad and fruit dessert you will have created a low GI meal in less than 20 minutes!
- Top a homemade tomato and basil soup with floating ravioli and grated Parmesan cheese.

SPAGHETTI

GI 44 (plain)
GI 42 (wholemeal)

Probably the most popular pasta of all, spaghetti's round, long strands are available fresh and dried and in a variety of flavours such as spinach and wholemeal. With its sturdy texture, spaghetti's versatility is endless. It blends beautifully with cooked and raw vegetables; any mixture of herbs and spices; meats, poultry, fish and shellfish; sauces containing olive oil, margarine, butter or light cream; and even nuts such as walnuts, pine nuts and sunflower seeds – all of which fit in a healthy, balanced diet.

All the low GI virtues of regular spaghetti apply to wholemeal spaghetti and they can be used interchangeably in any recipe with the same sauces and accompaniments. Just keep in mind that you'll be taking in more than double the amount of dietary fibre when you opt for wholemeal spaghetti.

Serving suggestions

- Serve spaghetti with a low fat meat sauce made from lean cuts of beef, pork or veal plus chopped tomatoes, carrots, onions, celery and fresh herbs.
- Toss al dente spaghetti with smoked salmon, capers and a little olive oil and finish with a twist of two of lemon juice.
- Make a spaghetti and tomato salad – enjoy as a light meal and use leftovers for lunch the next day. Dice 3 medium tomatoes and combine in a bowl with 1 tablespoon of olive oil, 1 tablespoon of capers, 1 crushed garlic clove, the juice of a lemon, a sprinkle of chilli powder (or to taste), a few pitted black olives, freshly ground black pepper to taste and a handful of torn basil leaves. Combine with a cup of cooked spaghetti and serve cold or warm. Serves 2.

SPIRALI

GI 43

There are so many dried pasta shapes – from spirals (spirali), shells (conchiglie), bows (farfalle, literally butterflies), quill-shaped tubes (penne and penne rigate), small wheels (rotelle), twists (gemelli, literally twins) to round tubes such as cannelloni which are stuffed then baked. Everyone has their favourites. The great news for pasta lovers is that they all have a relatively low GI. Whether you serve them with tomato- or vegetable-based sauces, simply fold through your favourite vegetables or use them in salads, they are ideal for creating healthy, balanced meals in minutes.

Serving suggestions

- Serve your favourite shapes with lightly steamed cauliflower or broccoli florets and diced lean crispy bacon (pancetta is even better) cooked with a sliced red chilli. Top with chopped parsley and a little grated Parmesan.
- Enjoy a quick pasta and red bean salad. Combine 200 grams (7 oz) of cooked pasta shapes with 200 grams (7 oz) of canned red kidney beans (drained), 3 finely chopped spring onions and a tablespoon of chopped fresh parsley. Toss with an oil and vinegar dressing made from 1 tablespoon of olive oil, 1 tablespoon of white wine vinegar, 1 teaspoon of Dijon mustard, a crushed clove of garlic and freshly ground black pepper. Serves 4.

TORTELLINI

GI 50 (cheese)

Tortellini are a small, crescent-shaped, filled pasta available in a range of fillings – including spinach and ricotta, chicken, veal, ham, mushrooms and cheese in a variety of combinations. The overall nutrient content will vary depending on the fillings. You can usually buy it fresh, frozen or vacuum packed and all you have to do is cook and serve.

Serving suggestions

- Toss cooked tortellini with fresh chopped herbs such as parsley and basil, a minced garlic clove and a little olive oil.
- Try this time-saving tortellini meal. Cook spinach and cheese tortellini according to the packet instructions until al dente and serve with bought or homemade tomato sauce topped with a little grated Parmesan cheese. Serve with a big garden salad for a complete meal in minutes.

VERMICELLI

GI 35

Rather like cappellini, vermicelli is a thin type of spaghetti that's available fresh and dried. Because it is so fine it cooks quickly, so watch the times. Serve with light sauces or add to soups and stir-fries.

Serving suggestions

Toss *al dente* vermicelli with:

- lightly steamed strips of courgette, finely chopped parsley, a few walnut halves, a twist of black pepper and a little grated Parmesan cheese
- a bought or homemade tomato sauce with yellow and red marinated pepper slices, anchovies, flaked canned tuna, olives, capers and basil

Pasta makes a quick and easy meal with many prepared pasta sauces on the market (although it's easy to make your own). Stick to tomato-based sauces or toss with vegetables rather than the creamy ones laden with fat. And use a modest sprinkle of cheese on top.

RICE

Carb-rich rice is one of the world's oldest and most culti- vated grains – there are some 2000 varieties worldwide – and the staple food for over half the world's population. A soup, salad or stir-fry based around rice with a little fish, chicken, tofu or lean meat and plenty of vegetables will give you a healthy balance of carbs, fat and protein plus some fibre and essential vitamins and minerals.

Rice can have a very high GI value, or a low one, depending on the variety and its amylose content. Amylose is a kind of starch that resists gelatinisation. Although rice is a wholegrain food, when you cook it, the millions of microscopic cracks in the grains let water penetrate right to the middle of the grain, allowing the starch granules to swell and become fully 'gelatinised', thus very easy to digest.

So, if you are a big rice eater, opt for the low GI vari- eties with a higher amylose content such as basmati or Koshihikari (Japanese sushi rice). These high-amylose rices that stay firm and separate when cooked combine well with Indian, Thai and Vietnamese cuisines.

Brown rice is an extremely nutritious form of rice and contains several B vitamins, minerals, dietary fire and protein. Chewier than regular white rice, it tends to take about twice as long to cook. The varieties available in Britain that have been tested to date have a high GI, so enjoy it occasionally, especially combined with low GI foods. Arborio risotto rice releases its starch during cooking and has a medium GI. Wild rice (GI 57) is not actually rice at all, but a type of grass seed.

As with pasta and noodles, it's all too easy to overeat rice, so keep portions moderate. Even when you choose a low GI rice, eating too much can have a marked effect on your blood glucose. A cup of cooked rice combined with plenty of mixed vegetables can turn into three cups of a rice-based meal that suits any adult's daily diet.

> ### Why 'gelatinisation' means high GI
>
> The starch in raw carb-rich foods such as rice grains is stored in hard, compact granules that make the food difficult to digest unless you cook it. This is why eating raw potatoes can give you a stomach ache. During cooking, water and heat expand starch granules to different degrees; some actually burst and free the molecules. This happens when you make gravy by heating flour and water until the starch granules burst and the gravy thickens. If most of the starch granules have swollen during cooking, we say that the starch is fully gelatinised. It is now also easy to digest, which is why the food will have a high GI.

BASMATI RICE
GI 58

Basmati is a long grain aromatic rice grown in the foothills of the Himalayas and is especially popular in India. When cooked the grains are dry and fluffy, so they make the perfect bed for curries and sauces. You can buy brown or white basmati rice – brown basmati has more fibre and a stronger flavour, but it takes twice as long to cook. It also has a higher GI.

Serving suggestions

- Toss rice in an oil and vinegar dressing with sultanas, chopped red and green peppers, sweetcorn kernels and finely sliced red onion and celery to make a simple salad.
- Rice on the run is great for lunch the next day, too. Pour a lightly beaten egg into an oiled frypan and cook over a medium heat until bubbly. Flip over to cook on the other side, turn onto a board and chop into slices. Sauté a finely diced courgette and a red pepper, a stick of thinly sliced celery and a grated carrot in a little oil

Freshly cooked rice has a higher GI than cold, reheated rice. This is one of the reasons for sushi's low GI.

in the pan. Add minced garlic, ginger and chopped shallots, stir till aromatic, then add 100 grams (3½ oz) of cooked basmati rice and stir until heated through. Sprinkle with soy sauce to serve.

SUSHI
GI 48–55

Ideal for snacks and light meals, these bite-sized parcels are usually made with combinations of raw or smoked fish, chicken, tofu and pickled, raw and cooked vegetables and wrapped in dried seaweed and rice seasoned with vinegar, salt and sugar. Even though the rice used to make sushi is short grain and somewhat sticky, sushi still has a low GI, possibly because of the vinegar (acidity puts the brakes on stomach emptying) and the viscous fibre in the dried seaweed. In addition, sushi made with salmon and tuna boosts your intake of healthy omega-3 fats. Sushi served with miso is a delicious light and low GI lunch.

In Japan, sushi is made with Koshihikari rice (GI 48), a short grain rice also called sushi rice with an appetising aroma, sweet flavour, a lightly sticky, soft texture when cooked and a low GI. Use it whenever a softer textured rice is required such as in desserts. You can also use it as a low GI substitute for arborio rice when making a risotto.

Serving suggestions

- It is perfect for sushi, rice balls and other Japanese and Korean dishes, but Koshihikari also goes well with all Asian food.
- Koshihikari makes delicious rice puddings or creamed rice. Boil ½ cup of rice with 1 cup of water for 5 minutes until the water is absorbed. Add 2 cups of low fat milk and cook over a low heat for 20–25 minutes until the rice is tender. Stir in sugar, honey or other sweetener to taste.

WHOLE CEREAL GRAINS

Wholegrain simply means grains that are eaten in nature's packaging – or close to it – traditional rolled oats, cracked wheat and pearl barley, for example. The slow digestion and absorption of these foods will trickle fuel into your engine at a more usable rate and therefore keep you satisfied for longer.

There are countless reasons to include more whole cereal grains in your diet, but it's hard to go past the fact that because you are eating the whole grain, you get all the benefits of its vitamins, minerals, protein, dietary fibre and protective anti-oxidants. Studies around the world show that eating plenty of wholegrain cereals reduces the risk of certain types of cancer, heart disease and type 2 diabetes.

A higher fibre intake, especially from whole cereal grains, is linked to a lower risk of cancer of the large bowel, breast, stomach and mouth. Eating these higher fibre foods can help you lose weight because they fill you up sooner and leave you feeling full for longer. They improve insulin sensitivity, too, and lower insulin levels. When this happens, your body makes more use of fat as a source of fuel – what could be better when you are trying to lose weight?

BARLEY
GI 25 (pearl)
One of the oldest cultivated cereals, barley is nutritious and high in soluble fibre, which helps to reduce the post-meal rise in blood glucose – it lowers the overall GI of a meal. In fact barley has one of the lowest GI values of any food. Look for products such as pearl barley to use in place of rice as a side dish, in porridge or to add to soups, stews and pilafs. You can also use barley as a substitute for rice to make risotto. Barley flakes, or rolled barley,

which have a light, nutty flavour, can be cooked as a cereal and used in baked goods and stuffing.

Serving suggestion

To make a zesty and satisfying chunky lentil and barley soup, cook a finely chopped onion gently in a little olive oil for about 10 minutes, or until soft and golden. Add 2 crushed cloves of garlic, ½ teaspoon of turmeric, 2 teaspoons of curry powder, ½ teaspoon of ground cumin and a teaspoon of minced chilli (or to taste) then add 1 litre (32 fl oz) of chicken stock or water. Stir in 110 grams (3 ¾ oz) of pearl barley, 100 grams (3½ oz) of red lentils and a 400 gram (14 oz) can of tomatoes. Bring to the boil, cover and simmer for about 45 minutes or until the lentils and barley are tender. Season to taste and serve sprinkled with chopped fresh parsley or coriander. Serves 4.

> **Wholegrains on the side**
>
> Try barley, buckwheat, bulghur or quinoa as a change from rice – vegetarian or wholefood cookbooks will give you some tasty recipes.

What's the difference?

❑ *Wholegrain foods* contain the whole grain – the bran, germ and endosperm. Even when processed much of the grain is intact – 'whole' or 'cracked'. It's these grainy bits that slow down the rate of digestion. A rule of thumb: if you can't see the grains then it's probably not low GI.

❑ *Wholemeal foods* contain all the components of the grain, but they have been milled to a finer texture and we digest them faster. Wholemeal foods usually have the same GI as their white counterparts. For example, white bread's GI is 70, wholemeal's is 71. Wholemeal foods are an important source of fibre and nutrients in a balanced diet.

BUCKWHEAT
GI 54

Gluten-free buckwheat is not a type of wheat or a true cereal at all – it's a herbaceous plant that produces triangular seeds. However, because the seeds are used in exactly the same way as cereal grains, that's what people think they are. Buckwheat has a rather nutty flavour and is a good source of protein, B vitamins, magnesium, potassium and soluble fibre.

It is easy to cook and you can use it in place of rice or other wholegrain cereals such as bulghur or add it to soups, stews and casseroles. Buckwheat flour is widely used for making pancakes, muffins, biscuits, and is an indispensable ingredient for Russia's blini and Japan's soba noodles.

Serving suggestion
To make buckwheat and buttermilk pancakes with berries, combine 130 grams (4½ oz) buckwheat flour, 35 grams (1¼ oz) wholemeal flour, 1½ teaspoons baking powder and 2 tablespoons of raw (demerara) sugar in a mixing bowl. Make a well in the centre and pour in 2 lightly beaten eggs, 250 ml (9 fl oz) buttermilk and 1 teaspoon of vanilla essence and whisk until smooth. Add a little more milk if the pancake batter is too thick. Heat a frypan over medium heat and lightly spray with olive oil. Pour 60 ml (2 fl oz) of the mixture into the pan and cook for 1–2 minutes each side, or until the pancakes are golden and cooked. Repeat with the remaining mixture. Top the pancakes with a spoonful of yoghurt and some blueberries. Serves 4 – two pancakes per person.

BULGHUR
GI 48
Also known as cracked wheat, bulghur is made from whole wheat grains that have been hulled and steamed before

grinding to crack the grain. The wheat grain remains virtually intact – it is simply cracked – and the wheat germ and bran are retained, which preserves nutrients and lowers the GI. With its wheaty flavour you can use bulghur instead of rice or other grains in a range of recipes. Use it as a breakfast cereal, in tabbouleh, or add it to pilafs, vegetable burgers, stuffing, stews, salads and soups.

Serving suggestions

- Try this super-nutritious, high fibre mushroom and bulghur salad. Make a marinade with 3 tablespoons of lemon juice, 3 tablespoons of olive oil, a crushed garlic clove and a tablespoon each of freshly chopped parsley and mint (or more if you like). Marinate 125 grams (4½ oz) of sliced button mushrooms and 2 chopped spring onions in the mixture for about an hour. Place 200 grams (7 oz) of bulghur in a bowl, cover with hot water and let it stand for about 20–30 minutes until the water is absorbed and the bulghur softens. Drain well, squeezing out excess water. Toss the bulghur with the marinated mushrooms and spoon into a serving dish. Serves 4.
- To make tabbouleh, cover 90 grams (3 oz) of bulghur with hot water and soak for 20–30 minutes to soften. Drain well and squeeze out the excess water. Add 4 tablespoons finely chopped flat leaf parsley, 3 or 4 chopped spring onions, 2 tablespoons of chopped mint and a chopped tomato. Stir in a dressing made with 2 tablespoons each of lemon juice and olive oil. Tabbouleh is best made ahead of serving time to let the flavours develop. Serves 4.
- Pilaf made with bulghur has a far lower GI than rice pilaf. Serve it with casseroles or as a meal on its own with chopped vegetables. Sauté a thinly sliced brown onion in 1½ tablespoons of olive oil until it is translucent. Add a handful of crushed dry egg noodle vermicelli and stir

until it is pale gold in colour. Add 90 grams (3 oz) of bulghur and 250 ml (9 fl oz) of hot chicken stock. Cover and simmer on low heat for about 7 minutes or until it looks dry. Cover and stand for 10 minutes before serving. Serves 4 as a side dish.

QUINOA

GI 51

Quinoa (pronounced keen-wah) is a small, round, quick-cooking grain somewhat similar in colour to sesame seeds. It's a nutritional powerpack – an excellent source of low GI carbs, fibre and protein, and rich in B vitamins and minerals including iron, phosphorus, magnesium and zinc. You can also buy quinoa flakes and quinoa flour, but the GI of these products has not yet been published.

Health and organic food stores and larger super-markets are the best places to shop for quinoa. You may find it's a little more expensive than other grains. The wholegrain cooks in about 10–15 minutes and has a light, chewy texture and slightly nutty flavour and can be used as a substitute for many other grains. It is important to rinse quinoa thoroughly before cooking – the grains have a bitter-tasting coating designed by nature to discourage hungry hordes of birds.

Serving suggestion

- Make the most of this super grain – substitute gluten-free quinoa for rice, couscous, cracked wheat or barley in soups, stuffed vegetables, salads, stews and even in 'rice' pudding.
- To serve as a side dish, thoroughly rinse 1 cup of quinoa (if not pre-washed). Drain, place the grains in a medium-sized pot with 2 cups of water and bring to the boil. Reduce to a simmer, cover and leave to cook until all the water is absorbed.

- If you want a richer flavour, toast quinoa (but don't let it burn) in a dry pan for a few minutes before cooking as above.
- Give your day a hearty start with quinoa 'porridge' by adding 1 small apple, finely sliced, and a couple of tablespoons of sultanas to the pot while the quinoa is simmering. Add ½ teaspoon of cinnamon for extra flavour if you like. Serve with low fat milk and sweeten with honey or sugar to taste.

RYE
GI 34
Whole kernel rye is used to make bread, including pumpernickel and some crispbreads. It's an excellent source of fibre and also a good source of vitamins and minerals. It is more usually sold as rye flakes, which are the hulled, steamed and rolled rye grains. Like rolled oats, you can eat the flakes as a porridge or sprinkle them over bread before you bake it.

Serving suggestion
To make spicy stuffed tomatoes, gently cook 1 chopped onion in 1 tablespoon of olive oil for a minute or two. Add 2 crushed cloves of garlic and continue cooking until the onion is soft and golden. Add 1 diced medium-sized aubergine, 90 grams (3 oz) of rye flakes, 250 ml (9 fl oz) of water and 1 tablespoon of curry powder (or to taste). Stir, cover and simmer about 30 minutes or until the aubergine and rye flakes are tender and water is absorbed. Cut the tops off 4 large tomatoes and scoop out the insides; set the 'cups' aside. Chop the remaining tomato and add to the curry mixture. Remove the mixture from the heat and stir in a 150 gram (5½ oz) pot of plain low fat yoghurt and season with salt and freshly ground black pepper to taste. Spoon the curry mixture into the tomato cups and serve.

SEMOLINA
GI 55 (cooked)

Semolina is the coarsely milled inner part of the wheat grain called the endosperm. It is granular in appearance. The large particle size of semolina flour (compared with fine wheat flour) limits the swelling of its starch particles when cooked, which results in slower digestion, slower release of glucose into the blood stream and a lower GI.

You'll find durum wheat semolina in most supermarkets. You can use it to make homemade pasta or gnocchi or simply cook it and eat it as a hot cereal or make it into a traditional milk pudding. Use semolina to thicken sauces and gravies instead of plain flour.

Serving suggestion

To make semolina porridge, mix about 1 tablespoon of semolina with 3 tablespoons of low fat milk or water into a smooth paste. Slowly stir in 200 ml (7 fl oz) of semi-skimmed milk. Cook over a low heat, stirring continually for about 10 minutes to the desired consistency. Sweeten with a little honey or maple syrup, or serve with chopped fresh or canned fruit.

WHOLE WHEAT KERNELS
GI 41

As the most important cereal crop in the world, wheat – mainly in the form of bread and noodles – nourishes more people than any other grain. The bulk of the world's wheat is milled into flour – usually white flour. But there are forms of wheat, with their bran and germ intact, that can be eaten as a main or side dish. Whole wheat kernels (also called 'groats' or wheat berries) are a highly nutritious food, packed with B vitamins, protein and minerals including iron, magnesium and manganese. Think of them as the wheat version of rice – but allow for much longer cooking times. They have a strong, nutty flavour. Add them to hearty soups and stews, or use them when baking bread.

> ## Couscous
>
> Semolina is also used to make couscous (GI 65), a coarsely ground semolina pasta that's quick and easy to prepare. With a GI in the medium range, we suggest you enjoy this convenient food in moderation. Alternatively, adding low GI pulses such as chickpeas to couscous recipes is not only delicious, it reduces the overall GI of the dish. For a change, why not try barley couscous?

Serving suggestion

To cook whole kernel wheat, wash 200 grams (7 oz) of wheat then soak in 500 ml (17 fl oz) of water overnight. Place the rehydrated wheat in a pan with a little extra water if necessary and bring to the boil. Turn down the heat and simmer gently for about an hour until soft and the water is mostly absorbed. The cooked wheat will keep in a covered container in the refrigerator for about two weeks. Prepared this way, whole wheat kernels can be used for many dishes such as pilafs, tabbouleh, to bulk up meat dishes, and side dish substitutes for rice or noodles.

PULSES, INCLUDING BEANS, PEAS & LENTILS

For a low GI food that's easy on the budget, versatile, filling, low in calories and nutritious, look no further than pulses – beans, chickpeas and lentils.

Humans have long known about the benefits of eating pulses. Not only do they keep in the cupboard for a year or more, they are an excellent source of protein, easy to prepare and cost very little. When you cook them, they more than double in weight – 200 grams (7 oz) of dry beans makes 500 grams (1 lb 2 oz) of cooked beans – and when you eat them, you'll feel satisfied for longer.

So, what are they? Also known as legumes, pulses are the edible dried seeds found inside the mature pods of leguminous plants. Pulses include various types of beans, peas, chickpeas and lentils. Green peas are pulses but we most often eat them fresh as a green vegetable, so we have included them in the vegetable section. Peanuts are pulses, too, but since they are usually thought of as nuts we have included them in that section.

Whether you buy them dried, or opt for canned

convenience, you are choosing one of nature's lowest GI foods. They are high in fibre and packed with nutrients, providing protein, carbohydrate, B vitamins, folate and minerals. When you add pulses to meals and snacks, you reduce the overall GI of your diet because your body digests them slowly. This is primarily because their starch breaks down relatively slowly (or incompletely) during cooking and they contain tannins and enzyme inhibitors that also slow digestion.

Although they have an excellent shelf life, old beans take longer to cook than young, which is why it's a good idea to buy them from shops where you know turnover is brisk. Once home, store them in airtight containers in a cool, dry place – they will keep their colour better.

What about wind?

Pulses of all sorts, including baked beans, are renowned for producing flatulence (gas) and many jokes. The components responsible are indigestible sugars called raffinose, stachyose and verbascose that reach the large bowel intact where they are fermented by resident flora. Believe it or not, this is good for colonic health, increasing the proportion of good bifidobacteria and reducing potential pathogens. However, not all pulses will make you windy, and not everyone has the problem to the same extent. If you are worried about the social implications, cooking pulses in fresh water (not the water you soaked them in) reduces the problem, as does eating small amounts regularly – your body becomes used to them. Alternatively, to prevent the problem, add a minute amount of powdered asafoetida spice to the pot during cooking – no more than a quarter of a teaspoon per cup of dried beans or lentils. We have also been told that adding a teaspoon of powdered gelatine to the pot during cooking will help – but we haven't tried this one ourselves.

Canned bean convenience

Don't feel guilty about using canned beans – the main aim is to enjoy these low GI superfoods. The only disadvantage with canned beans is that they generally tend to be soft. If you like a firmer texture, especially in salads, you'll probably need to cook your own.

How much?

Pulses are an important part of a low GI diet which is why it's a good idea to try to include them in your meals at least twice a week as a starchy vegetable alternative – more often if you are vegetarian. One serving is equivalent to 100 grams (3½ oz) of cooked beans, lentils, chickpeas or whole dried or split peas.

Serving suggestions

You can substitute one 400 gram (14 oz) can of beans for 150 grams (5½ oz) of dried beans.

- Drain and rinse canned beans and add them directly to soups, stews, salads or curries.
- Top lettuce with kidney beans or chickpeas marinated in an oil and vinegar dressing.
- Add beans or chickpeas to vegetable soups or minestrone.
- Make a puréed bean dip and serve with carrot or celery sticks, blanched mangetouts or cucumber strips.
- Create your own bean filling for tacos and burritos by mashing canned chilli beans with a fork.
- Purée cooked yellow split peas or canned navy beans to use as a base for soups or chowders.

Preparing dried pulses

1. **Wash** Wash thoroughly in a colander or sieve first, keeping an eye out for any small stones or 'foreign' material (especially with lentils).
2. **Soak** Soaking plumps the beans, makes them softer and tastier and reduces cooking times a little. Place them in a saucepan, cover with about three times their volume of cold water and soak overnight or for at least four hours. As a rule of thumb, the larger the seed, the longer the soaking time required. There's no need to soak lentils or split peas.
3. **Cook** Drain, rinse thoroughly, then add fresh water – two to three times the volume of the pulses. Bring to the boil then reduce the heat and simmer until tender. Generally, you will need to simmer lentils and peas for 45–60 minutes and beans and chickpeas for 1–2 hours, but check the recipe instructions. A couple of points to keep in mind:
❏ Adding salt to the water during cooking will slow down water absorption and the pulses will take longer to cook.
❏ Make sure that pulses are tender before you add acidic flavourings such as lemon juice or tomatoes. Once they are in an acid medium they won't get any softer no matter how long you cook them.

Time-saving tips
❏ If you don't have time to soak pulses overnight, add three times the volume of water to rinsed beans, bring to the boil for a few minutes then remove from the heat and soak for an hour. Drain, rinse, add fresh water then cook as usual.
❏ Cooked pulses freeze well. Prepare a large quantity of beans or chickpeas and freeze in meal-sized batches to use as required.
❏ Store soaked or cooked beans in an airtight container in the fridge. They will keep for several days.

Where to buy beans?

These days supermarkets stock a wide range of dried and canned beans. For the more unusual beans, check out your local health food store or Greek, Turkish, Middle Eastern, South American or kosher delicatessen or produce market.

BAKED BEANS

GI 48 (canned in tomato sauce)

Baked beans are a popular ready-to-eat form of pulse, an easy way to introduce children to the world of beans, and available in convenient single-serve cans. Haricot (navy) beans are most commonly used for baked beans. If you make your own baked bean recipe, it will have a lower GI.

Serving suggestions

* Top half a jacket potato cooked in the microwave with a scoop or two of canned or homemade baked beans sprinkled with a little grated cheese.
* A scoop or two of baked beans is a healthy addition to any meal or a satisfying breakfast or light meal served on grainy toast.

BLACK BEANS

GI 30 (home-cooked)

The black bean or black kidney bean is the small, shiny bean with an earthy sweet flavour often used in South and Central American and Caribbean cooking, and Mexican dishes such as refried beans. Add them to chilli con carne or to bean soups and salads for extra flavour and texture. In Latin-American-style dishes, a spicy bean mix made with black or red kidney beans is often served over rice.

Serving suggestion

Use leftover chicken and rice to make these tasty burritos. Preheat the oven to 180°C (350°F, Gas mark 4). Wrap 6 large tortillas in foil and warm in the oven. Cook 1 chopped onion and 1 crushed clove of garlic in a tablespoon of vegetable oil, stirring occasionally until softened. Add 200 grams (7 oz) of chopped cooked chicken, 200 grams (7 oz) of cooked or canned black beans, 200 grams (7 oz) of cooked basmati rice and 1 can of diced tomatoes. To serve, spoon about 3–4 heaped tablespoons of the filling into the centre of the warmed tortilla. Sprinkle 1 tablespoon of grated low fat cheese on top, fold in the ends, then roll the tortilla around the filling. Place in a large shallow baking dish. Sprinkle 100 grams (3½ oz) cup of grated low fat cheese on top of burritos, then cover with foil and heat in the oven for about 10 minutes, or until the cheese is melted and the filling is hot. Serve topped with chopped coriander. Makes 6.

BLACK-EYED BEANS
GI 42

Also known as cowpeas, Southern peas and black-eyed peas, these beans are medium-sized, kidney-shaped and cream-coloured with a distinctive black 'eye' and a subtle flavour. They are a popular 'soul food' in the southern states of the US where they are traditionally served with pork. Add black-eyed beans to soups and stews or serve as a side dish.

Serving suggestions

- Cook chopped leeks, onions and carrots with crushed garlic in a little olive oil. Add cooked or canned black-eyed, kidney and borlotti beans, canned tomatoes plus fresh thyme and bay leaves and a chopped red chilli to make a Mediterranean-style vegetable casserole.
- Soak a cup of black-eyed beans overnight then simmer in fresh water for about 30 minutes until tender. Drain and cool, then add chopped tomato and celery. Toss with a dressing of 2 tablespoons chopped parsley, 1 tablespoon seeded mustard, 1 crushed clove of garlic and 3 tablespoons each of olive oil and wine vinegar.

BORLOTTI BEANS

GI 41 (canned)

This medium-sized bean has a creamy texture, slightly nutty flavour and reddish-black to magenta streaks that fade to brown during cooking. It is widely used for soups, stews, casseroles and in salads and the delicious pasta and bean soup you will find served all over Italy (although they tend to use cannellini beans in the south).

Serving suggestions

- Combine a cup of cooked beans with 2–3 tablespoons of semi-dried tomatoes and a handful of baby spinach leaves in a balsamic dressing.
- Add borlotti beans to a salad of tuna chunks, onion rings, tomato slices, olives and chopped fresh parsley.
- Mash cooked or canned borlotti beans with sweet potato, 125 ml (4 fl oz) of heated semi-skimmed milk and some freshly grated nutmeg. Leave some of the beans whole for texture.

BUTTER BEANS

GI 31 (home cooked)

GI 36 (canned)

Sometimes called large lima beans, butter beans are a flat-shaped white bean with a smooth, creamy, slightly sweet flavour. Add to soups, stews and salads or simply heat and serve as a side dish topped with finely chopped fresh herbs.

Serving suggestions

- Add a cup of cooked butter beans and a crushed clove of garlic to steamed sweet potato (or yam) and mash as usual. Season to taste with a little salt and freshly ground black pepper and add enough water or low fat milk or soya milk for a creamy consistency.

- Dip pitta crisps into a butter bean purée. Purée a drained can of butter beans (or any white bean) with a crushed clove of garlic in the food processor slowly, pouring in just enough oil and lemon juice to create the desired consistency.

CANNELLINI BEANS

GI 31 (canned)

Also known as white kidney beans, cannellini beans are large, smooth-textured, mild-flavoured, kidney-shaped beans with a creamy white skin. They are used in soups, salads, stews, casseroles, bean pots such as the French cassoulet and in many Italian dishes.

Serving suggestions

- Add cannellini beans to puréed vegetable soups for a creamy texture. Simmer cauliflower florets until tender in chicken stock then blend with a cup of cooked beans and season to taste with salt and freshly ground black pepper. Top with freshly grated nutmeg and finely chopped parsley and serve.
- Make a salad of cannellini beans and finely sliced fennel tossed in a tangy lemon, oil and vinegar dressing and top with finely chopped flat leaf parsley.

CHICKPEAS

GI 28 (home cooked)

GI 40 (canned)

Also known as garbanzo beans or ceci, these versatile caramel-coloured pulses have a nutty flavour and firm texture. Popular in Middle Eastern, Mediterranean and Mexican cooking, they are the main ingredient in special-ties such as hummous and felafel and the basis for many vegetarian dishes. Keep a can in the cupboard or cooked chickpeas in the refrigerator and add them to soups, stews and salads or to a tomato-based sauce served with couscous or rice. After soaking, whole chickpeas can be roasted with salt and spices to make a crunchy low GI snack that's every bit as more-ish as crisps!

Serving suggestions

- Combine 2 oranges separated into segments, a drained and rinsed 400 gram (14 oz) can of chickpeas and a finely sliced fennel bulb (or two if small ones). Toss in a dressing made with olive oil, vinegar and orange juice for a tangy salad.
- To make a spicy pilaf, simmer a finely chopped onion in a little olive oil until soft, then add a cup of chopped button mushrooms and a crushed clove of garlic. Stir in 150 grams (5½ oz) of basmati rice, a teaspoon of garam masala and a cup of cooked chickpeas. Pour over 375 ml (13 fl oz) of chicken stock, bring to the boil then reduce the heat to very low, cover and simmer gently for 10–12 minutes or until the rice is tender and all the liquid is absorbed.

CANNED MIXED BEANS
GI 37 (canned)

Canned bean mixes which include red kidney beans, chickpeas and lima and butter beans make it easy to add protein and boost flavour and fibre to meals including soups and stews. You can also add canned mixed beans to your salad wraps, sandwiches and rolls for a lunch that lasts.

Serving suggestions

- For a meal in minutes, combine drained and rinsed mixed beans with baby spinach leaves, chopped spring onions, cucumber, yellow pepper, sliced radishes, finely sliced celery and halved or quartered cherry tomatoes and toss in a light lemony oil and vinegar dressing.
- Boost the flavour and fibre of a home-made tomato soup by adding a can of drained, rinsed four bean mix.

HARICOT BEANS
GI 33 (home-cooked)
GI 38 (canned)
These small, white, oval-shaped beans, sometimes called navy beans, are the ones most often used in the manufacture of commercial baked beans. They have a mild flavour and combine well in soups and stews.

Serving suggestion
Make your own baked beans to serve for breakfast on grainy toast or as a side dish. Combine a small chopped onion, 2 small diced peppers (red or green) and 600 grams (1 lb 3 oz) of cooked or canned haricot beans in a large casserole dish. Add 4 tablespoons of pure floral honey, 2 tablespoons of Dijon mustard, 1 tablespoon of white wine vinegar, 125 ml (4 fl oz) of tomato sauce and a few twists of freshly ground black pepper. Mix well then cover and cook in a preheated oven (180°C, 350°F, Gas mark 4) for about 45 minutes to an hour. Serves 6–8 as a side dish.

HUMMOUS
GI 6 (regular)
Hummous – puréed chickpeas, lemon juice, tahini, olive oil, garlic and sometimes ingredients such as roasted red peppers – is one of the most popular foods to emerge from the Middle East. It can be served as part of a mezze platter or used as a dip with pitta bread, or raw or blanched vegetables such as carrot and celery sticks. It's widely available in the refrigerator section of supermarkets and fresh produce stores, in specialist delis, or as a takeaway from Lebanese or Turkish restaurants.

Serving suggestions
* Use hummous as a spread for sandwiches, as a topping on grilled fish, chicken, with baked potatoes, or in a wrap with kebabs and salad or a falafel roll.

- To make your own, combine a 400 gram (14 oz) can of chickpeas (drained, reserving the liquid), 135 grams (4½ oz) of tahini (sesame seed paste), a large clove of garlic, chopped, 80 ml (2½ fl oz) lemon juice, plus a little salt and freshly ground black pepper to taste. Process in a blender or food processor, adding enough of the reserved chickpea liquid to make a smooth consistency.

LENTILS

GI 26 (red, home cooked)
GI 30 (green, home cooked)
GI 48 (green, canned)

Lentils are one food that people with diabetes should learn to love – they can eat them until the cows come home. In fact, we have found that no matter how much of them people eat, they have only a small effect on blood glucose levels. They are one of nature's superfoods – rich in protein, fibre and B vitamins and often used as substitutes for meat in vegetarian recipes.

All colours and types of lentils have a similar low GI value, which is increased slightly if you opt to buy them canned and add them towards the end of cooking time. Lentils have a fairly bland, earthy flavour that combines well with onions, garlic and spices. They cook quickly to a soft consistency and are used to make Indian dhal, a spiced lentil purée. Lentils also thicken any kind of soup or extend meat casseroles.

Serving suggestions

- Make a meal of lentil soup and low GI bread – you will feel completely satisfied. Canned lentil soup (GI 44) is a convenient, quick meal when you don't have time to prepare your own.
- To make a vegetarian lentil burger, simmer a chopped onion in olive oil for a few minutes to soften. In a bowl

thoroughly combine 400 grams (14 oz) of canned and drained lentils with the onion mix and 400 grams (14 oz) of mashed potato or sweet potato, season to taste with salt and freshly ground black pepper, adding a dash of Tabasco or chilli sauce for flavour. Form into patties and cook them on both sides until browned in the oven, on the barbecue or in a pan and combine with salad, tomato slices, chutney and grainy rolls.

- For an easy alternative to mashed potato, bring to the boil 250 ml (9 fl oz) of chicken or vegetable stock, 150 grams (5½ oz) of split red lentils and 1 bay leaf, then simmer until the lentils are mushy and thick. Season with salt and freshly ground black pepper. You may also like to add a teaspoon of curry powder for extra flavour.

LIMA BEANS
GI 32 (baby frozen)
The lima bean, a larger variety of the butter bean, comes from Peru. Baby lima beans, also called sieva beans, cook faster. They are popular in the US where they are served as a vegetable side dish. Dried and canned lima beans have a buttery flavour and are used in soups, stews and salads. If you are cooking your own, bring them to the boil slowly to prevent the skin from slipping off.

Serving suggestions

- Toss a cup of cooked beans with 3–4 tablespoons of sun-dried tomatoes, 30 grams (1 oz) of sultanas and 30 grams (1 oz) of chopped pecan nuts in a dressing made with the juice of a lemon and 2 tablespoons of olive oil. Season to taste and serve with finely chopped fresh dill.
- Gently warm 200 grams (7 oz) of cooked or canned lima beans in a pan with 60 ml (2 fl oz) of freshly squeezed lemon juice, a tablespoon of olive oil, 2 finely

chopped cloves of garlic and 2 teaspoons of fresh thyme (leaves picked) until just heated through. Toss in a salad bowl with 8 cooked baby beetroot cut into quarters, and a handful each of rocket and baby spinach leaves. Top with crumbled feta and serve.

Marrowfat or 'mushy' peas

Marrowfat peas (GI 39) are a completely different variety from the green or garden pea. They are large yellow peas that, like all pulses, are rich in nutrients and have a low GI. The maro pea was introduced to the UK from Japan over 100 years ago because the climate was suitable for pea growing. It then became known as 'marrowfat' because of its plump shape. You can buy marrowfat peas dried, in cans or as canned 'mushy peas'. They make delicious pea soup.

MUNG BEANS
GI 39 (home cooked)

Also known as green gram or golden gram, dried mung beans are small, olive-green beans that are used in many Asian cuisines for savoury dishes such as India's green gram dhal or to make a paste for popular sweets. The starch from mung beans is used in making bean thread and cellophane noodles. Like all pulses, they are a good source of fibre, iron and protein. You can buy sprouted mung beans in punnets – a useful source of vitamin C.

Serving suggestions

- Add mung bean sprouts as an extra vegetable to a stir-fry or fried rice at the end of cooking.
- Combine 100 grams (3½ oz) of mung bean sprouts, 100 grams (3½ oz) of baby spinach, 100 grams (3½ oz)

of baby rocket, 1 sliced cucumber, 1 punnet of baby tomatoes, halved, ½ an avocado, sliced, 1 small finely sliced red onion and 100 grams (3½ oz) of pitted black olives in a large salad bowl with a dressing made from olive oil, balsamic vinegar and a dash of lemon juice. Serves 4.

PEANUTS

See page 200

PEAS

GI 22 (whole dried, home cooked)
GI 32 (yellow or green split peas)
Like other pulses, dried peas are a nutritional storehouse and because they are slowly digested, a little goes a long way. Whole dried or blue peas are the dried version of garden peas and traditionally used in English dishes such as 'pease pudding' and mushy peas. Soak them before cooking.

Yellow or green split peas come from a variety of garden pea with the husk removed. They tend to disintegrate and are traditionally used for pea and ham soup and yellow split peas for making Indian dhal.

Serving suggestions

* Your local Indian takeaway will sell prepared dhals. Combined with flat bread and basmati rice, dhal makes a delicious low GI light vegetarian meal. To make your own dhal, rinse and drain 200 grams (7 oz) of red lentils and place in a saucepan with ½ a teaspoon of turmeric and a pinch of chilli powder. Add 375 ml (13 fl oz) of boiling water and cook for 15 minutes or until the lentils are very soft, but still retain their shape. Season to taste with salt. Heat 1 tablespoon of margarine or olive oil in a small frypan and gently cook a small finely chopped onion until soft and golden – about

---

Dhal (or dal)

Dhal can refer to dried pulses (Bengal gram, split peas, channa and lentils) as well as the purée that's usually served with Indian meals.

10 minutes. Stir 1 teaspoon of garam masala into the onion mixture, stir briskly for 30 seconds, then add 1 teaspoon of coriander and combine with the lentils. Season to taste with salt and freshly ground black pepper. You may also like to add a squeeze of lime.

- Make a thick pea soup with 350 grams (12 oz) of split peas, 2 finely chopped onions, 2 finely chopped carrots, 2 finely sliced sticks of celery and 2 litres (3½ pints) of stock or water. Add a bay leaf for flavouring, season with freshly ground black pepper and, for extra oomph, add a bacon bone or two while the soup is cooking.

See also Green peas, page 134.

PINTO BEANS
GI 39 (home-cooked)
GI 45 (canned)
This medium-sized mottled bean ('pinto' means painted) turns pinkish-brown when cooked. It's a staple in Latin-American cooking and used whole or made into refried beans as a filling for burritos or tacos.

Serving suggestion

- Make a colourful and crunchy bean mix for tacos. Combine 2 cups of cooked pinto beans with a finely diced green pepper, a cup of juicy red chopped tomatoes, 2 sliced spring onions, 1 cup of sweetcorn kernels (straight off the cob is best), ½ teaspoon of ground cumin and salt and freshly ground black pepper to taste. Serve with tacos and bowls of guacamole, shredded lettuce and grated low fat cheese. Serves 4.
- To make refried beans, heat a little olive or sesame oil in a frypan over medium heat. Add 1 finely sliced onion and 2 cloves of crushed garlic and cook very gently until soft and golden (about 10 minutes). Stir in 2 cups of cooked pinto (or black) beans, 2 teaspoons of cumin

and 125 ml (4 fl oz) of water or vegetable stock. Mash the beans into the liquid, adding more stock if the mixture seems too dry. Season to taste with salt and freshly ground black pepper.

RED KIDNEY BEANS
GI 36 (canned)

These tasty red beans are a popular addition to vegetarian and meat chilli dishes and nachos, tacos and burritos. Not only do red kidney beans play a leading role in Mexican and 'Tex-Mex' cuisines, a scoop is a sustaining side dish with main meals and adds substance to soups, stews and salads.

Serving suggestions

- Stir into a homemade or bought tangy tomato salsa to add a Mexican flavour.
- Create a colourful bean salad by combining a 400 gram (14 oz) can of kidney beans (drained) in a serving bowl with 200 grams (7 oz) each of cooked green beans and cooked yellow beans sliced on the diagonal. Finely slice half a red pepper, half a green pepper and 2 stalks of celery. Toss the beans and vegetables in a light dressing made with balsamic vinegar and olive oil. Coat the salad well – you will need about 125 ml (4 fl oz) of dressing. Serves 4–6 as a side dish.

ROMANO BEANS
GI 46 (home-cooked)

Sometimes referred to as Italian flat beans, romano beans can be eaten as a snap bean when very young or as a dried bean during later stages of maturity. They are used in a wide variety of bean and chilli dishes, soups and salads.

Tofu

Tofu has little or no carbs. It's a cheese-like curd made from soyabeans, and although it is not high in fibre, it's a low-cost, high-protein, low fat bean food that will surprise you with its versatility. By itself, tofu is bland, so marinate it in soy sauce, ginger, chilli and garlic or try it as part of a well-seasoned dish such as a stir-fry.

Serving suggestion

To make a spinach and bean stir-fry, gently cook 2 chopped spring onions and a finely chopped clove of garlic in a little olive oil. Add a seeded and diced red pepper and toss to heat through for 2–3 minutes. Stir in 150 grams (5½ oz) of baby spinach leaves, 2 tablespoons of chopped fresh chives and 400 grams (14 oz) of cooked romano beans. When heated through, season to taste, and serve topped with freshly grated nutmeg alongside bulghur, quinoa or low GI rice. Serves 4.

SOYABEANS

GI 14 (canned)

GI 18 (home cooked)

Soyabeans and soya products are the nutritional power-house of the pulse family. They have been a staple part of Asian diets for thousands of years and are an excellent source of protein. They're also rich in fibre, iron, zinc and vitamin B. They are lower in carbohydrate and higher in fat than other pulses, but the majority of the fat is polyunsaturated. Soyabeans are a rich source of phytochemicals, especially phytoestrogens, and have been linked with improvements in blood cholesterol levels, relief from menopausal symptoms and lower rates of cancer in many studies.

Serving suggestions

- Use canned soyabeans in place of other beans in any recipe.
- Make a quick soyabean and vegetable curry with chopped onions, garlic, carrots, tomatoes, cauliflower and broccoli using vegetable stock and your favourite curry paste.

NUTS

People who eat nuts once a week have less heart disease than those who don't eat any nuts. There are probably several reasons. Nuts contain a variety of anti-oxidants, which keep blood vessels healthy; arginine, an amino acid that helps keep blood flowing smoothly; folate; and fibre, which can both lower cholesterol levels. Although nuts are high in fat (averaging around 50 per cent), it is largely unsaturated, so they make a healthy substitute for foods such as biscuits, cakes, crisps, pastries and chocolate. They also contain relatively little carbohydrate, so most do not have a GI value.

> **How do you halve your risk of developing heart disease? By eating a small handful of nuts five to seven times a week!**

Nuts are one of the richest sources of vitamin E, with a small handful of mixed nuts providing more than 20 per cent of the recommended daily intake. The vitamin E content may explain the findings from a recent study from Harvard University School of Public Health which found that increased nut consumption, including natural peanut butter, may improve the body's ability to balance glucose and insulin.

How much?

One serving provides 10 grams of fat and is equivalent to:

- 15 grams (½ oz) – about 10 small or 5 large – nuts or a tablespoon of seeds
- 3 teaspoons (15 ml) peanut butter or Nutella®

How much a day?

Aim for a small handful (no fingers) of nuts most days.

- Smaller eaters: 1 serving most days
- Medium eaters: 1 serving a day
- Bigger eaters: 1–2 servings most days

Serving suggestions

- Use nuts and seeds in food preparation. Try toasted cashews in a chicken stir-fry; sprinkle walnuts over a pear and radicchio salad with a light blue cheese dressing; or top fruit desserts or muesli with natural almonds.
- Add toasted pine nuts to your favourite pasta dish.
- Sprinkle a mixture of chopped nuts and linseeds over cereal or salads, or add to baked goods such as muffins and slices.

CASHEWS

GI 22

Cashews, like all nuts, are cholesterol free and high in protein. Their carbohydrate content is quite low, which accounts for their low GI value. They do have a high fat content (almost half their total weight) but it is less than any other type of nut and three-quarters of it is heart-healthy polyunsaturated and monunsaturated fat. Cashews are also rich in several B vitamins and the minerals copper, magnesium and zinc. Because of their high nutrient content and energy density (calories/kilojoules) you can eat cashews several times a week, but keep the amounts you eat small and look for unsalted varieties.

Serving suggestion

Cashews make a healthy addition to salads, rice dishes and desserts and are a popular ingredient in Asian stir-fries.

NUTELLA®
GI 33

Nutella® is a sweetened chocolate spread based on hazelnuts, cocoa, skimmed milk powder and peanut oil and is a favourite even with non-chocoholics. About half its sugar content is milk sugar (lactose). Its fat content is high but the fats are mainly mono- and polyunsaturated (just like peanut butter), so it can be a healthy addition to the balanced diet of any active person.

Serving suggestions

- Add to banana smoothies, or stir a little through plain yoghurt for a chocolate fix.
- Soften a little Nutella® in the microwave and serve with a scoop of low fat ice-cream sprinkled with crunchy natural or toasted muesli.

PEANUTS
GI 14

A low carb but high fat, high protein food (50 per cent fat and 25 per cent protein), peanuts grow under the ground – they are also known as groundnuts. Technically a pulse, they are an excellent source of vitamins B and E and so low in carbohydrate that their GI doesn't really count – although their fat content does! Because peanuts are such a tasty and convenient finger food they are easily overeaten, so give yourself a specific ration. And stick to it!

All processed peanuts are quality-controlled for the presence of fungus that produces a toxin called aflatoxin, one of the most carcinogenic substances known. Because peanuts in the shell are not screened, throw away any mouldy ones. And a word to the wise: choose dry roasted peanuts and avoid salt.

Peanut allergy is an increasingly common food allergy especially in children. It occurs in approximately 1 in 50 children and 1 in 200 adults and is the allergy most likely to cause anaphylaxis (which involves swelling in the gut, respiratory tract and/or cardiovascular system) and death. Symptoms of allergy include itching, especially around the mouth, swelling tongue, flushed face, cramping, difficulty breathing, diarrhoea and vomiting. If peanut allergy is suspected urgent medical attention should be sought. One-third of all peanut-allergic people are also allergic to tree nuts such as brazil nuts, hazelnuts, walnuts, almonds, macadamia nuts, pistachios, pecans, pine nuts and cashews.

Serving suggestions

- Make up trail mixes with peanuts, sultanas, dried fruit and sunflower seeds for a no-fuss snack on the run.
- Sprinkle crushed nuts over salads for flavour and crunch or stir crushed nuts and chopped dried fruit through low fat yoghurt.
- Add crushed peanuts to the mix when baking biscuits or slices.

PEANUT BUTTER
GI 14

This delicious treat is made from ground nuts. The healthiest type of peanut butter has no added salt and is made from fresh, unroasted peanuts. Peanut butter is an excellent source of niacin and a good source of magnesium. The best way to include more peanut butter in your diet is to use it in place of butter or margarine.

Serving suggestions

- Top toast with peanut butter and banana or grated apple.
- Make a salad sandwich with lettuce, tomato, grated carrot, sprouts and cucumber, using peanut butter as the spread.
- Use peanut butter to make a satay sauce and serve with vegetables and kebabs.

FISH & SEAFOOD

We can't measure a GI for fish because it doesn't contain any carbohydrate. However, it is an important part of a balanced diet and we now know that just one serve of fish or seafood a week may reduce the risk of a fatal heart attack by about 40 per cent. The likely protective components of fish are the very long chain omega-3 fatty acids. Our bodies only make small amounts of these fatty acids which is why we rely on dietary sources, especially fish and seafood.

Increased fish consumption is linked to a reduced risk of coronary heart disease, improvements in mood, lower rates of depression, better blood fat levels and enhanced immunity.

How much?

Eat fish, including fresh, frozen, canned and smoked, one to three times a week as an alternative to a serve of meat, chicken or egg.

One serving is equivalent to:

- 150 grams (5½ oz) raw fish or seafood
- 115 grams (4 oz) grilled or steamed fish
- 100 grams (3½ oz) canned fish (drained)

Which fish?

Oily fish, which tend to have darker coloured flesh and a stronger fish flavour, are the richest source of omega-3 fats.

- Fresh fish with higher levels of omega-3s are: Atlantic salmon; smoked salmon; Atlantic, Pacific and Spanish mackerel; sea mullet; southern bluefin tuna; and swordfish. Eastern and Pacific oysters and squid (calamari) are also rich sources.
- Canned pink and red salmon (including the bones),

sardines, mackerel and, to a lesser extent, tuna, are all rich sources of omega-3s; look for canned fish packed in water, canola oil, olive oil, tomato sauce or brine, and drain well.

A WORD ABOUT FISH AND MERCURY

While there are many benefits of eating fish, if you are pregnant you do need to be careful about the types of fish you eat. Some fish contain high levels of mercury which can be harmful to your baby.

FSA (Food Standards Agency United Kingdom) recently revised their guidelines on mercury in fish. They advise that pregnant women, women planning pregnancy and children under 16 should continue to consume a variety of fish as part of a healthy diet but should avoid certain species – shark (flake), marlin and swordfish, and possibly limit the amount of tuna they eat. As an alternative to tuna enjoy other oily fish such as mackerel, herring, pilchards, sardines, trout and salmon.

For more information consult the website www.food.gov.uk

FISH FINGERS
GI 38

Fish fingers have a measurable GI because of their breadcrumb coating. Although low GI, they may be high in saturated fat, depending on the oil used in their manufacture. Check the food label carefully. Oven baking or grilling are the healthiest ways to cook them and, of course, serve them with plenty of vegetables or salad.

LEAN MEAT, CHICKEN & EGGS

As with fish and seafood, GI is not relevant to protein-rich meat, chicken and eggs. These foods are valuable inclusions in a healthy diet, however, not only for protein, but also for essential vitamins and minerals. Red meat is the best dietary source of iron, the nutrient used in carrying oxygen in our blood, and the main source of zinc, which is a part of over 100 enzymes throughout the body. Good iron and zinc status can improve your energy levels and exercise tolerance.

> Lean meat, chicken and eggs are valuable additions to a healthy diet thanks to their protein, and nutrients such as iron, zinc, vitamin B12, niacin and other B vitamins.

A chronic shortage of iron leads to anaemia, with symptoms including pale skin, excessive tiredness, breathlessness and decreased attention span. Even mild iron deficiency can cause unexplained fatigue.

Although chicken contains about one-third as much iron as meat, it is readily absorbed, as it is from red meat, and provides a versatile, nutrient-rich alternative. Eggs also contain valuable amounts of the nutrients found in meat, although the iron is not as well absorbed. The cholesterol content of eggs is only a concern if you have high cholesterol levels and/or your total diet is high in saturated fat. Omega-3-enriched eggs, meat and chicken also make a significant contribution to long chain omega-3 fats which are so vital in human brain development and function.

How much?

Although nutritious, meat, chicken and eggs do not have to be a part of everyone's diet. After all, there are countless healthy vegetarians in the world! If you are not vegetarian, we suggest eating lean meat three times a week in addition to eggs or skinless chicken once or twice a week, accompanied by plenty of salad and vegetables. One serving is equivalent to:

- 100 grams (3½ oz) raw lean meat or chicken
- 2 medium eggs
- 1 small chop, fat removed
- 100 grams (3½ oz) cooked lean mince
- ½ skinless chicken breast
- 1 large chicken drumstick

How much a day?

One or two servings a day is appropriate for most people; bigger eaters may want a little more.

- Smaller eaters: 1–2 servings a day
- Medium eaters: 2–3 servings a day
- Bigger eaters: 3 servings a day

Shopping tips

- Choose lower fat meat products such as pastrami, leg ham and rolled turkey breast.
- Choose lean cuts of meat.
- Cut visible fat including skin from meat and poultry and drain away the fat after cooking.

Serving suggestions

- Marinate skinless chicken or lean meat to add flavour and moisture before grilling or baking. Try combinations of olive oil, red wine and garlic or lemon juice, olive oil, fresh herbs and pepper.
- Try cooking fresh fish in the microwave for a quick meal, basted with soy sauce, lemon juice or yoghurt and seasoned with fresh dill, paprika or curry spices. One fillet takes 60–90 seconds on full power.
- Pan-fry or stir-fry strips of lean meat or chicken in a

non-stick pan using small amounts of olive or rapeseed oil. Add flavour with ginger, garlic, chilli, lemon zest, adding sauces such as soy, oyster, hoi sin etc, after cooking.

- Enjoy poached eggs with grainy bread and baby spinach; scrambled eggs with salmon; or an omelette or frittata with lots of vegetables.

LOW FAT DAIRY FOODS & CALCIUM-ENRICHED SOYA PRODUCTS

Calcium is the most abundant mineral in our bodies. It builds our bones and teeth and is involved in muscle contraction and relaxation, blood clotting, nerve function and regulation of blood pressure. If we don't get enough calcium in our diet, our bodies will draw it out of our bones. Over a period of time, this can lead to osteoporosis, loss of height, curvature of the spine and peridontal disease (disease of the bones supporting our teeth).

> The key to strong, healthy bones is making sure we have plenty of calcium in our diet. Low fat dairy foods are among the richest sources and, for most of us, the easiest way to get the calcium we need.

Studies are now showing that calcium:

- can help lower high blood pressure
- may protect against cancer, particularly cancer of the bladder, bowel and colon, and possibly against breast, ovarian, pancreas and skin cancers
- can favourably influence blood fat levels and reduce the risk of stroke
- can reduce the risk of kidney stones
- can assist in weight regulation

Dairy foods

Dairy foods are recommended throughout childhood and beyond. Not only are they an important source of calcium, but they also provide energy, protein, carbohydrate and vitamins A, B and D. Virtually all dairy foods have low GI values – largely thanks to lactose, the sugar found naturally in milk, which has a low GI of 46.

By choosing low fat varieties of milk, yoghurt, ice-cream and custard, you will enjoy a food that provides you with sustained energy, boosting your calcium intake but not your saturated fat intake. Although cheese is a good source of calcium, it is not a source of carbohydrate as its lactose is drawn off in the whey during production. This means that GI is not relevant to cheese.

What about lactose intolerance?

Lactose, the sugar in milk, is a disaccharide ('double sugar') that needs to be digested into its component sugars before our bodies can absorb it. The two sugars (glucose and galactose) compete with each other for absorption. Once absorbed, the galactose is mainly metabolised in the liver and produces very little effect on our blood glucose levels. The remaining sugar, glucose, is present in a small enough amount not to cause a spike in blood glucose.

Some people are lactose intolerant because the enzyme lactase is not active in their small intestine. Children who are lactose intolerant often outgrow this by five years of age. If you are lactose intolerant, you should still be able to enjoy cheese – which is virtually lactose free – and yoghurt. The micro-organisms in yoghurt are active in digesting lactose during passage through the small intestine. Alternatively, try lactose-reduced or lactose-free milk and milk products, or low GI, low fat, calcium-enriched non-dairy alternatives such as soya milk. Note that rice milk has a high GI value (GI 92).

Non-dairy calcium sources

If you eat only plant foods or want to avoid dairy products, you may turn to soya beverages, yoghurts and desserts as an alternative. Soya products are not naturally high in calcium so look for calcium-fortified products if you are relying on them as a source of calcium.

Other non-dairy options that will boost your calcium intake are foods such as almonds, Brazil nuts, sesame seeds, dried figs, dried apricots, soyabeans, Asian greens such as bok choi, fish with edible bones such as salmon and sardines, calcium-enriched tofu and calcium-fortified breakfast cereals.

> ### Boning up
>
> We build our maximum bone strength by the time we reach about 20 years old. From our early 30s, bone calcium starts decreasing, but an adequate calcium intake, among other things, can help stop the decline.

How much?

One serving is equivalent to:

- 200 ml (7 fl oz) semi-skimmed milk
- 200 ml (7 fl oz) calcium-enriched low fat soya milk
- 150 grams (5½ oz) pot low fat yoghurt or calcium-enriched soya yoghurt
- 30 grams (1 oz) reduced fat hard cheese
- 200 ml (7 fl oz) low fat custard or 8 scoops (400 ml/ 14 fl oz) of low fat ice-cream are calcium-equivalent options but are higher in calories, so don't rely on them routinely.

How much a day?

Everyone should aim to eat or drink at least two or three servings of dairy foods or calcium-enriched soya products per day to meet calcium needs.

- Smaller eaters: 2 servings
- Medium eaters: 2 servings
- Bigger eaters: 3 servings

> ## Weight control
>
> Recent research suggests that people who include more dairy foods in their diet are better able to control their weight. Calcium is required to burn fat but it's also possible that some components of dairy inhibit fat absorption.

Serving suggestions

The experts tell us that it only takes 21 days to start building a new health habit. Here are some simple ways to get started and make sure you get two or three servings of dairy foods each day.

- Start your day with a fruit smoothie.
- Top your breakfast cereal with yoghurt.
- Relax with a café latte mid-morning.
- Add a slice of cheese or a dollop of ricotta to your sandwich.
- Reach for a glass of cool milk for a refreshing snack.
- Follow your main meal with a dairy dessert.
- End the day with warm milk and honey to ensure a good night's sleep.

Did you know?

In Britain at least two and a half million young people and women do not eat enough calcium, the building block for strong bones and teeth. Over time a diet low in calcium can increase the risk of developing brittle bone disease (osteoporosis). One of the easiest ways to meet your daily calcium requirement is to consume two or three portions of milk, yoghurt or cheese. It's easy. All you need is:

- ❏ 200 ml (7 fl oz) glass of semi-skimmed or skimmed milk—plain or flavoured
- ❏ 150 gram (5½ oz) pot of low fat natural or fruit yogurt
- ❏ 30 gram (1 oz) match-box-sized piece of cheese

For more information go to www.milk.co.uk

Cheese – a great source of calcium

Perfect for sandwich fillings, snacks and toppings for pasta and with gratin dishes, cheese also contributes a fair number of calories. Most cheese is around 30 per cent fat, much of it saturated.

Ricotta and cottage cheese are good low fat choices – usually less than 7 per cent fat. Use them as an alternative to butter or margarine for sandwiches. It's worth trying fresh ricotta from a deli – you may find its soft creamy texture and fresh flavour tastier than pre-packaged tub ricotta. When making lasagne, use creamy ricotta instead of white sauce. Flavoured cottage cheese or natural cottage cheese with freshly snipped chives or basil and a twist of black pepper make ideal low fat toppings for toast and crackers for snacks and light lunches.

Although there are a number of good reduced fat cheeses available, others can lose out in the flavour stakes for a relatively small reduction in fat. If you are a real cheese lover and having a hard time finding a tasty low fat one, try these tips for making the most of your higher fat cheese choices.

❑ Consider eating a little of a strong-flavoured cheese rather than a lot of something bland and tasteless.

❑ Shave a few strips of fresh Parmesan over pasta – a vegetable peeler does the job nicely. Grating and shaving helps a little cheese go a long way.

❑ Enjoy full fat cheeses in small amounts occasionally. This includes regular types of cheddar, blue vein, Swiss, brie, Camembert, gouda and havarti.

❑ Try some mozzarella cheese – whole milk or semi-skimmed – it may contain less fat than some reduced fat cheeses. Grate and sprinkle over stuffed vegetables such as aubergines or peppers, baked potatoes and pizzas before cooking.

Boning up

The best way to safeguard your bones is to pack in enough calcium before your mid to late 20s and thereafter eat a well balanced diet with plenty of weight-bearing activity like walking, running, aerobics, tennis, football and dancing, which will strengthen your bones.

CHOCOLATE MILK

GI 24 (low fat, sweetened with aspartame)
GI 34 (low fat, sweetened with sugar)

Flavoured milks are available in regular or low fat varieties with relatively modest amounts of added sugar (about 4 per cent) compared with soft drinks (11–12 per cent). Adding a moderate amount of sugar in the form of chocolate syrup or powder or other flavours does not significantly raise the GI of low fat milk. For many people, children and adults alike, who don't like the taste of plain milk or prefer something sweeter, this dairy choice can add some extra vitamins and minerals to the day's nutrient intake. However, the choice of a low fat type is important, as is a smaller, rather than larger, serve size if you're watching your calorie intake.

Although some parents might be concerned that flavoured milk simply adds extra sugar to their child's diet, it is a far more nutritious drink than a soft drink. A study in Canada has shown that children and teenagers who drink flavoured milk consume fewer soft drinks and fewer fruit drinks than those who do not, and have far better calcium intakes. This is significant when you consider that maximum bone strength is built up in our younger years and 82 per cent of our children aren't getting the recommended three daily serves of dairy foods they need.

Serving suggestions

- Make flavoured milk ice-cubes for snacks after school or on hot days.
- Blend flavoured milk with fruit and a dollop of low fat yoghurt for a quick smoothie.

CUSTARD
GI 43 (made with powder)

Custard is a good source of calcium and protein, especially for young children who don't like drinking milk. Packet custard based on wheat starch is quick and easy to prepare. Make it with semi-skimmed milk or low fat calcium-enriched soya milk and sprinkle a little freshly grated nutmeg on top for that traditional 'baked custard' look. Serve hot or cold with fresh or canned fruit – especially peaches or nectarines – or with a sliced banana stirred through.

Serving suggestions

* Refuel with a chilled single-serve pot of custard from the dairy dessert cabinet in the supermarket. Look for low fat varieties.
* Top winter warming desserts like apple and rhubarb crumble with a creamy custard sauce or use as a filling for pastries.
* For that special occasion, make a 'real' custard with milk, a vanilla pod and egg. Bring 500 ml (17 fl oz) of milk almost to the boil, remove from the heat, add a vanilla pod and set aside for 15 minutes to infuse. Meanwhile, whisk 5 egg yolks and 125 grams (4½ oz) of caster sugar in a bowl until thick and creamy. Remove the vanilla pod from the milk and pour the milk into the egg mixture, stirring vigorously. Place in a heavy-based saucepan and cook over a medium heat (do not allow to boil), stirring constantly, until the custard thickens. Strain if the custard becomes lumpy.

DAIRY DESSERTS
GI 32–48 (chilled, low fat)

From flavoured crème fraîche to mousse, rice pudding to tiramisu, today's refrigerated dairy cabinet is filled with tempting, ready-to-eat, light, creamy, even aerated, desserts packed in single-serve pots, packs and pouches. Without the effort needed to whip up a pudding from scratch, they provide a guilt-free after-dinner indulgence or a convenient snack on the run and without adding too many calories. Because they are milk based they can be a useful source of calcium and provide an alternative to yoghurt or ice-cream when you want something sweet. Choose low fat, low GI products and enjoy in moderation.

Serving suggestions

- Lightly grill fresh fruits and serve topped with a dollop of a chocolate or vanilla dairy dessert as an alternative to ice-cream or yoghurt.
- Enjoy single-serve dairy desserts as a satisfying snack when you need to refuel on the run or as an alternative to other morning or afternoon snacks.

FLAVOURED MILK POWDERS
GI 40 (Milo® made with semi-skimmed milk)
Milk is an important source of calcium throughout life. Adding a moderate amount of refined sugar in the form of Milo®, Ovaltine® or Horlicks® does not significantly raise the GI of semi-skimmed or skimmed milk. As with flavoured milks from the chilled dairy cabinet, this is an excellent dairy choice for children and adults that can help add some extra vitamins and minerals to the day's nutrient intake.

ICE-CREAM
GI 37–49 (low fat)
Ice-cream is not just a treat, it's a useful source of bone-building calcium plus some protein and the other essential vitamins and minerals found in milk. Because it contains added sugar, the GI generally tends to be a little higher than milk and yoghurt. Look for low fat varieties when you shop – you'll find that some taste as good if

not better than their full fat counterparts. Add a scoop to milkshakes and smoothies and enjoy a small portion as a snack or dessert with fruit.

Serving suggestions

For a satisfying snack or quick breakfast in a glass, whip up a nutritious smoothie. Start with your fruit combination and add about 250 ml (9 fl oz) of milk and a scoop of low fat ice-cream or yoghurt to make it creamy. Boost the vitamin and fibre content with a little wheat germ or bran. For a thicker texture, blend with frozen fruit. If you don't have time to freeze the fruit, simply whirl in some crushed ice until the smoothie is as thick as you like. Here are some combinations to try:

- Tangy banana and apple – blend until smooth: 1 frozen banana, 125 ml (4 fl oz) of orange juice, 1 gala apple, peeled and roughly cut into chunks, 125 ml (4 fl oz) of semi-skimmed milk and a scoop of low fat ice-cream or yoghurt.
- Raspberry and peach – blend until smooth: 125 ml (4 fl oz) of apple juice, 2 scoops of low fat ice-cream, 1 peeled, sliced and partially frozen peach and 6 or 7 partially frozen raspberries. Whirl in a few spoonfuls of crushed ice and serve.
- Creamy banana and strawberry – blend until smooth: 1 banana, 6 strawberries, sliced, 250 ml (9 fl oz) of semi-skimmed milk and 1 scoop of low fat ice-cream. Whirl in a few spoonfuls of crushed ice and serve.

INSTANT PUDDINGS
GI 40–47

Instant puddings, like custard, are useful in helping children and teenagers (and adults) achieve the three servings of dairy foods a day they need to build strong bones. These

Fat count

• Regular milk contains less than 4 per cent fat.

• Semi-skimmed milk contains less than 1.7 per cent fat.

• Skimmed milk contains no more than 0.3 per cent fat.

dried packet mixes come in a range of flavours and are the speediest way to whip up a nutritious, satisfying and economical dessert and because they are so easy to make, even young children can help in the kitchen. Choose low fat milk or low fat calcium-enriched soya milk for these dairy desserts and serve with fresh or canned fruit.

Serving suggestions

• Make instant pudding iced treats for after-school snacks. Combine pudding and milk in a deep bowl and beat with a mixer following the packet instructions. Spoon the mixture into individual cupcake containers and leave to set for about a minute. Insert ice-cream sticks into the centre and freeze.
• Whip up banana smoothies with extra flavour by blending a tablespoon of instant pudding mix per 250 ml (9 fl oz) of milk.

MILK

GI 27–34 (range of skimmed to regular fat milks)

Nutritionally, milk packs a punch. It's long been valued for protein, the bone-building minerals calcium and phosphorus and vitamins such as riboflavin (vitamin B2). Milk also has a low GI – a combination of the moderate glycaemic effect of its sugar (lactose) plus the milk protein, which forms a soft curd in the stomach and slows down the rate of stomach emptying. Regular whole milk is high in saturated fat, but these days there is a wide range of milk to suit everybody's needs, including semi-skimmed or skimmed varieties. So enjoy a glass of milk or a milkshake or smoothie and use milk in your cooking for desserts and sauces, but opt for the semi-skimmed and skimmed types.

We sometimes include buttermilk in our recipes. Despite its name, buttermilk isn't high in fat – it's made from skimmed milk. Specially chosen bacterial cultures are added in its manufacture to give the traditional texture and slightly sour taste that makes it popular for baking.

Serving suggestions

- Hot milk and honey makes a nutritious nightcap. Research shows that people do sleep more soundly after a warm milk drink at night. Warming the milk activates an amino acid called tryptophan, which the body converts to serotonin, the hormone associated with calmness and wellbeing.
- When you're out for a coffee choose a skimmed milk café latte (a 'skinny latte') or cappuccino and get a calcium boost!
- White sauce is used in dishes such as mornay, lasagne and savoury soufflés and is the base for many sauces. To make it, the traditional method is to melt 2 tablespoons of butter or margarine in a small saucepan over a low heat. Blend in 2 tablespoons of plain flour and cook over a low heat for 1–2 minutes, then slowly add 250 ml (9 fl oz) of milk, stirring constantly until smooth and thickened. Season to taste with salt and freshly ground black pepper, celery salt, nutmeg, or a few tablespoons of chopped chives or parsley. You can make a lower fat version by heating 250 ml (9 fl oz) of semi-skimmed milk with 1 whole peeled onion and a bay leaf. When hot, stir in 1 tablespoon of cornflour blended with a little cold milk and stir over a low heat until thickened. Remove the onion and bay leaf and discard and season as above.

SOYA MILK
GI 36–44 (reduced fat, calcium fortified)
Drinking this completely dairy- and lactose-free beverage is an easy way to include soya protein in your diet. Whole soyabeans – which are usually GM/GE free (check the label)

– are mixed with filtered water and flavourings to produce a milk-like product. Once enjoyed by vegetarians, soya milk has become increasing popular, possibly because it tastes good and is recognised to be rich in phytoestrogens, nutrients that are known to have health benefits.

Soya milk is available fresh from the chilled dairy cabinet, in long life packs and in powdered forms. You can also buy flavoured products. To ensure it is a suitable alternative to regular dairy milk, soya milk is often enriched with a range of vitamins and minerals including calcium and riboflavin (vitamin B12). Choose a low fat, calcium-enriched milk and use it exactly as you would regular milk – on your breakfast cereal, with hot or cold drinks or in your cooking when making desserts and sauces.

Serving suggestions

If you haven't tried calcium-enriched, low fat soya milk before, here are some easy ways to get started.

- Mix it in with mashed sweet potato, pumpkin or potato; or in a combination of all three vegetables.
- Try a soya latte or soya banana smoothie or use in other flavoured milk drinks.
- Use it to make white sauce for lasagne or moussaka.
- Make dairy desserts with soya milk.

SOYA YOGHURT

GI 50 (fruit flavoured, sweetened with sugar)

Soya yoghurt is usually made from soyabeans or soya protein rather than soya milk. Look for calcium-enriched, low fat varieties and use in exactly the same way as you would dairy yoghurts as a snack or dessert, or added to smoothies and shakes. Unflavoured soya yoghurt can be used in dips, sauces and spreads.

YOGHURT

GI range 14–43
GI 14–21 (low fat, flavoured, no added sugar)
GI 26–43 (low fat, flavoured, sweetened with sugar)
Yoghurt is a concentrated milk product rich in calcium, riboflavin and protein, and all varieties have low GI values, mainly due to the combination of acidity and high protein. Artificially sweetened, flavoured yoghurts have the lowest GI values and contain fewer calories than the naturally sweetened flavoured versions. Drinking yoghurts are also available and will have similar GI values. Low fat yoghurt provides the most calcium for the least calories (520 mg calcium in a 200 gram/7 oz pot).

People who are lactose intolerant can usually safely consume yoghurt without experiencing abdominal distress. Special types of bacteria added to some yoghurts (eg. Bifidobacteria) may colonise the large intestine and provide health benefits. Research in this area is still controversial.

Eating a 200 gram (7 oz) pot of yoghurt is equivalent to drinking a 250 ml (9 fl oz) glass of milk. As with other dairy products, choose the low fat varieties and enjoy throughout the day with breakfast cereals or as a snack or dessert.

Serving suggestions
Always keep a pot of low fat plain yoghurt in the fridge, trying different brands until you find one you like. It's a great base for dips, salad dressings and sauces – sweet and savoury.

- Serve chicken salad with a yoghurt dressing made from a 200 gram (7 oz) pot of low fat plain yoghurt, 2 tablespoons of lemon juice, a couple of teaspoons of a tangy mango chutney and 2 tablespoons of finely chopped mint.
- Spice plain yoghurt with a little ground cumin and

cardamom to make a sauce for topping burgers or falafel rolls. Add fresh mint for a finishing touch.

- Make a spicy Indian 'lassi' drink by blending 200 grams (7 oz) of low fat natural yoghurt with ½ teaspoon of ground cumin and a pinch of salt to taste. Chill. Just before serving, stir in 1/4 teaspoon of finely minced onion and a few strips of finely sliced green chilli. Pour into a tall glass over lots of ice-cubes and serve – delicious as an appetiser before an Indian meal.

- For a sweeter taste, mango lassis are a meal in a glass or a delicious way to finish a spicy dinner. You can make this lassi in about 5 minutes by combining in a blender 1 medium sized mango, diced, with 125 ml (4 fl oz) of freshly squeezed orange juice, a few spoonfuls of ice-cubes, 1 tablespoon of pure floral honey or a little more to taste, and 1 teaspoon of rosewater if you have it. Process for about 30 seconds until the ingredients are just blended. Add 300 grams (10½ oz) of low fat natural yoghurt and whizz for another 30–40 seconds until it's frothy. Makes 4 glasses (250 ml/9 fl oz each).

low gi eating made easy
Tables

Here's your easy and reliable reference to the GI of foods. Use these tables to choose the best carbs for your health and to enjoy low GI foods every meal, every day.

Remember, it is carb quality that counts.

We have categorised the foods A to Z under the following headings:

- Bakery products – including cakes and muffins
- Beans, peas and lentils – including split peas, lentils, chickpeas and baked beans
- Beverages – including fruit and vegetable juices, soft drinks, flavoured milk and sport drinks
- Biscuits – including commercial sweet biscuits, savoury crispbreads and plain crackers
- Bread – including sliced white and wholemeal bread, fruit breads and flat breads
- Breakfast cereals – including processed cereals, muesli, oats and porridge
- Cereal grains – including couscous, bulghur and barley
- Dairy products and alternatives – including milk, yoghurt, ice-creams, dairy desserts and soya products
- Fruits – including fresh, canned and dried fruit
- Miscellaneous – including various fast foods
- Pasta, noodles and rice
- Snack foods – including muesli bars, fruit sticks and straps and nuts
- Sweeteners and spreads – including sugars, honey and jam
- Vegetables – including green vegetables, salad vegetables, root vegetables and soups

All you need to do for everyday low GI eating is make **MOST** of your carbohydrate choices from the **EVERYDAY** foods, taking into account the serving sizes shown. Remember larger servings will increase the glycaemic load of the food and may change its ranking.

Note: We have organised the **EVERYDAY** foods into those you can eat according to your appetite and those where you need to exercise a bit of restraint and some sensible portion caution.

EVERYDAY foods

These 'eat according to your appetite' foods have a **low GI** and a **low GL** (depending on how much you put on your plate). They are slowly digested, long-lasting foods, which are the best sources of sustained energy. Their low GI gives them a high fill-up factor which means you can eat them according to appetite. Some of your EVERYDAY foods – granary bread, fresh fruit, low fat yoghurt, split peas, soya beans, rolled oats, pure floral honey and sourdough bread.

EVERYDAY CAUTION WITH PORTION foods

These foods have a moderate or low GI and a moderate to high GL, again, depending on your serving size. They're great sources of carbohydrate but it's sensible to give some thought to the quantity of these foods, because of their potential to have a high GL if you overload your plate or go back for seconds or thirds. Some of your **EVERYDAY CAUTION WITH PORTION** foods – fruit juices, noodles, pasta, rice, soft drinks, crumpets, flavoured milks, fruit breads, muesli bars and sultanas.

OCCASIONAL foods

These foods have high GI values but a moderate GL. Their high GI makes them rapidly digested and much less satisfying than the **EVERYDAY** foods so keep them occasional. Some foods that are higher in saturated fat have also been included in this group. Some of your **OCCASIONAL** foods – potatoes, scones, crackers and processed cereals.

KEEP FOR A TREAT foods

These are high GI and high GL or are high in saturated fat. Many of them are standard fare in our British diet but by stimulating blood glucose and insulin spikes they contribute to our risk of obesity, diabetes and heart disease. Don't be fooled by the low fat nature of some of them! Some of your **KEEP FOR A TREAT** foods – puffed cereals, white bread, bagels, jelly beans, chocolate.

BAKERY PRODUCTS

Everyday foods	Everyday caution with portion foods	Occasional foods	Keep for a treat foods
	Apple muffin, home-made 60 g	Angel food cake, plain 50 g	Banana cake, home-made 80 g
		Bran muffin, commercially made 125 g	Blueberry muffin, commercially made 125 g
		Carrot cake, commercially made 125 g	Chocolate cake, made from packet mix with icing 125 g
		Crumpet, white 50 g	Croissant, plain 60 g
		Scones, plain, made from packet mix 50 g	Cupcake, strawberry-iced 38 g
		Sponge cake, plain, unfilled 63 g	Pound cake, plain 50 g
			Vanilla cake made from packet mix with vanilla icing 125 g

BEANS, PEAS AND LENTILS

Everyday foods	Everyday caution with portion foods	Occasional foods	Keep for a treat foods
Baked beans, canned in tomato sauce 150 g	Black-eyed beans, soaked, boiled 150 g		
Black beans, boiled 150 g	Broad beans 80 g		
Borlotti beans, canned, drained 75 g	Haricot beans, cooked, canned 150 g		
Butter beans, canned, drained 75 g	Kidney beans, red, canned, drained 150 g		
Butter beans, dried, boiled 150 g			
Cannellini beans 85 g			
Chickpeas, canned in brine 150 g			
Chickpeas, dried, boiled 150 g			
Dark red kidney beans, canned, drained 150 g			
Four bean mix, canned, drained 75 g			
Green lentils, canned 50 g			

BEANS, PEAS AND LENTILS			
Everyday foods	**Everyday caution with portion foods**	**Occasional foods**	**Keep for a treat foods**
Green lentils, dried, boiled 150 g			
Haricot beans, dried, boiled 150 g			
Kidney beans, red, dried, boiled 150 g			
Lima beans, baby, frozen, reheated 150 g			
Mung beans 150 g			
Peas, dried, boiled 150 g			
Red lentils, dried, boiled 150 g			
Soyabeans, canned, drained 150 g			
Soyabeans, dried, boiled 150 g			
Split peas, yellow, boiled 20 mins 150 g			

BEVERAGES

Everyday foods	Everyday caution with portion foods	Occasional foods	Keep for a treat foods
Carrot juice, freshly made 250 ml	Apple juice, no added sugar 250 ml	Isostar® sports drink 250 ml	Milo® powder in full fat milk 250 ml
Coffee, black, no milk or sugar 200 ml	Coca-Cola®, soft drink 250 ml	Lucozade®, original, sparkling glucose drink 250 ml	
Diet soft drinks 250 ml	Cranberry Juice Cocktail, Ocean Spray 250 ml		
Milo® powder in skimmed or reduced fat milk 250 ml	Fanta®, orange soft drink 250 ml		
Tomato juice, no added sugar 250 ml	Grapefruit juice, unsweetened 250 ml		
	Orange juice, unsweetened 250 ml		
	Pineapple juice, unsweetened 250 ml		

BISCUITS			
Everyday foods	**Everyday caution with portion foods**	**Occasional foods**	**Keep for a treat foods**
Ryvita® crispbread 25 g		Crispbread, generic 25 g	
		Crispbread, gluten-free 21 g	
		Digestive biscuits, plain 25 g	
		Oatcakes 55 g	
		Rice cakes, puffed, white 25 g	
		Wafer biscuits, vanilla, plain 25 g	
		Water crackers, plain 25 g	

BREAD

Everyday foods	Everyday caution with portion foods	Occasional foods	Keep for a treat foods
Fruit & Muesli loaf, Bürgen® 40 g	Gluten-free low carbohydrate 30 g	Bun, hamburger, white 53 g	Bagel, white 70 g
Fruit Loaf, thick sliced 30 g	Gluten-free multigrain brown, sliced 30 g	Dark rye bread 30 g	Baguette, white 30 g
Pumpernickel bread 30 g	Gluten-free mutigrain white, sliced 30 g	Gluten-free bread, white, sliced 30 g	Light rye bread 30 g
Rye bread, Bürgen® 40 g	Hibran, Bürgen 44 g	Stuffing, bread 30 g	Melba toast, plain 30 g
Sourdough bread, organic, stoneground, wholemeal 32 g	Multigrain sandwich bread 30 g	Sunflower Maltigrain, Allinson 47 g	
Sourdough rye bread 30 g	Pitta bread, white 75 g	White bread, regular sliced 30 g	
Sourdough wheat bread 30 g	Tasty wholemeal, Kingsmill 38 g		
Soya and Linseed, Bürgen 40 g			

BREAKFAST CEREALS

Everyday foods	Everyday caution with portion foods	Occasional foods	Keep for a treat foods
All-Bran®, Kellogg's® 30 g	Frosties®, Kellogg's® 30 g	Bran Flakes, Kellogg's® 30 g	Rice Krispies®, Kellogg's® 30 g
Oat bran, raw, unprocessed 10 g	Muesli, Natural 45 g	Cornflakes, Crunchy Nut, Kellogg's® 30 g	
Porridge, regular, made from oats with water 30 g	Special K®, regular, Kellogg's® 30 g	Cornflakes®, Kellogg's® 30 g	
Rolled Oats, raw 30 g		Porridge, instant, made with water 30 g	
		Puffed Wheat breakfast cereal 30 g	
		Shredded Wheat 30 g	
		Sultana Bran, Kellogg's® 30 g	

CEREAL GRAINS

Everyday foods	Everyday caution with portion foods	Occasional foods	Keep for a treat foods
Barley, pearl, boiled 150 g	Barley, rolled, raw 50 g		
Semolina, cooked 150 g	Buckwheat, boiled 150 g		
	Cornmeal (polenta), boiled 150 g		
	Couscous, boiled 5 mins 150 g		
	Quinoa, organic, raw, 50 g		
	Rye, raw 50 g		
	Wheat, cracked, bulghur, ready to eat 150 g		
	Whole-wheat kernels, raw 50 g		

DAIRY PRODUCTS – ICE-CREAM, CUSTARD AND DESSERTS			
Everyday foods	**Everyday caution with portion foods**	**Occasional foods**	**Keep for a treat foods**
Custard, vanilla, reduced fat 100 ml			Custard, home-made from milk, wheat starch and sugar 100 ml Ice Cream, Regular, full fat, average of several types 50 g

DAIRY PRODUCTS – MILK AND ALTERNATIVES

Everyday foods	Everyday caution with portion foods	Occasional foods	Keep for a treat foods
Milk, semi-skimmed, low fat (1.4%) 250ml			Milk (3.6% fat) 250 ml
Skimmed milk, low fat (0.1%) 250 ml			
Soya milk, full fat (3%) 250 ml			
Soya milk, low fat, calcium-fortified 250 ml			

DAIRY PRODUCTS – YOGHURT			
Everyday foods	**Everyday caution with portion foods**	**Occasional foods**	**Keep for a treat foods**
Yoghurt, Ski™, low fat, with sugar, strawberry 200 g	Soya yoghurt, 2% fat, with sugar, peach and mango 200 g		
Yoghurt, Ski™, no fat, with sugar, all flavours 200 g			

FRUIT FRESH			
Everyday foods	Everyday caution with portion foods	Occasional foods	Keep for a treat foods
Apple, fresh 120 g	Banana, raw 120 g		
Apricots, fresh 168 g	Watermelon, raw 120 g		
Avocado 120 g			
Cantaloupe, fresh 120 g			
Cherries, dark, raw 120 g			
Custard apple, fresh, flesh only 120 g			
Figs 50 g			
Grapefruit, fresh 120 g			
Grapes, fresh 120 g			
Kiwi fruit, fresh 120 g			
Lemon 40 g			
Lime 40 g			
Mango, fresh 120 g			
Orange, fresh 120 g			
Papaya (pawpaw), fresh 120 g			
Peach, fresh 120 g			
Pear, fresh 120 g			
Pineapple, fresh 120 g			
Plum, raw 120 g			
Raspberries 65 g			
Strawberries, fresh 120 g			

FRUIT – CANNED			
Everyday foods	**Everyday caution with portion foods**	**Occasional foods**	**Keep for a treat foods**
Peaches, canned, in heavy syrup 120 g	Apricots, canned in light syrup 120 g	Lychees, canned, in syrup, drained 120 g	
Peaches, canned, in light syrup 120 g			
Peaches, canned, in natural juice 120 g			
Pear halves, canned, in natural juice 120 g			
Pear halves, canned, in reduced-sugar syrup 120 g			

FRUIT – DRIED			
Everyday foods	Everyday caution with portion foods	Occasional foods	Keep for a treat foods
Apple, dried 60 g	Cranberries, dried, sweetened 40 g		
Apricots, dried 60 g	Dates, Arabic, dried, vacuum-packed 55 g		
Prunes, pitted 60 g	Figs, dried, tenderised 60 g		
	Raisins 60 g		
	Sultanas 60 g		

MISCELLANEOUS – FAST FOOD

Everyday foods	Everyday caution with portion foods	Occasional foods	Keep for a treat foods
Consommé, clear, chicken or vegetable 250 ml	Black bean soup, canned 250 ml		Chicken nuggets, frozen reheated in microwave 5 mins, 100 g
Lentil soup, canned 250 ml	Chicken Tikka Biryani 450 g		Pizza, Super Supreme, pan, Pizza Hut 130 g
Minestrone soup, Traditional, canned 250 ml	Chicken Tikka Masala & Pilau Rice, Be Good To Yourself range 400 g		Pizza, Super Supreme, thin and crispy, Pizza Hut 100 g
Tomato soup, canned 250 ml	Fish fingers 100 g		
	Green pea soup, canned 250 ml		
	Lamb Bhuna & Rice, 500 g		
	Split pea soup, canned 250 ml		
	Sushi, salmon 100 g		

PASTA			
Everyday foods	**Everyday caution with portion foods**	**Occasional foods**	**Keep for a treat foods**
	2 Minute noodles, 99% fat free, Maggi 80 g		2 Minute noodles, regular, Maggi 80 g
	Capellini pasta, white boiled 180 g		Rice pasta, brown, boiled 180 g
	Fettuccine, egg, boiled 180 g		
	Gnocchi, cooked 180 g		
	Linguine pasta, thick, durum wheat, boiled 180 g		
	Linguine pasta, thin, durum wheat, boiled 180 g		
	Macaroni, white, durum wheat, boiled 180 g		
	Mung bean noodles (bean thread), dried, boiled 180 g		
	Ravioli, meat-filled, durum wheat flour, boiled 180 g		
	Rice noodles, dried, boiled 180 g		

PASTA

Everyday foods	Everyday caution with portion foods	Occasional foods	Keep for a treat foods
	Rice noodles, fresh, boiled 180 g		
	Rice vermicelli, dried, boiled, Chinese 180 g		
	Soba noodles, instant, served in soup 180 g		
	Spaghetti, white, durum wheat 180 g		
	Spaghetti, whole-meal, boiled 180 g		
	Spirali pasta, white, durum wheat 180 g		
	Tortellini, cheese, boiled 180 g		
	Udon noodles, plain 180 g		
	Vermicelli, white, durum wheat, boiled 180 g		

RICE			
Everyday foods	Everyday caution with portion foods	Occasional foods	Keep for a treat foods
	Basmati rice, white, boiled 150 g		Instant rice, white, cooked 6 mins with water 150 g
	Wild rice, boiled 150 g		Jasmine rice, white, long-grain, cooked in rice cooker 150 g
			Risotto rice, Arborio, boiled 150 g

SNACK FOODS

Everyday foods	Everyday caution with portion foods	Occasional foods	Keep for a treat foods
Jelly, diet, made from crystals with water 125 g	Cashew nuts 30 g Marshmallows, plain, pink and white 25 g Muesli bar, chewy, with choc chips or fruit 31 g Muesli bar, crunchy, with dried fruit 30 g Peanuts, roasted, 50 g Pecan nuts, raw 50 g Popcorn, plain, cooked in microwave 20 g Taco shells, cornmeal-based, baked 40 g	M&M's®, peanut 30 g Pretzels, oven-baked, traditional wheat flavour 30 g	Cadbury's® Milk Chocolate, plain 30 g Chocolate, Milk, plain, Nestlé® 50 g Chocolate, Milk, white, Nestlé® 50 g Corn chips, plain, salted 50 g Dark chocolate, plain, regular 30 g Jelly beans 30 g Licorice, soft 60 g Mars Bar®, regular 60 g Milky Bar®, plain white chocolate, Nestlé® 50 g Polos®, pepper-mint 30 g Pop-Tarts™, chocotastic 50 g Skittles® 50 g Twix® bar 60 g

SWEETENERS AND SPREADS			
Everyday foods	**Everyday caution with portion foods**	**Occasional foods**	**Keep for a treat foods**
Honey, pure floral (various) 25 g	Glucose tablets 10 g		
Hummous, regular 30 g	Honey, blended, various 25 g		
Jam, strawberry, regular 30 g	Marmalade, orange 30 g		
Maple syrup, pure, Canadian 24 g	Sugar 20 g		
Nutella®, hazelnut spread 20 g			

VEGETABLES			
Everyday foods	**Everyday caution with portion foods**	**Occasional foods**	**Keep for a treat foods**
Alfalfa sprouts 6 g	New potato, canned 150 g	Desiree potato, peeled, boiled 150 g	French fries, frozen, reheated in microwave 150 g
Artichokes, globe, fresh or canned in brine 80 g	Pumpkin 80 g	Instant mashed potato 150 g	
Asparagus 100 g	Swede, cooked 150 g	New potato, unpeeled and boiled 150 g	
Aubergine 100 g	Sweet potato, baked 150 g	Parsnips 80 g	
Bean sprouts, raw 14 g	Yam, peeled, boiled 150 g		
Beetroot, canned 80 g			
Bok choi 100 g			
Broccoli 60 g			
Brussel sprouts 100 g			
Cabbage 70 g			
Carrots, peeled, boiled 80 g			
Cauliflower 60 g			
Celery 40 g			
Courgette 100 g			
Cucumber 45 g			
Endive 30 g			
Fennel 90 g			
Green beans 70 g			
Leeks 80 g			
Lettuce 50 g			

VEGETABLES			
Everyday foods	Everyday caution with portion foods	Occasional foods	Keep for a treat foods
Mangetout sprouts 15 g			
Mushrooms 35 g			
Onions, 30 g			
Peas, green, frozen, boiled 80 g			
Pepper 80 g			
Radishes 15 g			
Rhubarb 125 g			
Rocket 30 g			
Shallots 10 g			
Spinach 75 g			
Squash, yellow 70 g			
Sweetcorn, on the cob, boiled 80 g			
Sweetcorn, whole kernel, canned, drained 80 g			
Taro 150 g			
Tomato 150 g			
Turnip 120 g			
Watercress 8 g			

Acknowledgements

In thanking colleagues who have helped us with this book, we would like to single out Hachette Livre's Publishing and Production Director, Fiona Hazard, for making it all 'so easy', our editor, Jacquie Brown, for her attention to detail and eye for consistency and our project editor Anna Waddington for whom nothing is too much trouble.

We wanted to create special Low GI Eating Made Easy tables to make it really easy for readers to choose healthy low GI foods, and we could not have done so without the cheerful efforts and database wizardry of Associate Prof Gareth Denyer at the University of Sydney.

We would also like to thank Johanna Burani whose suggestions for the US edition of The Top 100 Foods we have incorporated into this book and for permission to include her Cherry Oat Crunchies recipe from Good Carbs, Bad Carbs (Marlowe & Company); Kate Marsh who checked the information on PCOS for us and dietitian, Penny Hunking, who has helped us with this UK edition.

Further Resources

For further information on GI
www.glycemicindex.com
This is the University of Sydney's glycemic index website where you can learn about GI and access the GI database which includes the most up-to-date listing of the GI of foods that have been published in international scientific journals.

http://ginews.blogspot.com
GI News is the official glycemic index newsletter published online each month by the University of Sydney's GI Group.

www.gisymbol.com.au
The Glycemic Index (GI) Symbol Program is a food labelling program with strict nutritional criteria that aims to help people make informed food choices. The site includes a complete listing of foods carrying the GI symbol.

For information on:

Food labelling and food additives
Food Standards Agency
www.food.gov.uk

Finding a dietitian
British Dietetic Association (BDA)
www.bda.uk.com

Diabetes
Diabetes UK
www.diabetesuk.co.uk

Heart health
Heart UK
www.heartuk.org.uk

British Heart Foundation
www.bhf.org.uk

PCOS
The main resource for women with PCOS in the UK
www.verity-pcos.org.uk

Information source for polycystic ovarian syndrome (PCOS),
diabetes and insulin resistance.
www.diagnosemefirst.com

Index

About the authors

Kaye Foster-Powell is an accredited practising dietitian with extensive experience in diabetes management: she provides consultancy on all aspects of the glycaemic index.

Jennie Brand-Miller is an internationally recognised authority on carbohydrates and health. She is Professor of Human Nutrition at the University of Sydney and President of the Nutrition Society of Australia.

Jennie and Kaye have co-authored 16 books in the worldwide bestselling New Glucose Revolution series, which has sold over three million copies and is changing the way the world views carbohydrates.

Philippa Sandall is an editor and writer who specialises in food, nutrition, health and lifesytle. She was closely involved in creating the first New Glucose Revolution title with Jennie and Kays in 1995, *The GI Factor*, and has played an integral role in developing and managing the series.

'Free Sea Creates Free People'

To George, Gabriel and Vanessa

T.M.C. ASSER INSTITUUT – THE HAGUE
INSTITUTE OF ECONOMIC AND INDUSTRIAL RESEARCH (IOBE) – ATHENS

The Common Shipping Policy of the EC

by

Dr. Anna Bredima-Savopoulou
Prof. John Tzoannos

N·H
P⌒C

1990
NORTH-HOLLAND
AMSTERDAM – NEW YORK – OXFORD – TOKYO

ISBN 0 444 88553 6

North Holland
Elsevier Science Publishers B.V.
P.O. Box 211
1000 AE Amsterdam
The Netherlands

Sole distributors for the U.S.A. and Canada:
Elsevier Science Publishing Company, Inc.
655 Avenue of the Americas
New York, N.Y. 10010
U.S.A.

T.M.C. Asser Instituut – Institute for Private and Public International Law, International Commercial Arbitration and European Law.
20-22 Alexanderstraat, 2514 JM The Hague, The Netherlands – tel.: (0)70-420300 – telex: 34273 asser nl, telefax: (0)70-420359

Director: C.C.A. Voskuil

Senior Staff: M. Sumampouw (Private International Law), Ko Swan Sik (Public International Law), J.J.M. Tromm and A.E. Kellermann (Law of the European Communities), J.A. Swartzburg-Freedberg (International Commercial Arbitration), G.J. de Roode, Institute Manager (General Affairs), J.A. Wade (Legal Translations), M.H. Bastiaans (Publications), J.S. de Jongh (Library and Information).

The T.M.C. Asser Instituut was founded in 1965 by the Dutch universities offering courses in international law to promote education and research in the fields of law covered by the departments of the Institute: Private International Law, Public International Law, including the Law of International Organisations, Law of the European Communities and International Commercial Arbitration. The Institute discharges this task by the establishment and management of documentation and research projects, in some instances in co-operation with non-Dutch or international organisations, by the dissemination of information deriving therefrom and by publication of monographs and series.

PRINTED IN THE NETHERLANDS

FOREWORD

When on October 10, 1988, the distinguished Greek-American scholar, Professor Speros Vryonis Jr. delivered his inaugural lecture as first Director of the Alexander S. Onassis Center for Hellenic Studies at New York University, he chose as his topic, 'The Greeks and the Sea'. Said Professor Vryonis, 'The intimate relation of the Greeks to the sea, so spectacular in our times, is nothing new but is rather only the most recent manifestation of a constantly recurring phenomenon throughout the history of the Greeks.'

It is, accordingly, fitting that the first major study of the common shipping policy of the European Community be produced by two Greeks. I must immediately note a relationship with one. Dr. Anna Bredima-Savopoulou is my cousin. Graduate, with first-class honors, of the Law School of the University of Athens, Dr. Bredima-Savopoulou earned her master's degree, also with first-class honors, in maritime law and her doctoral degree, in European Community law, from the University of London as well as a certificate in European Community law from the University of Paris. She brings not only a scholar's background but a practitioner's experience to this survey. Dr. Bredima-Savopoulou has since 1977 served as advisor to the Union of Greek Shipowners, since 1981 as a member of the Economic and Social Committee of the European Community and since 1987 as a member of the Board of Directors of the Comité des Associations d'Armateurs des Communautés Européennes (CAACE).

Professor John Tzoannos is a graduate with honors in economics from the University of Manchester and has earned a master's degree in economics and econometrics from the University of Southampton. He obtained his doctoral degree in industrial economics from the University of Birmingham. Professor Tzoannos has an extensive University teaching experience in business finance, quantitative methods and shipping economics. He also combines an in depth research experience in shipping economics as head of the Maritime Research Department at the Institute of Economic and Industrial Research in Athens with the practical knowledge of policy making on maritime issues as a member of the Board of Directors of the CAACE since 1987.

The analysis by these two scholars of the development of the law and regulations governing the common shipping policy of the EC and of the problems, prospects and implications of that policy seems to me (an American observer who despite his Hellenic origins pretends to no expertise in maritime matters) to be significant beyond its subject.

For surely the unified EC market, with all the celebration that will mark its formal inauguration in 1992, is an edifice that will be constructed over time. Indeed, the carpenters have already been at work and the observing world knows that the architects, political and economic, of the new Europe are still not agreed on the blueprints.

Yet, to reiterate, bricks are being laid and mortar placed. That there will be a European 'house' of some kind — certainly an office building, open for business in every sector — there can be no doubt. One of those commercial activities is shipping, and the authors discuss, with appreciation for the legal, economic and political dimensions of their subject, how EC common maritime policy has evolved, where it is now and where it is likely to go.

I have little doubt that it is in large part through the hammering out in the commercial, cultural and political arenas of national, European and even international debate and decision that the new Europe will be constructed, fitfully and unevenly, building block by building block. Dr. Bredima-Savopoulou and Professor Tzoannos have given us one example of the development of EC common policy in a field, shipping, crucial to the future of the Community. In so doing, they offer a model for the study of the forging of EC policies in other areas of commerce.

A final observation from a non-European may be in order. 1992 marks not only the Year of Europe but, of course, the 500th anniversary of the discovery, by a European, of America. With a market of over 320 million people and a combined gross national product exceeding $4 trillion, 'Europe' will now be discovered anew by many Americans — and by many others.

For the new Europe, itself a remarkable phenomenon, is taking shape at a remarkable moment. Look at the international stage on which Europe is so increasingly prominent an actor. The dramatic circumstances are evident: Gorbachev and *perestroika,* United States-Soviet rapprochement on arms control, rising demands for democracy in Eastern Europe, a Japan mighty in economic power but uncertain of its global political role, and a wide range of issues commanding concern across national boundaries: drugs, AIDS, environmental pollution, Third World poverty.

On such a stage, the European Community will be a protagonist of considerable force — in many ways. This book shows us one.

John Brademas
President
New York University
New York City
Autumn 1989

PREFACE

Despite the importance of shipping to European Community trade, both internal and external, to most people the maritime sector of the EC remains a *terra incognita*. Although the Community adopted the first set of common shipping policy measures in 1986, there has been no comprehensive study of the implications of the new maritime policy. It was this vacuum that prompted the authors to address the subject. Another reason the authors felt it imperative to shed more light on the existing armoury of EEC rules for maritime transport is that the process leading to 1992 has provoked discussion within the European Community about possible further measures affecting shipping policy as well as discussion abroad about the prospect of a 'Fortress Europe'. Europe '92 is looming larger and larger in the consciousness of leaders in Europe, North America and Japan.

The authors hope that their experience in the formulation of shipping policy, at both national and European Community levels, is adequately reflected in this study. They hope, too, in view of lack of information on shipping matters to both academics and practitioners, that this survey will be of wide interest.

Although both writers clearly have a liberal perspective on the subject – they strongly agree with Goethe's assertion that 'Free sea creates free people' (Faust, 2nd part, Act 5, 2nd scene) – they have attempted to be objective in their analysis. The authors are dedicated to the idea of 'Europe' and hope that this study – which emanated from Greece, the largest maritime nation in the European Community – will serve as a stimulus to debate and further studies from other Member States. After all, diversity of views is the essence of the European Community.

The book is the product of an interdisciplinary approach. Shipping policy lends itself to this methodology *par excellence* in that it is a subject that encompasses aspects of law, economics and policy making.

The authors are deeply indepted to Dr. John Brademas for his Foreword. The authors express appreciation as well to the Institute of Industrial and Economic Research (IOBE) of Athens for its cooperation. A special thanks must also be extended to the T.M.C. Asser Instituut of The Hague, which was responsible for the academic supervision of the text and particularly to Dr Jacques Tromm and Ms Marjolijn Bastiaans. Research for the manuscript was completed in December 1988.

Finally, responsibility for drafting and for any faults in Chapters 4, 5, 6, 7 and 8 rests on Dr Anna Bredima-Savopoulou and in Chapters 1, 2, 3, 9, 10, 11 and 12 on Professor John Tzoannos.

Athens, Summer 1989

TABLE OF CONTENTS

Chapter 4

Chapter 5

Chapter 6

ATTITUDES VIS-A-VIS COMMON SHIPPING POLICY PROPOSALS BY VARIOUS INTEREST GROUPS

Chapter 7

POSITIONS BY COMMUNITY INSTITUTIONS

Chapter 9

THE IMPLICATIONS OF THE 1986 PACKAGE OF MEASURES FOR THE INDIVIDUAL EC MEMBER STATES

XVI

LIST OF ABBREVIATIONS

ACP	African, Caribbean and Pacific (countries)
A.J.I.L.	American Journal of International Law
CAACE	Comité des Associations d'Armateurs des Communautés Européennes
CCAF	Comité Central des Armateurs de France
CENSA	Council of European and Japanese National Shipowners Associations
CJEC	Court of Justice of European Communities
CIF	Cost, Insurance, Freight
COMECON	Council of Mutual Economic Assistance
COST	Coopération Europeénne dans la domaine de la recherche Scientifique et Technique
CSC	International Convention for Safe Containers
CSG	Consultative Shipping Group
dwt	deadweight tonnes
EC	European Community
ECU	European Currency Unit
EEC	European Economic Community
EP	European Parliament
ESC	Economic and Social Committee
ESC	European Shippers Council
EUA	European Unit of Account
FMC	Federal Maritime Commission
FOB	Free on Board
FRG	Federal Republic of Germany
GCBS	General Council of British Shipping
grt	gross registered tonnes
GDP	Gross Domestic Product
HMSO	Her Majesty's Stationary Office
ILO	International Labour Organisation
IMCO	Intergovernmental Maritime Consultative Organisation
IMO	International Maritime Organisation
ITF	International Transport Workers' Federation
LIBOR	London Inter-Bank Offered Rate
MARPOL	International Convention for the Prevention of Pollution by Ships
MOU	Memorandum of Unterstanding
OECD	Organisation of Economic Cooperation and Development
OJ / O.J.	Official Journal (of the European Communities)
SAR	International Convention on Maritime Search and Rescue

SOLAS	International Convention on the Safety of Life at Sea
UGS	Union of Greek Shipowners
U.K.	United Kingdom
UN	United Nations
UNCTAD	United Nations Conference on Trade and Development
UNICE	Union des Industries des Communautés Européennes
U.S.A.	United States of America
U.S.S.R.	Union of Soviet Socialist Republics
VTS	Vessel Traffic Management Services

CHAPTER 1

INTRODUCTION

The year 1985 must be considered a turning point for policy making in the European Community (EC) with respect to its maritime sector, since it was then that the Commission submitted to the Council for the first time a comprehensive memorandum and set of proposals for interlinked measures in support of that sector[1]. Following extensive deliberations and bargaining some of these proposals became Community law with the adoption by the Council of a package of four maritime Regulations in December 1986[2].

The present study's prime target is to assess the effects of that package on existing institutional arrangements and policy making concerning maritime activity on various fronts such as the national shipping policies of Member States, the integration of maritime policy at EC level, and international maritime relations. To this purpose the study attempts an interdisciplinary analysis of policy formulation for the shipping sector in the EC taking into account the interaction of play by all key actors, prior to and following the adoption of the 1986 package of Regulations.

This exercise should be of interest to practitioners, researchers and students of the European integration process for a number of reasons: Here we have a sector for which no explicit provisions exist in the Treaty of Rome as far as the development of a common policy and the harmonisation of supply side conditions are concerned. In fact it was only after 1973 that the governments of Member States started adhering to the view that the general provisions of the Treaty do apply in this sector. Hence, it is much more difficult for the key actors in Community policy making, notably the Commission and the governments of Member States, to come to an agreement on what set of elements should constitute EC maritime policy.

Shipping is predominantly an international activity. The merchant fleets of Member States apart from serving domestic or intra-Community

trades are also involved in the carriage of goods
between Member States and third countries, or only
between third countries. Thus, maritime policy
formulation at EC level unavoidably has to take into
account the Community's international economic and
political relations with third countries as well as
those of its individual Member States. It has also
to be consistent with their commitments in the
international maritime order.

Notwithstanding those complexities, policy
formulation in the maritime sector has been trying
to strike the right balance between the interests of
its key actors, shipowners, seafarers and shippers
at a time of a prolonged depression in the
international shipping markets. Hence, the present
analysis can also be viewed as a study of the
initiatives for greater interdependence of activity
in a specific sector within the Community under the
pressure of economic recession.

The analysis examines a number of issues that
characterise maritime policy making such as (a) the
degree of protection afforded by governments on
their national shipping sector vis-a-vis external
competition, (b) the use of government subsidies,
(c) the relative weights given to the interests of
shipowners, and users of shipping services, and (d)
the institutional arrangements concerning the
employment of factors of production, especially
labour, in the production of maritime services.

In relation to these issues the study also
examines the extent to which the Community
involvement with the maritime sector constitutes a
substitute for national policies pursued by
individual Member States, through their
harmonisation.

Given the international character of shipping
activity, the study pays special attention to
international maritime relations and their role in
the formulation of EC maritime policy. It also
assesses the impact of the 1986 package on the
international maritime scene.

For the purpose of obtaining a full insight into
the process of European integration in maritime
transport the study attempts to identify the key

factors involved and assesses their implications in terms of the direction and speed of that process. Such factors include the changing environment for maritime activity both internally within the Community and externally, the activities of interested pressure groups, and the response of the Community institutions as well as of the governments of Member States to those activities.

One point of clarification: for the purposes of the present analysis, shipping is viewed as an activity per se, not linked in anyway to shipbuiling or ports. The latter are considered as distinct sectors from the maritime transport sector, having their own characteristics and being subject to different considerations. Hence, the study concentrates on policy concerning only the maritime transport sector and there are only occasional references to shipbuilding or ports.

ORGANISATION OF THE STUDY

The study begins with an examination of the position of EC shipping in the context of shipping trends worldwide. In particular, it highlights the developments in the shipping capacity of the fleets of EC Member States in comparison to other fleets, the age profile and the role of EC interests in open registry fleets. These are all presented in Chapter 2 which also includes the developments in international seaborne trade. Thus, this Chapter contains the necessary background material for the assessment of maritime policy developments.

Chapter 3 concentrates on the description of the philosophy and key characteristics of national maritime policy in the EC Member States. It examines in detail their position on questions of protectionism afforded to the national shipping industry, employment of seafarers, development of parallel or off-shore registries, international conventions and rules on shipping matters, links of shipping activity with shipbuilding and competition rules.

The study then turns its attention to the course of EC initiatives in the area of shipping prior to the publication of the 1985 Commission Memorandum and proposals for a Common Maritime policy. These initiatives are discussed in Chapter 4.

Chapter 5 presents the 1985 Commission Memorandum and proposals and highlights their salient features.

The response from various interest groups generated by the above common shipping policy proposals of the Commission is analysed in Chapter 6. The groups covered consist of shippers, shipowners and trade unions.

Chapter 7 discusses the positions adopted vis a vis the Commission proposals by the Community institutions. In particular, it analyses the Transport Council deliberations, the Opinion and Report adopted by the Economic and Social Committee and the debate and Resolution adopted by the European Parliament.

The actual package of measures adopted in 1986 as well as the Statements on Community shipping policy by the Council are examined in detail in Chapter 8.

The analysis then proceeds to identify and assess the implications of the package at three levels: (a) the individual EC Member States, (b) the Community as a whole, and (c) at the international level.

The implications for the individual Member States of each of the four Regulations and the package as a whole are discussed in Chapter 9. The emphasis of the discussion is on the likely adjustments that are expected in the Member States maritime policy.

In assessing the implications of the package at Community level Chapter 10 examines in detail its contribution towards the integration of maritime markets, the harmonisation of the EC external maritime relations and its effects on competition policy. The same chapter also identifies points within the package that are likely to cause friction within the Commission itself.

The implications at international level are examined in Chapter 10. The analysis centres upon the key questions whether the package is likely (a) to strain international maritime relations and (b) to lead to a more liberal or protectionist international maritime order.

The analysis in Chapter 9, 10 and 11 takes into account all the relevant information on the way that the four Regulations have been implemented until the time of the completion of the study. Thus, the assessment of the implications reflects actual developments in policy application.

Given that the Council in December 1986 stated that the four Regulations constituted only a first stage in the elaboration of the Community's maritime policy, the present study would not have been complete without an assessment of future trends and prediction of the likely course of future measures. This is done in Chapter 12 as a conclusion to the study. The assessment of future trends is highly conditioned by the experience obtained from the actual application of the four Regulations in the first test cases faced by the Community institutions and the interplay of various pressure groups in lobbying for future measures.

NOTES

1 Commission of the European Communities "Progress Towards a Common Transport Policy: Maritime Transport" Commission Communication and Proposals to the Council Transmitted on the 19th March 1985. Bulletin of the European Communities. Supplement 5/85, and O.J. No C212 of 23rd August 1985, pp. 2-21 (proposals only).

2 Regulations 4055/86, 4056/86, 4057/86, and 4058/86. O.J. No L378 of 31st December 1986.

CHAPTER 2

THE EC MARITIME INDUSTRY IN THE CONTEXT OF WORLD SHIPPING TRENDS

THE FORTUNES OF EC AND WORLD SHIPPING

The joint Community action in the maritime field in the form of the package of the December 1986 regulations would not have materialised but for the prolonged crisis in international shipping and the relative decline in the total capacity of the fleet under Community flags. The institutional pressures concerning the application of the EC common rules to shipping would not have been sufficient (as the preceding decades' experience has demonstrated) to produce the package of concrete measures represented by the December 1986 regulations.

The decline in the relative overall position of the EC fleets vis a vis other principal world fleets between 1970 and 1987 can be traced on Tables 2.1 and 2.2.

Table 2.1 presents capacity in each fleet in terms of number of ships and Table 2.2 in terms of tonnage (gross registered tonnes).

Countries have been classified into groups as follows:

■ EC: All the 11 member states excluding Luxembourg which has no national flag fleet.
■ OECD: The above 11 EC member states as well as Australia, Austria, Canada, Finland, Iceland, Japan, New Zealand, Norway, Sweden, Switzerland, Turkey, and U.S.A.
■ COMECON: Albania, Bulgaria, Cuba, Czechoslovakia, German Democratic Republic, Hungary, Poland, Romania, U.S.S.R., Vietnam.
■ Far East: Taiwan, People's Republic of China, Hong-Kong, South Korea.
■ Open Registries: Bahamas, Bermuda, Cyprus, Liberia, Panama, Somali Republic.

Table 2.3 expresses the figures on Table 2.1 in percentage terms taking 1970 as the base year.

The figures in both tables reveal that until
1980 there had been considerable growth in shipping
capacity in all the principal fleets.

Growth in terms of tonnage was more pronounced
than in terms of number of ships showing that, on
average, ship sizes had increased. This may be
attributed to technological change which offers
possibilities of economies of scale in ship
operation.

The total size of the combined EC fleets grew by
a much smaller percentage than the corresponding
size of the world total would or the other principal
fleets, indicating that the decline in the relative
position of the EC fleet had started long before the
recent crisis.

The most impressive growth rates had been
experienced by the fleets of the Far Eastern and the
open registry countries, as well as those in the
"Rest of the World" whilst the Comecon fleets had
grown by less than the world total.

These trends imply a significant improvement in
the competitive advantage enjoyed in operating ships
under Far Eastern and open registry flags.[1] On the
other hand, the slower rates of growth in the
Comecon fleets might be due to resource constraints.

One reason for these different rates of growth
must undoubtedly have been the ability to employ
factors of production at a significantly lower cost
as well as more efficiently.

Another important factor must have been the
resort to protectionism by various countries in
favour of their national flag ships. Protectionism
involves both acts of cargo reservation and flag
discrimination as well as granting various subsidies
from the public purse to ship operators.[2]

It is worth noting in this respect that all the
principal fleets experienced significant growth
between 1975 and 1980 in spite of the world economic
recession brought about by the first oil shock of
1973, and its negative effects on the volume of
seaborne trade.

This phenomenon must be attributed to the "income effects" resulting from the various instruments used by governments to protect their national shipping industry.[3] Because of cargo reservation and subsidies the national shipowner operates on a higher production function than would be justified by the state of the freight and factor markets, by purchasing new tonnage, replacing his existing one with more productive units, or by refraining from disinvestment.

The above phenomenon is also due to "substitution effects" of capital for labour resulting from subsidies, such as accelerated depreciation allowances, investment grants and tax free reserves, because these subsidies change the relative prices of these factors in favour of capital.

Similar substitution effects must have also resulted from the soft loans granted by shipyards to their prospective customers for new buildings. These were made possible by the desire of many governments to either develop or preserve a substantial national shipbuilding capacity.

The development of world seaborne trade in the 70's and 80's in terms of various categories of cargo can be seen on Table 2.4. It will be noted that there was a drop in the volume of crude oil transported by sea in 1974 and 1975 in comparison to 1973 and in the volume of oil products in 1974, 1975 and 1976. Similarly, the volume of iron ore, which is used in the steel industry was below the 1973 level for five consecutive years.

It will be seen from the same table that the effects of the second oil crisis on seaborne trade were more pronounced. From 1980 onwards its total volume has been continuously below the 1979 level.

The demand for shipping capacity is not, however, only a function of the volume of trade but also of the average haul per voyage.

Considerable changes have taken place during the last decade in the geographical patterns of trade (eg. the discovery of new oil reserves in the North Sea and Mexico which are close to key consumption

areas) which have resulted in a substantial decrease
in average haul per voyage.

These developments are reflected on Table 2.5
where the effective demand for shipping capacity is
measured in terms of tonne-miles.

It is clear from that table that the decrease in
total effective demand for shipping capacity since
1979 had been more pronounced than implied by the
figures in the previous table.

On the other hand, the supply of total world
shipping capacity, as seen from the figures on
Tables 2.1, 2.2 and 2.3, did not adjust to the falls
in effective demand. A more clear picture
concerning the imbalance between total world supply
and demand for shipping capacity is presented on
Table 2.6. Figures on total world tonnage available
and tonne-miles have been translated into index form
taking 1976 as a base year, separately for liquid
and dry cargoes.

It is worth noting that in the liquid bulk
trades both the capacity of the relevant fleet and
effective demand (in tonne-miles) decreased between
1976 and 1987. However, the decrease in effective
demand was much more substantial (standing in 1987
at nearly a half of its 1976 level) than the
decrease in capacity.

On the other hand, both effective demand and
capacity in the dry bulk trades experienced a
significant increase but the increase in capacity
outstripped the corresponding increase in demand.

The effects of the imbalance between supply and
demand on the freight markets for shipping are
reflected on representative freight rate figures for
key bulk commodities, presented on Table 2.7. These
figures are also presented on Table 2.8 in index
form taking 1976 as the base year, so as to
demonstrate more clearly the trends in gross
earnings of shipping companies. That same table
presents also in index form the price deflator of
GDP in the EC 10 countries (excluding Spain and
Portugal) as well as the LIBOR for three month
deposits in U.S. dollars. These variables are

intended to demonstrate as proxies trends in operating costs and the cost of capital.

On the basis of the figures on Tables 2.7 and 2.8 it can safely be inferred that the cash flow position of shipping companies world-wide must have been under considerable strain during the last years.

However, turning back to Tables 2.1, 2.2 and 2.3 it becomes clear that the strain on the cash flow position of shipping companies has not resulted in a uniform downward adjustment of shipping capacity world wide.

In fact since 1980 there has been a very clear divergence in the fortunes among various principal fleets: The total EC (11) fleet has declined sharply both in terms of number of ships and tonnage. A small decrease in capacity has also been experienced in the Comecon fleets. At the same time the total world tonnage has decreased but the number of ships has increased.

On the other hand, the fleets of the Far East, the open registries and the rest of the world have continued on the growth path, in spite of the recession following the second oil shock.

This clear divergence in the fortunes of the various fleets following the second oil crisis in 1979 must be attributed to the fact that the prolonged depression in the freight markets accentuates the impact of protectionism and subsidies, the accessibility to factors of production at a lower cost and the efficiency of operations on the ability of shipowners to compete for cargoes.

The same remark can be made about the fortunes of the individual national fleets within the EC which have not moved in a uniform way. Eg. the Belgian fleet is still bigger than its 1975 level both in terms of tonnage and number of ships. The Greek fleet remained bigger in terms of tonnage compared to its 1975 level but smaller in terms of number of ships.

Overall it can be observed that the relative decline in the size of the EC fleets has been bigger in terms of number of ships rather than tonnage. Thus there has been a trend towards exploiting economies of scale which must have resulted in a proportionately bigger decrease in the number of seafarers employed than the decrease in capacity.

DEFINITION OF THE SHIPPING INDUSTRY

When examining the maritime industry it is immediately realised that this term covers a number of diverse activities which are only linked together by a common characteristic, i.e. the carriage of goods and passengers by vessels over the surface of water. As seen from the angle of the EC maritime policy formulation, and in particular Article 84 of the Treaty of Rome our analysis concentrates on "the business of transporting goods and persons in ships from a dockside point across the sea for commercial return".[4]

Thus, it excludes the operation of vessels in inland waterways, the fishing industry, research vessels, etc. Furthermore, our analysis does not extend to the shipbuilding and shiprepair industries per se which are really part of the manufacturing sector. However, the interaction of shipping and shipbuilding policies will be examined later on, since in many instances these overlap considerably.

One way of classifying the diverse shipping activities into more homogeneous sub-sectors is to use the criterion of the type of good or passenger being transported. The main entities that can be distinguished according to this criterion are as follows:

(a) The transportation of cargoes in bulk form which usually represent raw materials to be used in various manufacturing processes. These cargoes can further be subdivided into

(i)   liquid bulks, consisting mostly of oil and oil products, and

(ii) dry bulks, eg. iron ore, grain, coal, etc.

(b) The carriage of general cargo, which mostly consists of finished manufactured products.

(c) The transportation of containers.

(d) The carriage of passengers by sea, and

(e) The production of tourist services on board ships, i.e. cruising services.

A second criterion for classifying shipping activities concerns the regularity of service offered, i.e. whether the ship involved operates in the liner, or tramp trades.

In the liner trades the ships are operated by companies which provide regular, scheduled, services to shippers or forwarders between specific ports. A key feature in the liner trades is the organisation of shipping companies into conferences ostensibly for the purpose of rationalising services and capacity utilisation.[5]

Tramp vessel services on the other hand involve "any transport of cargo in ships which are hired wholly or partly for the carriage of cargoes on the basis of a voyage or time charter or any other form of contract against rates of freight which are established in free competition in accordance with conditions of supply and demand".[6]

A third criterion classifies shipping activity according to whether the cargoes carried are related to the economy of the country where the ship is registered or not. Three main classes can be distinguished here: (a) coastal trades within one country, (b) trades between the country of registration and another country (bilateral trades), and (c) trades between third countries (cross-trading).

The above distinctions should be borne in mind when analysing shipping policy priorities in each country, since they explain to a large extent the position enjoyed by each specific maritime sector in its respective national economy.

The structure of the combined fleets of the EC Member States as well as of other major world

groupings of fleets in terms of the type of goods or
passenger being transported as it has changed since
1970 can be seen on Table 2.9. In particular that
table presents total tonnage in grt under each
category of ship for each country or groups of
countries for the years 1970 and 1987. The relevant
figures for each category are also expressed in
percentages in terms of the total tonnage under the
particular flag.

It will be noted that in addition to the major
world groupings of fleets, table 2.9 presents
separately the fleet of Greece since the latter
differs significantly in structure from the other EC
fleets, with a heavy emphasis on bulk carriers, and
is by far the largest fleet.

In fact whilst the percentage in bulk carriers
in the total EC fleet was in 1987 well below the
corresponding percentage in the total world fleet,
in the Greek fleet was much higher.

The first point to note is that in line with the
trends in international trade there has been a
significant change in the structure of the major
fleets between 1970 and 1987. Tanker and general
cargo fleets represent in terms of tonnage a much
smaller percentage of the total shipping capacity.

However, the degree of that decrease is not
uniform in all fleets. Eg. in Greece the percentage
of total tonnage in tankers has remained the same
whilst its general cargo fleet represented in 1987
only 11% of the total fleet as opposed to 42% in
1970.

Significant decreases in the proportionate
contribution to total shipping capacity of the
tanker sector were experienced in the Comecon and
Far Eastern fleets. A decrease in corresponding
percentage took also place in the open registry
fleets. Nevertheless, that percentage remains the
highest among these fleets.

An important development over that period
concerns the role of container ships, which are
normally employed in the liner trades. Between 1970
and 1987 the role of that type of ship has been
enhanced so as to represent 9.5% of total EC and

5.6% of the total world shipping capacity. This is
the result of technological change leading to
widespread containerisation of the carriage of many
goods (mostly finished manufactured ones) which were
formerly carried in general cargo ships.

The switch to containerisation requires a much
higher capital investment both with respect to the
type of vessel to be used and the port
installations. A prerequisite for such an
investment would in turn be a low degree of
uncertainty concerning the demand of shipping
services and accessibility to the relevant markets,
which in this case are those of the conference
dominated liner trades. In those trades access to
cargoes can be obtained either through the ability
to participate in a closed conference system or
through cargo reservation practices.

In the case of the EC, liner trades are
dominated by the closed conference system which
means that entry into it is restricted to those
shipping companies that existing member companies
wish to co-operate with. This system, which creates
a cartel in shipping services has developed with the
aim of preventing instability in the liner shipping
markets at the expense of free competition. The
fact that many governments of EC member states
either tolerate or support must be attributed to a
strong wish on their part to have stability in the
shipping trades serving the export markets for their
manufactured goods.

It should also be remembered that traditional
liner companies serving Western Europe developed
originally to serve trade between their national
countries and its colonies. These strong trade ties
persist even today and are mirrored into bilateral
shipping agreements involving cargo sharing.[7]

It comes as no surprise, therefore, that the
highest percentage in container ships of total fleet
capacity is to be found among the combined EC fleet.
It will be noted, however, that the Greek merchant
fleet is an exception to this phenomenon, since its
proportion in container ships is insignificant.

The Greek fleet, which represents approximately
a third of total EC capacity, is primarily oriented

towards the carriage of raw materials in bulk form, both liquid and dry.

The volume of cargoes involved in Greece's external trade is very small compared to its fleets capacity and the latter serves cross-trades between third countries

AGE PROFILE

The prolonged shipping crisis and the resulting negative pressures on the cash flow position of shipping companies, referred to above, have discouraged investment activity in new ships.

Thus, whilst the total number of ships on order worldwide stood in September 1982 at 2428 representing approximately 60 million dwt, in September 1987 that number stood at only 846 ships corresponding to 33 million dwt.

As a consequence there has been a marked deterioration of the age profile of most merchant fleets in the world, as described by the frequency distributions according to age, either by tonnage or by number of ships. These distributions for the years 1982, 1986 and 1987 are presented for the EC and other major merchant fleets respectively on Tables 2.10 and 2.11.

As it can be seen from these tables there has been a significant decrease in most fleets of the percentage of total tonnage or the total number of ships under 10 years of age.

This decrease appears to be more pronounced among EC fleets, with the exceptions of Germany, Greece and the Netherlands, compared to most other fleets.

Given that the age of a ship and the embodiment of technological advances in it are closely linked, it can be inferred that the aging of most Community fleets represents in general a deterioration in their technical efficiency. This should in turn have affected adversely the cost effectiveness of those fleets.

   This development would seem to reinforce the
pressure for concerted Community action in the
maritime field and especially the call for positive
measures to improve the competitiveness of the EC
merchant fleets, as a follow-up to the 1986
regulations.[8]

Table 2.1

Principal Merchant Fleets of the World by

Number of Ships

	1970		1975		1980		1986		1987	
	No of ships	% of world total	No of ships	% of world total	No of ships	% of world total	No of ships	% of world total	No of ships	% of world total
Belgium	230	0.4	252	0.4	290	0.4	355	0.5	350	0.5
Denmark	1,210	2.3	1,371	2.15	1,253	1.7	1,063	1.4	1,256	1.6
France	1,420	2.7	1,393	2.2	1,241	1.7	984	1.3	954	1.3
FRG	2,868	5.5	1,964	3	1,906	2.6	1,752	2.3	1,414	1.9
Greece	1,850	3.5	2,743	4.3	3,922	5.3	2,255	3.0	1,948	2.6
Irish Republic	86	0.2	93	0.1	141	0.2	154	0.2	153	0.2
Italy	1,639	3.1	1,732	2.7	1,739	2.3	1,569	2.1	1,571	2.1
Netherlands	1,598	3	1,348	2.1	1,263	1.7	1,334	1.8	1,307	1.7
United Kingdom	3,822	7.3	3,622	5.7	3,181	4.3	2,256	3.0	2,165	2.9
Portugal	376	0.7	440	0.7	350	0.5	355	0.5	292	0.4
Spain	2,234	4.2	2,667	4.2	2,767	3.7	2,397	3.2	2,350	3.1
EC 11	17,333	33	17,625	27.6	18,053	24.4	14,474	19.3	13,760	18.3
Other OECD	17,946	34.2	20,739	32.5	22,594	30.6	23,264	30.9	22,984	30.5
Total OECD	35,279	67.3	38,364	60.2	40,647	55	37,738	50.2	36,744	48.8
Comecon	7,116	13.5	9,135	14.3	10,142	13.7	8,721	11.6	9,074	12
Far East	967	1.8	1,826	2.9	3,065	4.15	4,402	5.8	4,675	6.2
Open Registries	3,233	6.2	6,124	9.6	7,406	10	8,322	11.1	8,740	11.6
Rest of the World	5,849	11.15	8,275	13	12,572	17	16,083	21.4	16,007	21.3
World Total	52,444	100	63,724	100	73,832	100	75,266	100	75,240	100

Source: Lloyd's Register of Shipping, Statistical Tables

Table 2.2
Principal Merchant Fleets of the World by Tonnage (GRT)

	1970 Tonnage	1970 % of world total	1975 Tonnage	1975 % of world total	1980 Tonnage	1980 % of world total	1986 Tonnage	1986 % of world total	1987 Tonnage	1987 % of world total
Belgium	1,062,152	0.46	1,358,425	0.4	1,809,829	0.4	2,419,661	0.6	2,268,383	0.5
Denmark	3,314,320	1.45	4,478,112	1.3	5,390,365	1.3	4,651,224	1.1	4,873,465	1.2
France	6,457,900	2.8	10,745,999	3.1	11,924,557	2.8	5,936,268	1.5	5,371,273	1.3
FRG	7,881,000	3.5	8,516,567	2.5	8,355,638	1.9	5,565,214	1.4	4,317,616	1.1
Greece	10,951,993	4.8	22,527,156	6.6	39,471,744	9.4	28,390,800	7.0	23,559,852	5.8
Irish Republic	174,977	0.08	210,389	0.06	208,986	0.05	149,308	0.03	153,637	0.04
Italy	7,447,610	3.3	10,136,989	3	11,095,694	2.6	7,896,569	1.9	7,817,353	1.9
Netherlands	5,206,663	2.3	5,679,413	1.6	5,723,845	1.4	4,324,135	1.1	3,908,231	1.1
United Kingdom	25,824,820	11.3	33,157,422	9.7	27,135,155	6.5	11,567,117	2.8	8,504,605	2.1
Portugal	870,008	0.38	1,209,701	0.35	1,355,989	0.3	1,114,444	0.3	1,048,197	0.3
Spain	3,440,952	1.5	5,433,354	1.6	8,112,245	1.9	5,422,002	1.3	4,949,387	1.2
EC 11	72,632,395	31.9	103,453,527	30.23	120,584,047	28.7	77,436,747	19.1	66,771,999	16.5
Other OECD	75,813,484	34	95,319,081	28.4	95,324,387	23.3	84,456,264	20.8	78,794,190	19.5
Total OECD	148,445,872	65.9	198,772,608	58.6	215,908,434	52	161,893,011	39.9	145,566,189	36.1
Comecon	18,604,643	8.18	25,378,328	7.4	31,990,937	7.6	35,233,053	8.7	36,627,858	9.1
Far East	3,554,661	1.6	6,320,291	1.8	14,974,075	3.6	31,194,056	7.7	32,102,964	7.9
Open Registries	41,409,494	18.2	86,162,197	25.2	108,423,500	25.8	111,945,221	27.6	121,905,415	30.2
Rest of the World	15,475,187	6.1	25,528,939	6.9	48,613,705	11	64,644,926	15.9	67,295,696	16.7
World Total	227,489,864	100	342,162,363	100	419,910,651	100	404,910,267	100	403,498,122	100

Source: Lloyd's Register of Shipping, Statistical Tables

Table 2.3
Index of Size of Merchant Fleets (1970=100)

	1970		1975		1980		1986		1987	
	In No of ships	In ton-nage	In No of ships	In ton-nage	In No of ships	In ton-nage	In No of ships	In ton-nage	In No of ships	In ton-nage
Belgium	100	100	109.5	128	126	170	154	228	152.2	213.6
Denmark	100	100	113.3	135	104	163	88	140	103.8	147
France	100	100	98	166	87	185	69	92	67.2	83.2
FRG	100	100	68	109	103	106	61	71	49.3	54.8
Greece	100	100	148.3	205	212	360	122	259	105.3	215.1
Irish Republic	100	100	108.1	120	164	119	179	85	177.9	87.8
Italy	100	100	105.7	136	106	149	96	106	95.8	105
Netherlands	100	100	84.3	109	79	109	83	83	81.8	75.1
United Kingdom	100	100	94.8	128	89	105	59	45	56.6	32.9
Portugal	100	100	117	139	93	156	94	128	77.7	120.5
Spain	100	100	119.4	158	124	236	107	158	105.2	143.8
EC 11	100	100	100.6	142.5	103	166.1	84	107	79.4	91.9
Other OECD	100	100	115.5	125.7	125.9	125.7	130	111	128.1	103.9
Total OECD	100	100	108.7	133.9	115.2	145.4	107	109	104.1	98
Comecon	100	100	108	138.8	115.45	145.6	123	189	127.5	196.9
Far East	100	100	188.8	177.8	316.9	421.2	455	877	483.4	903.1
Open Registries	100	100	189.4	208.1	229	261.8	275	270	270.3	294.3
Rest of the World	100	100	141.5	165	214.9	314.1	275	418	273.7	434.9
World Total	100	100	121.5	150.4	140.8	184.6	144	178	143.5	177.4

Table 2.4

Development of World International Seaborne Trade
Figures in million metric tons (tonnes)

Years	Crude Oil	Oil Pro-ducts	Iron Ore	Coal	Grain	Other Cargo Estim.	Total Trade Estim.
1970	996	245	247	101	89	804	2482
1971	1070	247	250	94	91	825	2577
1972	1185	261	247	96	108	866	2763
1973	1366	274	298	104	139	940	3121
1974	1361	264	329	119	130	1045	3248
1975	1263	233	292	127	137	995	3047
1976	1410	260	294	127	146	1075	3312
1977	1451	273	276	132	147	1120	3399
1978	1432	270	278	127	169	1190	3466
1979	1497	279	327	159	182	1270	3714
1980	1320	276	314	188	198	1310	3606
1981	1170	267	303	210	206	1305	3461
1982	993	285	273	208	200	1240	3199
1983	930	282	257	197	199	1225	3090
1984	950	297	306	232	207	1320	3312
1985	871	288	321	272	181	1360	3293
1986	958	305	311	276	165	1370	3385
1987	963	302	309	272	182	1390	3418

Source: Fearnley's Review 1987

Table 2.5

International Seaborne Trade in Tonne-Miles
Figures in thousand million

Years	Crude Oil	Oil Pro- ducts	Iron Ore	Coal	Grain	Other Cargo Estim.	Total Trade Estim.
1970	5598	890	1093	481	475	2118	10655
1971	6555	900	1185	434	487	2169	11730
1972	7720	930	1156	444	548	2306	13104
1973	9207	1010	1398	467	760	2562	15404
1974	9661	960	1578	558	695	2935	16387
1975	8885	845	1471	621	734	2810	15366
1976	10199	950	1469	591	779	3035	17023
1977	10408	995	1386	643	801	3220	17453
1978	9561	985	1384	604	945	3455	16934
1979	9452	1045	1599	786	1026	3605	17513
1980	8219	1020	1613	952	1087	3720	16611
1981	7193	1000	1508	1120	1131	3710	15662
1982	5212	1070	1443	1094	1120	3560	13499
1983	4478	1080	1320	1057	1135	3510	12580
1984	4450	1140	1631	1270	1157	3720	13368
1985	4007	1150	1675	1479	1004	3750	13065
1986	4640	1265	1671	1586	914	3780	13856
1987	4610	1295	1650	1567	1002	3840	13964

Source: Fearnley's Review 1987

Table 2.6
Development of the Volume of Seaborne Trade in Index Form

Year	Volume of Trade in Crude Oil & Oil Products	Capacity of World Tanker Fleet	Volume of Trade in Iron Ore, Coal and Grain	Capacity of World Dry Bulk Fleet
1976	100	100	100	100
1977	101	104	100	110
1978	94	105	103	116
1979	94	106	120	118
1980	83	107	129	119
1981	73	105	132	123
1982	56	103	129	130
1983	50	98	124	136
1984	50	93	143	140
1985	46	88	146	146
1986	54	82	139	145
1987	53	81	145	143

Source: Fearnley's Review

Table 2.7

Highest and Lowest Rates Recorded in Three Representative Dry Bulk Trades

Year	Grain US Gulf-Antwerp/ Rotterdam		Coal Hampton Roads- Japan		Iron Ore Brazil- N.W.Europe		LIBOR %
	High	Low	High	Low	High	Low	
1976	8.50	4.00	8.00	5.50	5.00	3.15	5.58
1977	7.00	3.95	7.45	6.25	4.25	3.35	6.00
1978	10.85	4.75	11.00	5.30	3.85	3.10	8.85
1979	19.00	7.50	20.00	8.25	14.50	6.50	12.09
1980	24.15	14.25	29.00	15.50	13.00	9.50	14.19
1981	22.00	8.75	28.50	17.50	15.00	7.00	16.87
1982	12.00	5.75	19.60	10.80	7.00	4.45	13.29
1983	9.00	7.00	17.50	12.35	6.50	5.95	9.72
1984	10.75	7.75	11.25	9.50	5.60	5.50	10.94
1985	11.59	5.65	10.95	8.575	6.05	3.62	8.40
1986	8.25	4.50	9.00	6.00	4.50	2.70	7.40
1987	10.25	7.00	10.10	6.95	7.25	3.00	

Table 2.8

Indices (1976=100) of Freight Rates, Cost of Capital and Inflation in the EC (10)

Year	Grain US Gulf-Antwerp/ Rotterdam		Coal Hampton Roads- Japan		Iron Ore Brazil- N.W.Europe		LIBOR %	Price Deflation of GDP
	High	Low	High	Low	High	Low		
1976	100	100	100	100	100	100	100	100
1977	82	99	93	114	85	106	108	110
1978	128	119	138	96	77	98	159	119
1979	224	188	250	150	290	206	217	130
1980	284	356	363	282	260	302	254	144
1981	259	219	356	318	300	222	302	157
1982	141	144	245	196	140	141	238	171
1983	106	175	219	225	130	189	174	182
1984	126	194	141	173	112	175	196	191
1985	136	141	137	156	121	115	151	202
1986	97	113	113	109	90	86	133	210
1987	97	112.5	112.5	109	90	86		

Table 2.9

Distribution of Major Fleets by Type of Vessel

Source: Lloyds Register of Shipping: Statistical Tables

	GREECE				EEC 11				O.E.C.D.			
	1970		1987		1970		1987		1970		1987	
	Tonnage 000 GRT	%	Tonnage 000 GRT	%	Tonnage 000 GRT	%	Tonnage 000 GRT	%	Tonnage 000 GRT	%	Tonnage 000 GRT	%
Oil Tankers	3,872	36.4	9,247	39.5	29,050	42.4	23,298	36.9	54,724	37.2	47,346	34.6
Ltg.Gas Carriers	8	0.07	63	0.3	417	0.6	1,136	1.8	1,050	0.7	4,690	3.4
Chemical Tankers	–		3	0.01	136	0.2	488	0.8	399	0.3	1,051	0.8
Other Tankers	–		22	0.09	–		81	0.1	–		161	0.1
Total Tankers	3,880	36.5	9,335	39.9	29,603	43.2	25,004	39.6	56,173	38.2	53,248	38.9
Bulk/Oil Carriers	152	1.4	1,016	4.3	1,183	1.7	2,941	4.7	5,296	3.6	5,478	4.0
Ore/Bulk Carriers	2,032	19.1	9,540	40.8	10,774	15.7	16,426	26	26,997	18.3	35,831	26.2
Total Bulk Carriers	2,184	20.5	10,557	45.1	11,957	17.5	19,367	30.7	32,293	21.9	41,309	30.2
General Cargo	4,451	41.8	2,755	11.8	24,330	35.5	9,744	15.5	54,256	36.9	22,443	16.4
Container Ships	–		169	0.7	601	0.9	5,997	9.5	1,889	1.3	11,708	8.5
Ferries, Passenger & Other Types	123	1.2	585	2.5	1,990	2.9	2,991	4.7	2,455	1.7	8,033	5.9
Total Gen.Cargo & Other Types	4,574	43.0	3,509	15	26,921	39.3	18,732	29.7	58,600	39.9	42,184	30.8
Total All Types	10,638		23,401		68,480		63,103		147,066		136,741	

Table 2.9 Continued

	COMECON				FAR EAST			
	1970		1987		1970		1987	
	Tonnage 000 GRT	%	Tonnage 000 GRT	%	Tonnage 000 GRT	%	Tonnage 000 GRT	%
Oil Tankers	3,936	30.2	5,493	20.1	727	21.2	4,344	14
Liq.Gas Carriers	7	0.05	202	0.7	-		239	0.8
Chemical Tankers	1	0.01	15	0.06	3	0.1	104	0.3
Other Tankers			15	0.05	-		19	0.06
Total Tankers	3,944	30.3	5,725	20.9	730	21.3	4,705	15.2
Bulk/Oil Carriers	49	0.4	767	2.8	-	-	2,201	7.1
Ore/Bulk Carriers	902	6.9	7,042	25.7	530	15.5	13,922	45.0
Total Bulk Carriers	951	7.3	7,809	28.5	530	15.5	16,123	52.1
General Cargo	7,918	60.8	12,141	44.3	2,150	62.8	6,790	21.9
Container Ships	-		806	2.9	-	-	2,696	8.7
Ferries, Passenger & Other Types	203	1.6	898	3.3	10	0.3	614	2.0
Total Gen.Cargo & Other Types	8,121	62.4	13,845	50.5	2,160	63.1	10,100	32.6
Total All Types	13,016		27,379		3,420		30,928	

Source: Lloyds Register of Shipping: Statistical Tables

Table 2.9 Continued

	OPEN REGISTRIES				WORLD			
	1970		1987		1970		1987	
	Tonnage 000 GRT	%	Tonnage 000 GRT	%	Tonnage 000 GRT	%	Tonnage 000 GRT	%
Oil Tankers	23,414	57	49,700	41.3	86,140	40.6	127.660	33.7
Liq.Gas Carriers	248	0.6	2,554	2.1	1,350	0.6	9,784	2.6
Chemical Tankers	33	0.08	1,666	1.4	451	0.2	3,465	0.9
Other Tankers	-	-	26	0.02	-	0.1	251	0.07
Total Tankers	23,695	57.7	53,946	44.8	87,940	41.4	141,159	37.2
Bulk/Oil Carriers	2,658	6.5	8,828	7.3	8,317	3.7	20,471	5.4
Ore/Bulk Carriers	8,195	19.9	35,226	29.2	38,334	18.1	110,557	29.1
Total Bulk Carriers	10,853	26.4	44,054	36.5	46,652	22.0	131,028	34.5
General Cargo	6,319	15.4	15,349	12.7	72,396	34.2	71,629	18.9
Container Ships	19	0.04	3,704	3.1	1,908	0.9	21,089	5.6
Ferries, Passenger & Other Types	212	0.5	3,431	2.8	2,991	1.4	14,248	3.7
Total Gen.Cargo & Other Types	6,550	15.9	22,484	18.6	77,295	36.5	106,966	28.2
Total All Types	41,098		120,484		211,887		379,153	

Source: Lloyds Register of Shipping: Statistical Tables

Table 2.10
Age Distribution of Principal Fleet by Tonnage

EEC Countries	UNDER 5 YEARS 1982	1986	1987	5-10 YEARS 1982	1986	1987	10-15 YEARS 1982	1986	1987	15-20 YEARS 1982	1986	1987	20+ 1982	1986	1987	UNDER 10 YEARS 1982	1986	1987	CHANGE IN PERCENTAGE 1987/1982	1986/1982
BELGIUM	44	42	NA	35	39	NA	9	14	NA	10	3	NA	2	2	NA	79	81	NA	NA	2
DENMARK	22	28	28	60	26	19	11	36	41	4	6	6	3	4	6	82	54	47	-35	-28
FRANCE	10	17	14	65	23	18	19	52	59	3	4	5	3	4	4	75	40	32	-43	-35
FRG	23	36	NA	46	31	NA	20	18	NA	8	10	NA	3	5	NA	69	67	NA	NA	- 2
GREECE	7	11	13	21	21	15	29	38	41	25	19	19	18	11	12	28	32	28	0	4
HOLLAND	20	35	NA	33	29	NA	25	23	NA	12	6	NA	10	7	NA	53	64	NA	NA	11
IRELAND	22	12	NA	61	44	NA	9	24	NA	3	8	NA	5	12	NA	83	56	NA	NA	-27
ITALY	12	6	7	40	19	14	16	38	43	15	19	18	17	18	18	52	25	21	-31	-27
PORTUGAL	14	22	NA	39	2	NA	23	37	NA	10	23	NA	14	16	NA	53	24	NA	NA	-29
SPAIN	23	12	NA	47	32	NA	20	38	NA	5	11	NA	5	7	NA	70	44	NA	NA	-26
UNIT. KINGDOM	16	13	10	49	27	26	22	39	36	8	12	15	5	9	13	65	40	36	-29	-25

NON EEC Countries	UNDER 5 YEARS 1982	1986	1987	5-10 YEARS 1982	1986	1987	10-15 YEARS 1982	1986	1987	15-20 YEARS 1982	1986	1987	20+ 1982	1986	1987	UNDER 10 YEARS 1982	1986	1987	CHANGE IN PERCENTAGE 1987/1982	1986/1982
BAHAMAS	NA	10	10	NA	27	23	NA	48	53	NA	13	10	NA	2	4	NA	37	33	NA	NA
BRAZIL	43	22	19	31	40	40	15	25	26	3	6	8	8	7	7	74	62	59	-15	-12
CHINA	12	18	16	20	14	14	17	22	23	25	16	17	26	30	30	32	32	30	- 2	0
TAIWAN	33	32	36	6	25	23	41	18	12	10	24	27	10	1	2	39	57	59	20	18
CYPRUS	7	3	4	5	10	9	29	44	42	21	33	37	38	10	8	12	13	13	1	1
HONG-KONG	42	38	25	28	22	29	20	33	34	7	6	11	3	1	1	70	60	54	-16	-10
INDIA	15	20	24	41	17	16	18	39	38	18	15	12	8	9	10	56	37	40	-16	-19
JAPAN	26	31	34	39	24	27	30	35	27	4	9	10	1	1	2	65	55	61	- 4	-10
S. KOREA	17	19	24	24	15	14	37	34	29	14	25	24	8	7	9	41	34	38	- 3	- 7
LIBERIA	12	13	14	52	22	16	24	52	53	9	12	14	3	1	3	64	35	30	-34	-29
N. ZEALAND	21	11	NA	52	40	NA	10	35	NA	7	6	NA	10	8	NA	73	51	NA	NA	-22
NORWAY	18	24	23	55	29	25	23	35	36	2	7	10	2	5	6	73	53	48	-25	-20
PANAMA	14	30	31	28	17	17	21	29	30	16	14	14	21	10	8	42	47	48	6	5
PHILIPPINES	9	34	32	24	13	19	33	26	25	15	21	17	19	6	7	33	47	51	18	14
SINGAPORE	22	22	20	40	25	21	17	42	45	8	9	12	13	2	2	62	47	41	-21	-15
SWEDEN	30	33	NA	49	34	NA	13	19	NA	5	10	NA	3	4	NA	79	67	NA	NA	-12
TURKEY	7	7	NA	25	15	NA	33	41	NA	18	23	NA	17	14	NA	32	22	NA	NA	-10
U.S.S.R.	16	15	14	21	20	20	21	20	21	26	21	19	16	24	26	37	35	34	- 3	- 2
U.S.A.	20	11	13	22	27	23	13	20	23	7	10	12	38	32	29	42	38	36	- 6	- 4

Source: Lloyd's Register of Shipping: Statistical Tables

CHAPTER 2

Table 2.11
Age Distribution of Principal Fleet by Number of Ships

EEC Countries	UNDER 5 YEARS			5-10 YEARS			10-15 YEARS			15-20 YEARS			20+			UNDER 10 YEARS			CHANGE IN PERCENTAGE	
	1982	1986	1987	1982	1986	1987	1982	1986	1987	1982	1986	1987	1982	1986	1987	1982	1986	1987	1987/1982	1986/1982
BELGIUM	21	21	NA	22	20	NA	16	15	NA	14	12	NA	27	32	NA	43.4	41	NA	NA	- 2.39
DENMARK	13	16	16	30	15	13	16	21	13	15	17	15	26	31	34	43	31	29	-14	-12
FRANCE	11	11	11	25	15	14	17	26	24	12	12	13	30	36	38	34	26	25	- 9	- 8
FRG	21	24	NA	21	22	NA	19	12	NA	16	12	NA	23	30	NA	42	46	NA	NA	4
GREECE	11	11	8	13	27	10	21	38	21	18	19	18	42	11	43	19	32	18	- 1	13
HOLLAND	26	24	NA	28	27	NA	19	22	NA	14	12	NA	13	15	NA	54	51	NA	NA	- 3
IRELAND	NA	NA	NA	NA	13	NA	NA	NA	NA	16	NA	NA	NA	NA	NA	NA	20	NA	NA	NA
ITALY	10	7	7	13	13	14	18	19	43	16	20	18	43	41	18	23	20	21	- 2	- 3
PORTUGAL	11	NA	NA	11	NA	NA	21	NA	NA	21	NA	NA	36	37	NA	22	NA	NA	NA	NA
SPAIN	12	7	6	27	14	12	17	25	25	18	17	15	26	37	42	39	21	NA	NA	-18
UNIT. KINGDOM	13	11	10	24	15	15	18	20	19	15	16	16	30	38	40	37	26	25	12	11

NON EEC Countries	UNDER 5 YEARS			5-10 YEARS			10-15 YEARS			15-20 YEARS			20+			UNDER 10 YEARS			CHANGE IN PERCENTAGE	
	1982	1986	1987	1982	1986	1987	1982	1986	1987	1982	1986	1987	1982	1986	1987	1982	1986	1987	1987/1982	1986/1982
BAHAMAS	NA	14	12	NA	23	27	NA	28	32	NA	15	15	NA	20	14	NA	37	39	NA	NA
BRAZIL	24	17	16	23	24	25	16	20	20	6	8	11	31	31	28	47	41	41	- 6	- 6
CHINA	16	13	11	23	17	18	13	22	17	15	16	41	33	32	13	39	30	29	-10	9
TAIWAN	16	11	11	16	17	18	45	24	17	21	37	41	2	21	13	32	28	29	- 3	- 4
CYPRUS	3	5	5	6	10	12	16	27	32	20	35	35	55	11	16	9	13	17	8	4
HONG-KONG	24	33	22	29	19	24	19	29	30	11	8	12	17	11	12	53	52	46	- 7	- 1
INDIA	17	24	28	23	19	17	19	22	21	11	16	15	21	19	19	40	43	45	5	3
JAPAN	28	21	21	26	31	32	30	22	21	11	19	18	5	7	8	54	52	53	- 1	- 2
S. KOREA	14	8	8	15	15	14	24	20	12	33	26	21	14	31	38	29	23	22	- 7	- 6
LIBERIA	17	17	16	39	27	22	25	38	41	12	15	17	7	3	4	56	44	38	-18	-12
N. ZEALAND	30	23	NA	24	27	NA	21	23	NA	7	12	NA	17	15	NA	54	50	NA	NA	- 4
NORWAY	17	11	9	18	17	15	17	17	16	17	17	16	30	38	44	41	28	24	-17	-13
PANAMA	12	20	19	10	17	17	20	20	22	18	18	17	34	25	25	30	37	36	6	7
PHILIPPINES	9	12	10	27	21	16	23	15	15	25	25	24	40	36	35	19	24	26	7	5
SINGAPORE	18	23	17	20	18	23	21	30	31	18	18	21	23	8	8	45	44	40	- 5	- 1
SWEDEN	18	11	NA	25	19	NA	15	15	NA	11	15	NA	32	41	NA	38	29	NA	NA	9
TURKEY	15	13	NA	17	15	NA	16	21	NA	9	17	NA	35	32	NA	40	32	NA	NA	- 8
U.S.S.R.	12	15	13	17	15	15	20	19	20	21	23	21	30	28	31	29	30	28	- 1	1
U.S.A.	25	8	5	22	31	29	15	17	20	10	14	13	28	30	33	47	39	34	-13	- 8

Source: Lloyd's Register of Shipping: Statistical Tables

CAPACITY UNDER OPEN REGISTRY FLAGS

The above picture on the fortunes of the fleets of the EC Member States is considerably modified if one takes into account the shipping capacity under open registry fleets which is beneficially owned by Community nationals.

Although this capacity cannot strictly speaking be considered as coming under the Community "umbrella", EC beneficial ownership of shipping under open registry flags constitutes a complement of the fleets under the flags of member states. Furthermore, the recourse by Community shipowners to open registry flags is a means to remaining competitive while retaining economic control of the operation.[9]

Information on the beneficial ownership of ships under open registry flags has been published by the UNCTAD Secretariat on data supplied by A and P Appledore Ltd, for the years 1981 and 1987.

In respect to Community countries this information covers only those with beneficially owned tonnage exceeding 1 million dwt. For 1981 these countries are France, Germany, Greece, Italy, the Netherlands and the United Kingdom. For 1987 the list includes the same countries except Italy.

The relevant information is reproduced on tables 2.12 and 2.13 covering respectively 1981 and 1987. In addition these tables present information on capacity owned (national flags plus open registry flags).

A comparison of the above tables with table 2.2 reveals that open registry tonnage controlled by Community owners represents a much higher percentage of total open registry tonnage than the percentage of total national flag tonnage out of the world total tonnage.

Shipowners in only five of the Community countries (France, Germany, Greece, the Netherlands and the United Kingdom) owned nearly 30 per cent of total open registry tonnage.

This percentage confirms the key role of Community shipowners in the development of open registry shipping and makes the latter an important issue in maritime policy formulation at EC level.

Between 1981 and 1987 shipowners in France, Germany, Greece, and the United Kingdom increased their share of total open registry tonnage and only Dutch owners experienced a decrease.

The biggest increase in percentage share was that of Greek shipowners, who beneficially own nearly 21% of total open registry tonnage.

If open registry tonnage is added to national flag tonnage we note that the percentage share of total world capacity by Greek interest has remained the same, nearly 14 per cent, despite the prolonged crisis.

The German and Dutch shipowners appear to have weathered the storm well since their corresponding percentages have not decreased dramatically, as has been the case for the French and British shipowners.

The most important point emerging from the information on tables 2.12 and 2.13 is that shipowners in five Community countries, namely, France, Germany, Greece, the Netherlands and the United Kingdom controlled 21% of the total world tonnage in dwt, either under their national flags or open registry flags.

If to that percentage figure we add the percentages from table 2.2 on world tonnage represented by the national flags of the remaining EC member countries (excluding the percentages under open registry flags for which no information is available) it can safely be inferred that EC nationals controlled more than 28% of total world capacity in dwt.

Table 2.12
Total Beneficially Owned Capacity
under National and Open Registry Flags in 1981

	National Flag		Open Registry Flags		% of total Dwt of open re-gistries	Total Owned		% of total world Dwt
	Number	Dwt(000)	Number	Dwt(000)		Number	Dwt(000)	
FRANCE	1199	20112	33	1250	0.6	1232	21362	3.1
FRG	1820	12409	308	5774	2.9	2128	18183	2.6
GREECE	3710	73514	707	22586	11.4	4417	96100	13.8
ITALY	1677	17429	84	2195	1.1	1761	19624	2.8
NETHER-LANDS	1271	8600	117	2483	1.2	1388	11083	1.6
UNITED KINGDOM	2975	41273	141	3140	1.6	3116	44413	6.3

Source: Lloyd's Register of Shipping, Statistical Tables UNCTAD on data
supplied by A and P. Appledore Ltd.

Table 2.13
Total Beneficially Owned Capacity
under National and Open Registry Flags in 1981

	National Flag		Open Registry Flags		% of total Dwt of open re-gistries	Total Owned		% of total world Dwt
	Number	Dwt(000)	Number	Dwt(000)		Number	Dwt(000)	
FRANCE	954	8407	38	1768	0.8	992	10175	1.6
FRG	1414	5659	427	7340	3.4	1841	12999	2.0
GREECE	1948	42776	1311	45155	20.9	3259	87931	13.7
ITALY	1571	12178	N/A		N/A	N/A	N/A	N/A
NETHER-LANDS	1307	5123	146	2004	0.9	1453	7127	1.1
UNITED KINGDOM	2165	11676	257	5676	2.6	2422	17352	2.7

Source: Lloyd's Register of Shipping, Statistical Tables UNCTAD on data
supplied by A and P. Appledore Ltd.

N O T E S

1 Metaxas B. "Flags of Convenience", Gower,
   England, 1985.

2 See OECD Maritime Transport, Paris, 1984.
   Appendix 1, and US Department of Transportation
   Maritime Administration, Maritime Subsidies,
   Washington, DC, 1983.

3 Tzoannos, J. "The Fiscal Regime for Shipowning
   Firms in the EEC", Institute of Economic and
   Industrial Research, Athens, 1980. See also
   Chapter 3.

4 Committee of Inquiry into Shipping, Chairman: The
   Rt.Hon. the Viscount Rochdale, "Report". HMSO
   London 1970, Cmnd 4337.

5 The literature concerning the welfare effects of
   the conference system is very extensive. See eg.
   J.A.Zerby and R.M. Conlon, "An Analysis of
   Capacity Utilisation in Liner Shipping" Journ of
   Transport Economics and Policy, January 1983, pp.
   27-46 and "Editorial: The Case of Rochdale versus
   Rochdale" Maritime Policy and Management, Vol.
   12, No 3, 1985, pp. 177-179.

6 Economic and Social Committee of the EC "EEC
   Maritime Transport Policy" Brussels, 1986.

7 A good example is the plethora of bilateral
   maritime agreements between France and the
   francophone West African states reported in the
   Journal de la Marine Marchande, 21 January 1988.
   See also chapter 3.

8 See Chapter 8.

9 On the question of open registries see Commission
   of the European Communities, "Progress towards a
   Common Transport Policy; Maritime Transport",
   Com(85) 90 final, paras 79-85, Metaxas, B.N.
   "Flags of Convenience", Gower, England 1985, and
   Giannopoulos G.N., "The Economics of Flagging
   Out", Journal of Transport Economics and Policy,
   Vol. 22, May 1988.

CHAPTER 3

MARITIME POLICY IN THE EC MEMBER STATES

There are many factors that influence government maritime policy in each country. First of all, the orientation of maritime policy depends on whether government philosophy is for liberalism in economic activity especially in trade relations with third countries or for interventionism. In practice this distinction is not clear. Another key element is the weight given to shipping relative to other industries. Sometimes, shipping is viewed as a trunk industry subservient to other sectors of the economy. In other instances it is treated as a key industry on its own merits.

The relative weight attached to shipping depends on the economic magnitude of the sector in the context of the national economy, the strategic importance attached to it for defence purposes and the political pressure that interested parties (eg. maritime trade unions) can exercise.

It should also be pointed out that in some countries maritime policy is inextricably linked to policies pursued for shipbuilding whilst in others the shipping industry is treated in isolation from other sectors of the national economy.

Quantitative information on the value added by maritime activity in each national economy is not available through published sources. However, an indication of the relative importance of shipping in each national economy can be given by the size of the labour force employed in the maritime sector. This force should be defined to include not only those employed on board ships at any one time but back-up personnel as well as those employed in the ancillary industries.

Figures on the number of seafarers employed on board Community flag vessels at a specific point in time are presented on Table 3.1. The same table also presents the size of the total civilian labour force in each country so that the relative weight of shipping can be ascertained in each country in terms of generation of jobs.

Similarly, the same table presents figures on the employment generated by the shipbuilding sector.

The figures on the persons employed in the merchant marine and shipbuilding cover the year 1986 and those on total civilian population the year 1985. Bearing in mind that the annual charge in the latter is very small this difference in the time periods should not present any problems in making comparisons.

In making comparisons with other sectors it should be borne in mind that the number of persons employed in the merchant marine presented on Table 3.1 underestimate the magnitude of employment generated by shipping activity, since it does not include seafarers that are on leave or unemployed, or other back up personnel. Nor does it include employment in ancillary industries to shipping.

Unfortunately, there are no relevant data available and crude estimates can be made only on hearsay. In Greece eg. the average length of service of a seafarer on board a vessel is 6 1/2 months per annum. Given that on a specific date there were 31 935 on board its merchant fleet the actual manning requirements on an annual basis would be approximately 59 000 persons. To this figure one should add the number of seafarers serving on board foreign flag vessels and shore based personnel.

Even if the figures in the first column of Table 3.1 were to be multiplied by a factor of 3 to arrive at an approximation of the true number of jobs generated by maritime activity, it does not appear in general that shipping for most EC countries is a major sector in their national economy. The exceptions are Denmark and Greece for which it could safely be inferred that respectively 1.2% and 2.8% of their total civilian population is directly involved with maritime activity.

Table 3.1

Personnel Employed in the Merchant Marine, Shipping and Total Civilian Labour Force

Country	Persons Employed in the Merchant Marine in 1986	Persons Employed in Shipbuilding in 1986	Total Civilian Labour Force in 1985 In thousand	Persons in Merchant Marine as Percentage of Total Civilian Labour Force (%)	Persons in Shipbuilding as Percentage of Total Civilian Labour Force %
BELGIUM	2,928	3,871	3,577	0.09	0.1
DENMARK	9,779	12,260	2,522	0.4	0.5
FRANCE	6,807	13,498	20,916	0.03	0.06
FRG	20,470	38,118	25,011	0.08	0.02
GREECE	31,934	6,328	3,588	0.9	0.2
IRELAND	N/A	N/A	1,056	N/A	N/A
ITALY	N/A	13,809	20,509	N/A	0.07
NETHERLANDS	14,218	15,300	5,083	0.3	0.3
PORTUGAL	2,913(1985	14,150	4,029	0.07	0.4
SPAIN	19,873	22,996	10,623	0.2	0.2
UN. KINGDOM	29,781	11,694	24,089	0.1	0.5

Sources: OECD Maritime Transport, EEC Shipbuilders
Linking Committee.

Thus, one would expect that for the majority of the EC countries (with the exception of Denmark and Greece) shipping would receive special attention in the formation of government economic policy only as a trunk industry helping to promote the interests of other sectors such as manufacturing and agriculture or as a factor in national defence.

Shipbuilding is not a major force in the generation of employment opportunities either. Its relative position vis a vis shipping in that respect varies from country to country. Shipping appears to be more important than shipbuilding in Greece, Portugal and the U.K. whilst the relation is the reverse in Belgium, Denmark, France and Germany. The relative weight of the two sectors is about the same in the Netherlands and Spain.

The political clout of shipbuilding is enhanced in some countries (eg. France or the U.K.) by the fact that it is concentrated in certain regions, whithin which it represents a very high percentage of the labour force.

THE ELEMENTS OF MARITIME POLICY

The issues that characterise government maritime policy and are of relevance to European shipping policy can be summarised as follows:

1. Protectionism: Does government policy entail any acts of protectionism on (a) the supply side of maritime services in the form of subsidies and on (b) on the demand side in the form of cargo reservation and restraints on the operation of third country carriers.

2. Employment: What are the rules concerning the employment of non-national seafarers. Furthermore, is there a special treatment afforded to shipping in comparison to other sectors in relation to taxation of seafarers, social security and welfare provisions and training.

3. Development of new national ship registry in parallel to the existing one. This is a recent phenomenon and it allows shipping to develop as an off-shore activity not to be burdened by costs generated by the institutional arrangements in force in the national economy. The aim in this case is to retain under effective national control shipping capacity that would otherwise have flagged into open-registries.

4. International maritime affairs: What is the position adopted by the government in international maritime force and to what extent are international conventions and rules translated into national law.

5. Links with shipbuilding. Are there any specific government legislative provisions linking shipping activity with shipbuilding.

6. Competition policy: Are there any government attitudes vis a vis organisational arrangements in the production of maritime services, such as

the conference system, that might distort competition.

PROTECTIONIST ACTIVITIES

In general, EC member governments have shown through their actions a preference for a liberal regime for maritime transport. This preference has been translated into a common commitment to "safeguarding and promoting open trades and a situation of free competition on a fair and commercial basis in international shipping" through the OECD[1].

This commitment is not unique for the shipping sector but is in line with the trade policies pursued by the market economy countries, members of the OECD which aim at bringing down barriers to trade in both goods and services. However, this general attitude is qualified by protectionist measures which vary in degree of intensity from country to country.

A list of protectionist measures adopted in the various EC member countries concerning the supply side of maritime services is presented in Annex 3.1.

The information presented on these annexes is the result of collecting and collating data from a variety of sources.

Direct subsidies in the form of government grants towards the cost of acquiring a ship exist in France, Germany, Ireland, Italy, the Netherlands, and Spain.

Operating subsidies are given to shipping companies by their respective governments in France, Italy, Portugal and Spain. In those countries there exist additional subsidies to state controlled enterprises in shipping, in the form of covering up their losses with funds from the national exchequer.

In all countries there also exist special subsidies to shipping lines for the operation of services on certain unprofitable routes (eg. to remote islands) which are considered to be important for the national interest. Similar subsidies are given to other modes of transport, as well, and

should not be taken into account in evaluating
government maritime policy.

Indirect subsidies in the form of tax
concessions for the acquisition or operation of
ships are more widespread. It should be pointed,
however, that in many instances like the "business
expansion scheme" in the U.K. these are not unique
to the shipping industry, but also apply to other
economic activities like manufacturing.

The most common form of concession are the
accelerated depreciation allowances which exist for
shipowning enterprises in all EC countries except
Greece.

The effect of these allowances is to decrease
tax obligations and correspondingly improve the cash
flow resulting from an investment in ships in the
early years of its economic life, thus improving the
net present value of that investment.

In Greece, on the other hand, the system of
taxation for ocean going shipping is not based on
profits. Instead, shipping companies pay an annual
lump-sum, irrespective of whether they incurr
profits or losses, which is related to the size and
age of their vessels. Thus, no tax concessions are
granted to them, as under the profits based systems
of taxation.

Another form of tax concession is the ability of
shipping companies to create tax-free reserves from
operating profits or from book profits resulting
from a sale of vessel. Those reserves are to be used
to finance new investments in ships. Such reserves
are allowed in Denmark, France, Germany, the
Netherlands and Spain.

In some countries tax concessions are further
extended to include special reductions on corporate
tax rules on shipping revenues (in Germany, the
Netherlands and Spain), or a reduction in local
taxes (in Germany).

An important form of the concession, to be found
in all countries with a profits based system of
taxation involves the ability to carry forward
losses incurred in any one year to future years.
This instrument improves the cash flow stream for a

company by enabling it to take full advantage for tax purposes of deductible expenses against profits. It should be pointed out, however, that this instrument is also not unique to the shipping industry.

Government assistance is also given to shipowners in three countries through shipping finance in the form of interest rate subsidies and state guarantees for new shipping loans. The countries where such facilities exist are Belgium, Denmark and Germany. In Denmark these facilities are mainly for investment in small cargo ships and in Germany concern only guarantees from one coast Land to assist single-ship partnership.

In all EC member countries there exist also special finance packages for national shipowners who order vessels at national shipyards and register them at the home registy. These packages are known as home-credit schemes. These schemes constitute in effect indirect assistance to the national shipbuilding industry rather than to the shipowner, since their effect is to bring shipbuilding costs to the levels that the shipowner would achieve anyway at foreign yards.

On the demand side of shipping services protectionist activity[2] can be classified into (i) unilateral cargo reservation in the trade with third countries, (ii) bilateral cargo sharing agreements, (iii) multilateral cargo sharing agreements and (iv) cabotage.

(i)   Unilateral cargo reservation in international trade exists in France, Portugal and Spain for specific types of commercial cargo and all government cargoes including imports by state enterprises.

        France reserves under prewar legislation (laws of 1928 and 1935) 2/3 of hydrocarbon imports and 40 percent of coal imports for national flag carriers. Furthermore under a Decree Law of 1935 all cargoes shipped for account of the State or of state public services must be carried by French flag vessels.

        Portugal has introduced new regulations relating to cargo reservation under its

Decree-Law No 34/87 which modifies the extensive list of cargoes reserved to Portuguese flag carriers under previous legislation (Decree-Law No 75-u/77).

The new legislation still reserves 75 per cent by tonnage of items considered essential to the country to Portuguese flag carriers, but subjects this reservation to freight rates in line with international market rates.

Furthermore, there is still a 100 per cent reservation of goods imported or exported cif by the public administration or public enterprises to Portuguese flag vessels or foreign vessels chartered by Portuguese shipowners.

In Spain Regulation No 1382/1985 amending previous legislation still reserves an extensive list of commodities for Spanish flag vessels. That list includes crude oil, coal, lignite, coke, and various foodstuffs.

The new Spanish regulation has not modified the provision that all imports of government controlled cargoes must be carried in Spanish flag vessels.

Needless to say that all of the above cargo sharing provisions contravene EEC Regulation 4055/86 and it is surprising that the new Portuguese regulation was introduced after the relevant Community legislation had come into force.

In fact, it has become known that the Commission is taking action against the Portuguese government on this matter following a complaint from the Portuguese shippers' council.

(ii)   Bilateral agreements with third countries involving cargo reservation (usually on a 50-50 basis) for the fleets of the two countries involved are in operation in Belgium, France, Germany, Italy, Portugal and Spain.

A bilateral agreement instituting cargo sharing was also signed between Italy and Algeria in January 1987 after Regulation 4055/86 had come into force.

Following protests from Greece the issue was put before the Council, which in September 17th 1987 attempted to put the above agreement in a Community framework on an expost basis by agreeing that Italy could ratify the agreement with Algeria on the understanding that (a) the former would adhere to the UNCTAD Code as quickly as possible, (b) Algeria would be reminded that the agreement should conform to EEC legislation, and (c) the Commission and the member states would be informed on the position of the agreement within one year.

The Commission found this solution unsatisfactory on the basis that the Council should have invited Italy to modify the agreement, so as to state explicitly that there could be no discrimination between Italian ships and those of other EC member countries regarding access to the trade.

Consequently the Commission brought the Council's decision before the Court of Justice. The case was still pending at the time of writing.

(iii) The only multilateral cargo sharing agreement to which there is a commitment by the EC member countries is the UNCTAD Code of Conduct for Liner Conferences involving inter alia the 40-40-20 formula. This commitment originates from Regulation 954/79, which is discussed in Chapter 4. This institutionalisation of cargo sharing in the liner trades is a result of compromise, whereby developed, market economy countries gave in to the pressures of developing countries, which had long pressured for cargo sharing on a 50-50 basis.

Nevertheless, half of the EC member countries have not ratified the UNCTAD Liner Code yet, although it is now coming up for revision. These countries are Greece, Ireland, Italy, Luxembourg, Portugal and Spain.

The reluctance of Greece to ratify the Code
can be attributed to its strong opposition to
cargo sharing given the cross-trading
activities of its fleet. It can also be
attributed to the fact that Regulation 954/79
was presented to it as a fait accompli by the
nine countries just before its accession to
the EC.

Luxembourg is not a maritime country and has
had no active interest in this issue whilst
Italy, Portugal and Spain have shown through
their bilateral agreement a keeness to share
cargo on a 50-50 basis. Thus by not ratifying
the code these three Mediterranean countries
have avoided so far extending cargo
accessability under the UNCTAD Code formula in
their liner trades with third countries to
other EC operators.

In the case of Ireland the delay may be due to
the fact that there is no great involvement of
Irish shipping in the international liner
trades and therefore there is no great
political pressure for ratification.

(iv)   Cabotage restrictions are in force in France,
Germany, Greece, Italy, Portugal and Spain.
Also Denmark maintains cabotage restrictions
for trade with the Faroes. Furthermore trade
in Denmark involving vessels up to 500 grt is
allowed only for national flag carriers.

The main argument put forward by the
respective governments for justifying these
restrictions is a strategic one: Coastal
shipping provides vital links for the carriage
of goods and passengers to various parts of
the country and the production of maritime
services are considered in this case to entail
a national security dimension. Therefore,
this production should be in national hands
despite the costs that this form of
protectionism might generate for the consumers
of the relevant services.

It is noteworthy that in all of the above
countries except Germany cabotage involves to
a large degree service to islands (eg. the

Aegean, Madeira, the Balearies, Corsica, Sicily etc.).

The importance of coastal trade varies from country to country. This can be seen from Table 3.2 which presents separately the volume of international and domestic seaborne trade of each country. Unfortunately there are no data available on the volume of the domestic seaborne trade for Belgium, the Netherlands and Portugal.

The relative weight of coastal trade vis a vis the international trade of each country is big in Greece, Spain, Italy and the U.K., whilst it is very small in France, Germany and Ireland.

It is noteworthy, therefore, that there is no systematic relationship between the incidence of cabotage restrictions and the relative magnitude of demand for maritime services generated by the coastal trades of each country.

Table 3.2
International and National Seaborne Trade
in EC Countries in 1984

Country	International Trade Total of Goods Loaded and Unloaded in Million Tonnes	National Trade Total in Goods Loaded and Unloaded in Million Tonnes	National as Percentage of International %	Cabotage Restrictions
BELGIUM	120.3	N/A	N/A	NO
DENMARK	42.2	6.1	14.5	*
FRANCE	248.8	12.4	5.0	YES
FRG	128.6	3.7	2.9	YES
GREECE	47.8	18.4	38.5	YES
IRELAND	18.0	0.5	2.8	NO
ITALY	230.6	53.0	23.0	YES
NETHERLANDS	324.8	N/A	N/A	NO
PORTUGAL	121.3	N/A	N/A	YES
SPAIN	135.4	76.7	56.6	YES
UN.KINGDOM	297.5	98.4	33.1	NO

Source: Eurostat
* Denmark maintains cabotage restrictions for the trade with the Faroes. Also trade involving vessels up to 500 grt is allowed only for national flag carriers.

On the other hand, the relatively high
percentage of coastal trade vis a vis
international trade generated in Greece, Italy
and Spain could be taken to imply a high
resistance point to any proposals from the
Commission and other member countries for the
abolition of cabotage.

Bearing in mind the liberal orientation of the
maritime policies of the EC Member States, sprinkled
to varying degrees with the above measures of
protectionism, it is interesting to identify the
market shares of national flag carriers in the
external seaborne trade of each country.

The relevant information is presented in Tables
3.3 and 3.4 respectively for 1980 and the mid 80s.
Unfortunately, no information is available on the
activity of Portuguese flag carriers and on the
external trade of Denmark in both periods, and of
Italy and Portugal in the mid 80s.

A big share of the national external trade is
carried by national flag carriers in France, Greece
and the U.K., both inwards and outwards. In Germany
a big share is to be found on the export side while
in Spain the presence of national flag carriers is
strong in the carriage of imports.

On the other hand, in Belgium and the
Netherlands the corresponding shares of national
flag carriers are not impressive.

The big shares of national shipowners in the
carriage of imports of France and Spain could be due
to cargo reservation or sharing practices in the
trade of basic raw materials, such as oil or
minerals. On the export side which is dominated by
finished industrial goods the cases of France,
Germany and the U.K. the big shares could be due to
the closed conference system in the liner trades.

The case of Greece could be attributed to the
existence of a big fleet operating under competitive
conditions. This explanation gains ground by the
fact that the presence of Greek flag carriers is
strong in the trade of other EC countries as well.

An additional explanation of the high shares of national flag carriers in the imports of France, which is also relevant to the imports of the U.K. could be the existence of tanker fleets operated by oil companies based in those countries for the carriage of their own products.

It appears, therefore, from the above that there is no clear-cut connection between the degree of protectionism afforded to national shipping and flag shares in the external trade of EC countries.

It is interesting also to note that in the mid 80s about half of the total volume of seaborne trade of EC countries was carried by EC flag carriers. This market share by Community flags has materialised despite the lack of cargo reservation at Community level (Community cabotage) taking the whole of the EC as one economic entity, except for the provisions of the UNCTAD Code of Conduct on liner conferences, or the liberal orientations of the relevant policies in the individual member states. The Code cannot be taken to explain the above phenomenon, given that it covers only part of the liner trades (i.e. a small percentage of total seaborne trade), and that by the mid 80s it had not been ratified by all countries concerned.

Recipient of Service / Flag of Carrier	Belgium/ Luxembourg I	Belgium/ Luxembourg E	Denmark I	Denmark E	France I	France E	FRG I	FRG E	Greece I	Greece E	Italy I	Italy E	Netherlands I	Netherlands E	Portugal I	Portugal E	Spain I	Spain E	United Kingdom I	United Kingdom E
BELGIUM	5.0	3.1	N/A		0.3	0.9	2.1	0.8	0.0	0.0	0.6	0.1	0.9	0.9	0.2	0.0	0.2	0.4	0.8	2.6
DENMARK	0.8	2.3			1.5	1.7	3.2	6.5	2.1	0.6	0.7	1.2	1.6	4.0	2.1	5.7	2.3	3.9	2.5	2.3
FRANCE	1.6	2.1			26.7	19.4	1.5	0.9	0.3	0.9	3.2	2.0	3.6	1.9	2.0	1.1	1.1	1.8	5.8	4.4
FRG	4.4	10.4			4.1	4.6	13.4	24.4	0.8	0.7	2.4	4.1	6.6	10.8	5.1	24.9	2.4	5.1	7.6	10.0
GREECE	8.6	10.1			8.4	19.1	7.2	7.3	58.1	4.5	15.9	16.4	8.2	5.9	17.5	9.4	8.0	17.3	5.8	5.6
ITALY	1.5	1.0			2.5	4.1	2.2	0.3	4.5	2.8	24.1	17.7	2.6	2.1	1.3	1.1	2.5	3.5	1.0	2.5
NETHERLANDS	2.6	3.4			0.9	3.0	3.8	3.6	0.6	0.6	0.5	1.3	2.0	8.1	2.4	7.1	1.7	3.6	4.2	4.6
PORTUGAL	N/A	N/A			N/A	N/A	N/A	N/A	N/A	N/A	N/A	N/A	N/A	N/A	N/A	N/A	N/A	N/A	N/A	N/A
SPAIN	0.8	1.6			1.4	2.8	0.6	0.5	0.8	1.0	1.2	2.3	0.9	0.9	7.5	5.3	45.7	15.5	0.8	1.6
UNITED KINGDOM	20.4	22.8			10.7	11.6	13.8	6.6	1.4	3.6	4.8	5.4	13.0	25.3	4.0	7.3	3.4	5.0	30.9	36.9
TOTAL EC (excluding Portugal)	45.7	56.8			56.5	67.2	47.8	50.9	68.6	55.2	53.4	50.4	39.4	59.9	42.1	61.9	61.3	56.1	59.4	70.5
USSR	6.0	9.1			5.3	5.0	4.4	9.7	2.8	4.2	5.2	4.9	3.7	3.1	2.8	3.0	3.1	3.4	2.3	1.1
LIBERIA	8.4	3.7			16.1	4.6	18.0	3.2	9.1	7.9	17.4	7.4	25.5	5.5	13.0	1.9	11.6	8.2	12.4	7.2
PANAMA	3.1	3.7			1.0	2.4	2.4	2.7	4.8	3.7	3.5	8.5	2.1	3.0	3.9	6.6	1.7	5.1	4.1	1.5
CYPRUS	0.1	0.7			0.3	0.9	0.4	1.2	1.3	5.4	–		0.1	0.5	1.3	2.3	0.4	1.6	0.2	0.5
SINGAPORE	1.6	1.6			0.8	0.9	2.6	3.3	0.7	0.6	–		1.5	2.5	0.0	0.0	0.9	1.4	1.0	1.1

Source: OECD Maritime Transport

I = Imports
E = Exports

Table 3.4

Flag Shares in Total Seaborne Trade in Mid 80s in Percentages (%) of Tonnage

Flag of Carrier	Belgium/Luxembourg 1985		Denmark		France 1984		FRG		Greece 1983		Italy		Netherlands		Portugal		Spain		United Kingdom 1985	
Recipient of Service	I	E	I	E	I	E	I	E	I	E	I	E	I	E	I	E	I	E	I	E
BELGIUM	8.6	6.9			0.5	0.5	0.9	0.7	0.5	0.1	N/A		0.8	0.9		N/A	0.3	0.5	2.2	1.1
DENMARK	1.1	1.6			0.7	1.3	2.5	7.4	0.5	1.4			1.2	2.4			0.4	1.9	2.2	1.1
FRANCE	2.0	2.0			21.0	21.7	1.1	1.0	1.0	0.1			1.9	1.7			0.6	1.9	3.1	2.6
FRG	4.6	8.1			3.3	4.3	12.9	20.4	5.3	1.6			5.6	15.6			3.0	5.2	10.1	7.8
GREECE	5.7	7.0			8.6	10.2	6.0	4.7	32.3	43.3			6.6	3.5			3.5	3.7	5.4	6.2
ITALY	1.3	0.5			1.3	4.4	1.1	0.0	6.3	3.1			1.1	1.4			2.0	6.0	1.2	0.7
NETHERLANDS	4.0	3.7			1.9	3.2	4.2	3.1	1.5	1.0			2.4	8.7			1.3	2.7	4.3	5.2
PORTUGAL	N/A	N/A			N/A	N/A	N/A	N/A	N/A	N/A			N/A	N/A			N/A	N/A	N/A	N/A
SPAIN	1.4	1.7			3.4	3.5	0.7	0.6	3.1	0.6			1.2	1.5			43.7	9.0	1.2	2.0
UNITED KINGDOM	13.6	16.2			11.8	9.4	8.9	4.9	1.8	1.4			7.4	15.9			3.5	3.7	23.1	22.9
TOTAL EC (excluding Portugal)	42.3	47.7			52.5	58.5	38.3	42.8	52.3	52.6			28.2	51.6			58.3	34.6	52.8	49.6
USSR	6.0	5.6			4.0	8.5	6.2	10.0	4.9	5.5			5.0	2.9			2.2	4.7	2.4	1.2
LIBERIA	14.0	6.9			13.5	5.1	14.4	3.7	12.5	4.6			21.4	7.0			12.0	9.2	10.4	11.8
PANAMA	7.0	7.6			3.1	5.7	6.8	5.6	9.0	9.4			7.5	6.6			6.4	12.0	4.0	3.3
CYPRUS	2.0	3.7			0.9	2.2	1.3	1.8	9.1	7.0			1.5	1.8			1.6	4.7	1.2	0.6
SINGAPORE	2.9	2.9			2.4	1.1	2.3	2.0	5.4	1.0			2.4	1.9			1.9	1.6	1.6	6.6

Source: OECD Maritime Transport

I = Imports
E = Exports

In respect to operators from third countries it is noteworthy that Soviet vessels have not increased their shares whilst there is an important presence of open registry fleets especially of Liberia in seaborne imports.

Finally, comparing Tables 3.3 and 3.4 it is clear that there has been a decrease in the shares of national carriers with a notable exception the share in French exports, during the first half of the 80's. This phenomenon is related to the decrease in the capacity of the respective fleets discussed in the previous chapter.

It is noteworthy in those countries where some forms of protectionism exist, that these have not been sufficient to counterbalance the loss by national flag carriers of competitive advantage so as to preserve their market shares.

The above phenomenon can be also explained by the fact that governments have not deviated further away from liberal maritime policies, preferring not to impose extra costs to their national exchequer or the users of maritime services.

In any case despite the above decreases the fact that the percentages of Community generated trade carried by vessels of Member States remain high, would be expected to act as an additional constraint to any move towards protectionism, either at national or Community level.

EMPLOYMENT OF SEAFARERS

With respect to labour matters maritime policy in the Member States in general is characterised by special arrangements that differentiate the maritime sector from the treatment afforded to those employed in other sectors of the economy.

An area of clear cut distinction concerns the legality of employment of non-nationals on board national flag vessels.

Ever since the European Court's decision No 167/1973 the employment of other EC nationals on board a vessel flying the flag of a Member State should in principle be unimpeded as is the case in shore-based employment.

As from 1st January 1988 this principle should also apply to Greece, but not to the newest members of the Community, Portugal and Spain which are still under a transitional period concerning the free movement of labour.

However, none of the other Member States nor the Council of Ministers have taken any steps that would create the practical institutional framework needed for the operation of free movement of labour in seafaring within the Community, especially with respect to higher crew.

A big impediment is the mutual recognition of certificates for which no Community legislation exists, whilst all available information reveals widespread discrepancies between the practices followed by individual countries.

Denmark and Italy recognise certificates issued in other Member States as being equivalent to their national ones.

In France, the Netherlands and the U.K. national legislation specifies that those employed on board the national merchant fleet should hold certificates issued by the authorities in the respective countries. In the case of the U.K. the seafarer may alternatively hold certificates issued by the competent authorities in a British Commonwealth country.

Germany recognises the certificates issued in another EC member country, but requires a good knowledge of German.

Belgium, Greece and Ireland have not yet dealt with the issue of recognition of certificates.

The overall impression therefore, is that Member States are restrictive in their approach towards the employment of other Community nationals on board their national flag vessels.

This attitude may be attributed to worries that if free movement of labour within the Community were to be applied to seafaring without hindrance, unemployment among national seafarers would be exacerbated. It is important to remember that this issue has been raised at a time when Community shipping and its competitors are going through a big crisis coupled with technological change resulting in a significant loss of jobs.

Member States follow a very different approach vis a vis the employment of lower crews from developing countries. Special legal arrangements have developed over the years in some countries which permit the employment of those crews at wages and other conditions of employment which are different to those applicable to national seafarers.

This is arranged through bilateral agreements negotiated between Community shipowners and the seafaring unions of third countries (eg. Philippines, India, Bangla-Desh, South Korea etc.), under which the remuneration of crews reflects the opportunity cost of labour in those countries.

The aim of cource of those arrangements is to improve the competitive position of the national merchant fleets internationally, through labour cost savings, in line with the arrangements existing under open-registry flags.

Bilateral agreements are known to have existed for a number of years with the blessing or tolerance of national legislation, in Greece, the Netherlands and the U.K. Unfortunately details of these agreements are not available.

In some other EC countries governments permit the employment on non-nationals under ad hoc arrangements.

The extent of employment of non-nationals in the merchant fleets of the EC Member States can be seen on table 3.5. Personnel employed is classified into nationals, nationals of other OECD countries (including EC) and other countries. The latter category usually covers seafarers from the developing countries.

Among the EC fleets, five employ non-nationals to a significant degree. These are the fleets of

Table 3.5

Personnel Employed in the Merchant Marines of EC Member Countries

Country	1980				1986				Nationals as Percentage (%) of Total	
	Own Nationals	Other OECD	Other Countries	TOTAL	Own Nationals	Other OECD	Other Countries	TOTAL	1980	1986
BELGIUM	2,526	636	142	3.304	2.332	474	122	2.928	76	80
DENMARK	11,975	670	2,037	14,682	8,846	305	628	9,799	82	90
FRANCE	14,863	5	179	15,047	6,695	2	110	6,807	99	98
FRG	20,894	3,351	2,796	27,041	16,301	4,169		20,470	77	80
GREECE	52,518	1,074	25,867	79,459	28,791	3,143		31,934	66	90
IRELAND	1,839	29	3	1,871	N/A	N/A	N/A	N/A	98	N/A
ITALY	N/A	N/A	N/A	34,684	N/A	N/A	N/A	N/A	N/A	N/A
NETHERLANDS	6,139 *	1,863	1,910	9,912 *	10,071 **	4,147		14,218 **	62	71
PORTUGAL	5,856 *	0	0	5,856 *	2,913	0	0	2,913	100	100
SPAIN	22,928	0	0	22,928	19,873 **	0	0 *	19,873 **	100	100
UN. KINGDOM	64,668	13.411		78,079	28,980	3,021		32,001	83	91

Source: OECD: Maritime Transport

Figures with an * refer to 1979 and with ** to 1985

Belgium, Denmark, Germany, Greece, the Netherlands and the United Kingdom. Thus, for those countries it can be inferred that their governments have permitted over the years the employment of non-nationals in their merchant fleets.

On the other hand, in France, Ireland, Portugal and Spain it appears that there exists a very strict regime barring non-nationals from employment in the national merchant fleet.

For Italy no relevant information has been found.

It is also interesting to note that between 1980 and 1986 there has been a big drop in the percentages of non-domiciled seafarers out of the total number of persons employed.

Only in the Dutch and German fleets do non-domiciles represent now at least a fifth of the total labour force employed.

The decrease in the percentages of non-domiciled seafarers in the merchant fleets of Member States can be attributed to a large degree to the transfer of vessels beneficially owned by Community citizens to open registries or the new dual national registers.

In both instances these vessels are manned by low cost crews from third countries.

NEW REGISTRIES

In contrast to the above trend there is widespread employment of non-domiciles in the merchant fleets under the new parallel registers which three EC member countries operate, namely, France, the Netherlands and the United Kingdom.

These registers enable a shipowner to register his vessels under the national flag but operate it with a high degree of flexibility concerning choice and conditions of employment of factors of production, including labour. Thus, whilst the government of the particular state retains administrative control over the ships in the parallel register, the shipowner can operate under conditions similar to those found in the traditional open registries.

The oldest examples of parallel registries are those of the Dutch Antilles and Bermuda.

France has established such an "off-shore" national register in the Kerguelen islands. This is open to French shipowners for the registration of dry bulk carriers where they can employ up to 75 per cent non-French personnel.

The most notable of the British flag linked registers is that of the Isle of Man. That register involves low corporate and personal taxes as well as the ability to employ low cost crews from third countries.

At the time of writing (June 1988) a new parallel register was born in Denmark and additional ones were in the making in Germany and Luxembourg.

Thus many European countries are turning in increasing numbers to the invention of a parallel register for the operation of vessels under "off-shore" conditions as an answer to the loss of competitive advantage vis a vis third country fleets.

This practice is creating a two-tier regime for the operation of ships under the flag of the countries concerned; one with strict control of ship management including employment conditions, and a second with a high degree of flexibility in ship management.

It should be noted that the legal status in relation to the Treaty of Rome and the December 1986 regulations of the registries established in some dependent territories of Member States has not yet been clarified.

The Isle of Man and the Channel Islands eg. which are Crown dependencies, but not part of the United Kingdom, are covered in Protocol No 3 of the Act of Accession of the United Kingdom to the EC.

Article 2 of that Protocol states that Channel Islanders or Manxmen "shall not benefit from Community provisions relating to the free movement of persons and services".

On the other hand, vessels registered in the above territories fly the British flag. The question then arises whether such vessels could benefit from the provisions of Article 1 of Regulation 4055/86 concerning the freedom to provide services in intra-Community trade or transport to and from third countries.

INTERNATIONAL MARITIME AFFAIRS

The governments of the EC Member States have in general pursued over the years similar policies concerning the international regulation of maritime affairs. This is particularly evident in the context of UNCTAD where EC governments have joined forces with other OECD governments, forming the "Group B" of countries, to resist protectionist policies.

A similar convergence of policies is evident in the deliberations of the Consultative Shipping Group (CSG)[3] and its negotiations with the U.S. aiming at the adoption of common measures vis a vis third countries pursuing flag discrimination practices.

LINKS WITH SHIPBUILDING

In most EC member states governments look upon shipping and shipbuilding as being closely related industries. However, there exist wide differences between governments on how this view is translated into specific legislative measures.

In three countries, namely Italy, Portugal and Spain, national shipowners are compelled to place their orders of new vessels to national shipyards. In Belgium, Denmark, France, Germany, Italy and the Netherlands the only practical link between the two industries involves favourable terms offered to domestic shipowners to order in their home yards, if they so wish.

In Italy, the link concerns the two state owned groupings FINMARE (shipping) and FINCANTIERI (shipbuilding), whereby the former is obliged to place its orders with the latter.

In Portugal national legislation specifies that newbuilding orders by Portuguese owners have to be placed with the national shipyards.

In Spain prior to EC membership all vessels bought new or secondhand had to originate from Spain. This restriction has recently been replaced by a combination of import duties, waivers and quotas on imports from non EC countries which make it prohibitive for Spanish shipowners to place orders for newbuildings outside Spain.

Table 3.6

Favourable Terms Offered to Domestic Shipowners for Home Ordering

Country	% Loan	Interest	Repayment	Grants	Other
BELGIUM	70%	Up to 3% subsidy	15 years	Nil	Recoverable financial aid
DENMARK	80%	8% (2 yrs grace)	12 years	Nil	Loans for fishing vessels
FRANCE	Nil	Nil	Nil	7.5% or 15%	Nil
FRG	Nil	Nil	Nil	12.5%*	Extended low interest credit
ITALY	Nil	2.7%	12 years	Nil	Nil
NETHERLANDS	Nil	Subsiby 12% + premium 2.3%	5 years	Nil	Nil
NORWAY	80%	8%	8.5 years	Nil	Nil
SWEDEN	Depreciation loan of 25%				
JAPAN	50-60%	7.5% (3 yrs grace)	13 years	Nil	Additional loans available
SOUTH KOREA	50%	8-10% subsidy	8.5-11 yrs	Nil	Nil
TAIWAN	80%	8.5%	7 years	Nil	Nil
BRAZIL	85%	5-10%	15 years	Nil	Nil

Source: U.K. Department of Industry, 1987

* The Federal Government in Germany has recently replaced the 12.5 per cent grant to domestic owners by a direct subsidy to the shipbuilders of 20 per cent of the contract price.

It should also be noted that the shipbuilding
policies of Portugal and Spain have been given an
interim period of adjustment under the 6th Council
Directive of 26th January 1987[4] on aid to the
shipbuilding industry.

Given the much higher prices of newbuildings in
those countries compared to the prices that can be
obtained in Far Eastern yards[5] it is clear that the
governments concerned have opted for policies of
supporting their national shipbuilding industries by
imposing part of the cost of support on their
shipping industry.

In Spain and Portugal the shipping industries
are also obliged to insure their vessels in the
national insurance market, rather than having the
option of seeking the lowest insurance premia in
other insurance markets, like Lloyds in London.

This dirigiste framework is completed with the
forementioned cargo reservation practices,
ostensibly for the purpose of enabling the
shipowners to survive with the above cost burdens
through the creation of captive markets.

The home ordering schemes in existence in
Belgium, Denmark, France, Germany, Italy and the
Netherlands involve soft credit terms and in some
instances grants to domestic shipowners so as to
place orders in their national shipyards provided
the ships are then registered in their home
registry.

As can be seen from Table 3.6 which presents a
summary view home ordering schemes are not a unique
European phenomenon but can be found in other major
maritime nations.

The above schemes aim at encouraging rather than
compelling a national shipowner to order a new
vessel domestically by attempting to bring down the
cost of the new order to the level that can be
obtained in more competitive countries.

The two biggest maritime countries in the EC,
Greece and the U.K. have no measures in operation
linking the two industries.

The Greek government has announced an intention to bring into operation a domestic ordering scheme but has not yet introduced any relevant legislation. Such a scheme had been in force in the recent past but had not been successful in attracting any significant orders to Greek shipyards.

The U.K. government in accordance with its economic liberalism has been decreasing the amount of fiscal support to its shipbuilding industry.

It is clear from the above that most EC governments have refrained from imposing burdens on their shipping industries with the aim of supporting their shipbuilding industry.

Nevertheless, an analysis of new building orders placed with various shipyards according to the nationality of the registry to which each ship is destined, shows that shipyards in most EC countries tend to rely more heavily for new orders on their national shipowners than shipyards in third countries.

This analysis is presented in Table 3.7. Taking all EC shipyards together 61% of their total orders outstanding in October 1987 involved ships destined to be registered at home. The corresponding percentage taking the rest of the world as a whole was 42%.

There exists great variation of course between countries reflecting either the competitiveness of national shipyards or the effectiveness of the national home ordering schemes. In Greek shipyards there were no ships being built for national shipowners whilst in Belgium and Italy all ships on order were destined for the home market.

Table 3.7 also shows that intra-EC ordering of newbuildings represents a low percentage of total ordering: In October 1987 only 14% of total orders were for ships to be registered in other EC countries, other than the shipyards country.

Thus, although close links appear to exist in most EC countries between shipping and shipbuilding activity on a national basis (Greece, Portugal and the U.K. being notable exceptions) no such links are to be found at Community level.

This latter phenomenon could be attributed to a
number of factors such as (a) the non-existence of a
Community internal market for shipbuilding or
(b) the international character of most shipping
operations. Community shipowners order new ships in
their home shipyards either because they are ogliged
to or because they are presented with attractive
home ordering packages. Otherwise they place orders
with the most competitive yards in the Far East.

Table 3.7
Analysis of Orders of Ships by Nationality
of Customer for 1987

Country Shipyard	FLAG OF SHIPS BUILT							Open Registries
	Country flag	EEC countries' flag	Non EEC countries flag		Total built ships	Country flag per total built ships	EEC per total built ships	
			Open register	Others				
EEC Countries								
BELGIUM	4	0	0	0	4	100%	100%	0%
DENMARK	31	1	0	2	34	91%	94%	0%
FRANCE	3	0	2	5	10	30%	30%	20%
FRG	19	8	1	10	38	50%	71%	3%
GREAT BRITAIN	11	23	0	6	40	28%	85%	0%
GREECE	0	0	0	4	4	0%	0%	0%
ITALY	52	0	0	0	52	100%	100%	0%
NETHERLANDS	26	2	0	2	30	87%	93%	0%
PORTUGAL	1	0	3	10	14	7%	7%	21%
SPAIN	15	1	10	12	38	39%	42%	26%
TOTALS	162	35	16	51	264	61%	75%	6%

Source: Fairplay No 92, 8th October 1987

Table 3.7 Continued

FLAG OF SHIPS BUILT

Country Shipyard	Country flag countries' flag	EEC countries' flag	Non EEC countries flag — Open register	Non EEC countries flag — Others	Total built ships	Country flag per total built ships	EEC per total built ships	Open Registries
Non EEC Countries								
ALBANIA	1	0	0	0	1	100%	0%	0%
ARGENTINA	6	0	0	0	6	100%	0%	0%
BRAZIL	31	0	2	1	34	91%	0%	6%
BULGARIA	10	0	0	31	41	24%	0%	0%
CANADA	3	0	0	0	3	100%	0%	0%
CHILE	1	0	0	0	1	100%	0%	0%
CHINA	30	8	7	21	66	45%	12%	11%
EGYPT	3	0	0	0	3	100%	0%	0%
FINLAND	0	0	4	36	40	0%	0%	10%
GERMANY (EAST)	9	0	3	7	19	47%	0%	16%
INDIA	18	0	0	0	18	100%	0%	0%
INDONESIA	4	0	0	0	4	100%	0%	0%
JAPAN	74	12	55	26	167	44%	7%	33%
MALTA	0	0	1	0	1	0%	0%	100%
MEXICO	0	0	0	16	16	0%	0%	0%
NORWAY	3	0	0	0	3	100%	0%	0%
POLAND	26	1	7	47	81	32%	1%	9%
ROMANIA	23	0	0	12	35	66%	0%	0%
SINGAPORE	3	0	0	4	7	43%	0%	0%
SOUTH KOREA	19	8	51	43	121	16%	7%	42%
SWEDEN	2	0	0	1	3	67%	0%	11%
TAIWAN	8	0	0	1	9	89%	0%	0%
TURKEY	17	0	0	3	20	85%	0%	0%
USSR	25	0	0	0	25	100%	0%	0%
USA	7	0	0	0	7	100%	0%	0%
YUGOSLAVIA	0	0	20	25	45	0%	0%	44%
TOTALS	327	29	150	273	779	42%	4%	19%

Source: Fairplay No 92, 8th October 1987

COMPETITION POLICY

The distinctive issue of government competition policy in the maritime field is the system of liner conferences which although in practice takes various forms it commonly involves price-fixing and market sharing arrangements.

The extent to which liner conferences restrict competition depends on two conditions: (a) whether the conferences are "open" or "closed", and (b) whether in the case of closed conference independent operators can have competitive access to the relevant trade.

The welfare implications of the liner conference system have been the subject of controversy since the beginning of this century.[6]

Liner companies which are members of conferences argue that their system is a coordinating rather than a competitive device which guarantees regular and reliable services to shippers and achieves better capacity utilisation of resources.

On the other hand shippers and other users of maritime services have claimed that the behaviour of conferences is that of a monopolistic cartel, and have consequently pressed for government measures that would restrict its abuses.

The only qualification to this statement concerns the restrictive practices in the legislation of the U.K. (Protection of Trading Interests Act of 1980) which although it exempts international shipping from its scope it covers domestic and cross-Channel passage and car transports.

The EC member governments have not enacted any national anti-trust regulations governing specifically their maritime industries. Their policies have found expression in the formulation of relevant policies at international level, notably the UNCTAD code, the OECD and of course the EC.

This lack of national legislation could be attributed to a recognition on the part of the EC member governments of the peculiarities and complexities of shipping activity and consequently to a reluctance to impose on it a burdensome regulatory regime.

This attitude contrasts sharply to the attitudes that have prevailed on the other side of the Atlantic where the U.S. Shipping Act of 1916 had imposed the system of open conferences, and detailed regulations on their behaviour that would enable them to obtain anti-trust immunity.

More recently, the U.S. Shipping Act of 1984 simplified the regulatory regime but at the same time introduced the system of independent action for liner companies members of a conference so as to enhance competition.

American national legislation also prohibits restrictive practices to competition such as the recourse to exclusive patronage through the imposition by conferences of loyalty agreements to shippers. These make it difficult for a non-conference line to establish itself in a trade. The U.S. Shipping Act of 1984 has introduced instead the system of service contracts through which a shipper makes a commitment to provide a certain minimum quantity of cargo over a fixed period of time and the conference is committed to a certain freight rates and a defined service level.

The reluctance of European governments to get involved into the regulation of liner shipping was demonstrated as early as 1964 when they encouraged shipowners and shippers to establish their own self-regulatory regime under the "Note of Understanding" shigned between European conference lines and European shippers.

This "Note" led in turn to a series of Joint Recommendations agreed by the Council of European and Japanese National Shipowners Associations (CENSA) and the European Shippers Councils (ESC) covering the commercial relations of the two sides.

These Recommendations later evolved into the CENSA-ESC Code of Practice for Conferences which was established in 1971 following a request by the meeting of Ministers of Transport of Europe and Japan in Tokyo in February of that year.

In that meeting the ministers of transport expressed support for a self-regulatory regime for the conference system, as opposed to a government imposed one, that would curtail possible abusive practices on its part.

In the international fora and in particular the OECD and UNCTAD all EC member governments with the exception of Greece have charted a middle of the road course which on one hand accepts the usefulness of the existing liner conference system in ensuring regular and frequent services and on the other hand recognises the need for restrictions on their practices that limit the scope of competition.

It should be said however, that in the context of the UNCTAD Code these governments leaned towards the position of the closed conference system.[7]

These governments have not gone as far as to accept the "American" model of open conferences, independent action and service contracts.

On the other hand the Greek government has pressed for more stringent international rules that would enable all reasonably qualified shipping companies to join a conference.

The Greek attitude is determined by the insurmountable difficulties that Greek shipping companies have experienced in their attempts to join liner conferences or the problems they have faced as independent operators as a result of conference practices.

Nevertheless in respect to the treatment afforded to independent operators in various trades all EC member governments have pursued similar policies in line with all OECD governments aiming at keeping trades open to liner companies which are not members of conferences (known as outsiders).

The above governments were successful in introducing provisions (Articles 8 and 18) in the UNCTAD Liner Code Convention which attempt to safeguard the presence of non-conference lines in the regulated trades.

Furthermore, Conference Resolution 2 has resolved that the Code should not deny shippers an option in the choice between conference shipping liners and outsiders.

Also four EC member countries, Denmark, Germany, the Netherlands and the U.K., along with other OECD countries made a declaration to the effect that the presence of outsiders in the liner trades under conditions of fair competition should not be inhibited by other contracting parties to the Code.

Finally, it should be noted that all EC member governments have consistently taken the view that bulk shipping is a highly competitive activity and requires no government regulation.

ANNEX 3.1
List of Government Subsidies to Shipowners
in the EC Tax Concessions

	BELGIUM	DENMARK	FRANCE	FRG
Accelarating Depreciation Allowances	Declining Rates Method 20% in first year, 15% in subsequent 2 years and 10% in remaining five in an 8 year useful life. Depreciation is allowed on 113% of value of ship.	At the choice of ship-owner up to 30% in anyone year. Advance depreciation of 30% for ships under construction.	Reducing Balance Meth. 31.25% per annum in an 8 year useful life. For new ships 40% in first year. Alternatively straight line method.	Straight line or re-ducing balance methods 40% in first year. 12-14 years useful life.
Carrying Losses Forward Backward	5 years	5 years	5 years	5 years 2 years
Tax Free Reserves	Capital gains from the sale of a vessel which are reinvested within 3 years	25% of annual profits reinvested	To cover additional salary costs in case of expansion in re-evaluation of assets	Capital gains from the sale of a vessel which are reinvested
Other Concessions				Taxes halved on first 80% of profits
Operating Subsidies	Against operating costs		Against operating costs and for reinforcing company financial stru-ctures. Covering losses of nationalised compa-nies. Reimbursement of 66% of professional tax	Against cost of debt capital.
Investment Grants		Income tax relief for 20% of net income of an individual which is invested in new busi-ness	7.5%-10% of investment in new and second hand ships depending on type of ship.	12% of contract price of new ships. 20% for conversions
Provision of Cheap Credit		Guarantees of loans given by financial institutions for aqui-sition of smaller cargo ships.		Guarantees from coastal Lander governments on loans to single ship limited partnership.

ANNEX 3.1 Continued

	IRELAND	ITALY	NETHERLANDS	PORTUGAL
Accelerating Depreciation Allowances	100% initial allowance	Combination of reducing balance and straight line methods. 15% per annum in first 3 years. 10 years useful life.	Straight line or reducing balance methods 15 years useful life.	Straight line method in a 10 year useful life period. An increase of not more than 50% of applicable fixed not may be admitted.
Carrying Losses Forward Backward	Merchand shipping is treated as an export activity paying 10% profit tax instead of 50%.	5 years —	5 years 2 years	
Tax Free Reserves		Capital gains reinvested	Capital gains reinvested within 4y.	
Other Concessions				
Operating Subsidies		Covering losses of nationalised shipping companies		Against operating losses of nationalised shipping companies
Investment Grants	25% for new ships and second hand ships less than five years old.	5.5%-10% for new ships and second hand ships less than five years	11.5% for new ships and second hand ships less than five years old.	
Provision of Cheap Credit				Guarantees of loans to shipping companies

ANNEX 3.1 Continued

	S P A I N	U N I T E D K I N G D O M	GREECE
Accelarating Depreciation Allowances	Reducing balance method 8% per annum.	Reducing balance method 25% per annum	No subsidies given Greek ships pay tax according to their age and size independently of profits or losses realised.
Carrying Losses Forward Backward		Indefinitely 1 year	
Tax Free Reserves	Capital gains reinvested plus 50% of retained earnings		
Other Concessions	Tax credits on new investements & increase in number of employees		
Operating Subsidies	For companies operating in national interest & for making up losses incurred in the coastal trade. Compensation for extra costs faced in competition with other European ship.companies		
Investment Grants	5.5% plus additional subsidy up to 9.5% depending on type of ship.	Income tax relief under the Business Expansion Scheme for individuals investing up to 40000 pounds per annum in unquoted UK compan. owing or chartering new and second hand ships.	
Provision of Cheap Credit	Cheap loans for conversions and major repairs of ships. Assistance in financial restructuring of companies.		

Source: Commission of the European Communities: Inventory of Taxes.
        Lloyd's List, Fairplay, Seatrade Week.

NOTES

1   OECD, Code of Liberalisation of Current Invisible
    Operations, 12th December 1961 and Recommendation
    of the Council concerning Common Principles of
    Shipping Policy for Member Countries, 13th
    February 1987.

2   On the implications of protectionist activity see
    Goss R.O. "Some Economic Aspects of Flag
    Discrimination". Maritime Policy and Management,
    Vol.13, No.3, 1986.

3   The CSG consists of government representatives
    from Belgium, Denmark, Finland, France, the F.R.
    of Germany, Greece, Italy, Japan, the
    Netherlands, Norway, Portugal, Spain, Sweden, and
    the U.K.

4   87/167/EEC

5   Commission of the EC "A Comparison of
    Shipbuilding Costs and Prices in the EEC and Far
    East", October 1986.

6   House of Lords, Select Committee on the European
    Communities. "Competition Policy: Shipping".
    HMSO, London, 1983. Also see Maritime Policy and
    Management, "Editorial", Vol.12, No.3, 1985.

7   See Chapter 4.

CHAPTER 4

EC INITIATIVES IN SHIPPING 1958–1985

INTRODUCTION

Sea transport is mentioned in the Treaty of Rome only once. The last Article of Title IV (on transport) before its amendment by the European Single Act, Article 84 read[1] as follows:

"The provisions of the Title shall apply to transport by rail, road and inland waterway.
The Council may, acting unanimously, decide whether, to what extent and by what procedure appropriate provisions may be laid down for sea and air transport".

The insertion of the second paragraph was attributed to the Dutch who, as champions of the principle of freedom in maritime transport, aimed at excluding any Community intervention in shipping. The article was phrased in quite an original manner if compared with similar articles on other common policies. Instead of providing for a proposal of the Commission, opinions by the European Parliament and the Economic and Social Committee, for a timetable and the transition from unanimity to majority voting, Article 84, paragraph 2 only referred to a unanimous decision of the Council. Such a decision was not issued between 1958 and 1977. Therefore, prima facie under Article 84, paragraph 2 shipping seemed to be in a watertight compartment isolated from the rest of the Treaty. In fact, the phrasing of Article 84 paragraph 2, lent itself to various interpretations. According to the restrictive view, propounded by most governments and economic sectors involved, until the Council decided otherwise, air and sea transport were excluded not only from the application of the transport provisions of the Treaty but also from the application of the rest of the Treaty. According to the extensive view propounded by the Commission such an idea was untenable: if for the time being the transport provisions were inapplicable, the rest of the Treaty provisions did apply.

In spite of this divergence of views, the
subject remained in the limbo of a purely legal
controversy without any practical implications until
1973, when the scenario began to change for a number
of reasons justifying the characterisation of 1973
as the first turning point in the process towards a
common shipping policy.

EC INITIATIVES IN SHIPPING 1958-1973

In the pre-1973 period, EC involvement in
shipping policy measures was extremely low key or
virtually non existent. The following instruments
can be traced as either exempting the shipping
sector or paying lip service to it:

**Memorandum from the Commission to the Council on the
applicability of the competition rules in the Treaty
establishing the European Economic Community and the
interpretation of the Treaty's application to sea
and air transport.**[2]

This Memorandum took the line that, in the interest
of the economy as a whole and with a view to healthy
development of sea and air transport, the Community
institutions should take the decisions necessary to
ensure that these two modes are included in the
measures adopted in the field of transport in
furtherance of the Treaty's objectives (point 29).
A few months later the Commission presented a
further document, stating its position on maritime
transport.

**Memorandum on the basic approach to be adopted in
the common transport policy**[3]

According to the Commission, the provisions of
Articles 74 to 83 of Title IV (Transport) of the EEC
Treaty did not apply to sea and air transport. The
Treaty's general rules, however, were applicable in
principle to sea and air transport unless provision
was made to the contrary. However, it was obvious
that these two modes have specific characteristics;
they have much stronger ties with, and depend more
heavily on the world economy than the three modes of
inland transport. It was therefore in the
Community's interest to take this special situation
into consideration and not to interfere with these
modes' competitiveness outside the ambit of the

Treaty of Rome. Consequently, all the problems
raised by sea and air transport within the Treaty's
ambit should be examined and the measures required
to take their special situation into consideration
should be adopted under Article 84(2). It might
even prove expedient to suspend the application of
certain general Treaty rules to sea and air
transport for a period to be determined, until
suitable provisions had been adopted for these
modes.

**Action programme for a common transport policy
(Communication from the Commission to the Council).[4]**

The Commission confirmed the line taken by it in
1960 and 1961, but did not propose any concrete
measures. It merely stated that it was examining
whether it was necessary to apply special rules to
competition in the sea and air transport sectors
(point 237).

**Proposal for a Council Regulation regarding the
temporary non-application of Articles 85 to 94 of
the EEC Treaty to sea and air transport.[5]**

As certain Member States were against the
application to transport undertakings of Regulation
No 17, the first Regulation implementing the
competition Articles of the Treaty (Articles 85 and
86), the Council asked the Commission on 14 June
1962 to submit a proposal on this problem.

Regulation No 141 of the Council

This Regulation exempting transport from the
application of Council Regulation No 17[6] was
consequently enacted on 26 November 1962. The
Regulation also applied to sea transport.

As envisaged in Regulation No 141, this
Regulation was subsequently rescinded in respect of
inland transport modes by Regulation No 1017/68 of
the Council enacted on 19 July 1968.[7] However,
Regulation No 141 remained in force in respect of
sea transport until 1.7.87.

At the Council meeting of 20 October 1964 the
Commission pointed out that in the context of a
fully-fledged European Economic Community, two

sectors as important as sea and air transport could
not be left out of the integration process. The
inter-dependence of the transport modes called for
Community action in these two areas, so that the
measures for sea and air transport could be
coordinated with the measures for the other
transport modes. As regards sea transport, the
Commission considered it expedient to wait until
completion of the negotiations that were in progress
in other international institutions.[8]

At the Council meeting of 4 June 1970 the
Commission drew attention once again to the urgent
need for Community measures in the area of sea
transport and outlined several objectives. The
Commission announced that it would shortly be
submitting to the Council more concrete and more
detailed proposals regarding the action it
considered was most urgently required in this
sphere.[9]

EC INITIATIVES IN SHIPPING 1973-1985: CHANGES IN THE
EC AND INTERNATIONAL SHIPPING ENVIRONMENT

The legal controversy about the applicability of
the EEC Treaty to sea transport, which in practice
had led nowhere, was gradually transformed from 1973
onwards as a result of a series of events which gave
impetus to the development of a Community approach
to shipping matters:

- the first enlargement of the EC in 1973 brought
  sea transport more to the fore, in that not only
  were the United Kingdom and Denmark both important
  shipping nations but also that the United Kingdom
  and Ireland were both islands.

- the world-wide shipping crisis and the concomitant
  tonnage surpluses getting worse since 1973,

- the expansion of flag discrimination and
  protectionist practices,

- the expansion of state trading country shipping,
  particularly in the liner trades,

- several tanker disasters which led to extensive
  oil spillages such as the accident of the Amoco

Cadiz in March 1978 and to sensitizing of public
opinion on maritime pollution matters,

- the increasing number of questions, covering a
  wide range of shipping matters, submitted to the
  European Parliament and reflecting the revival of
  interest in shipping,

- the second enlargement of the Community in 1981
  with the accession of Greece, a leading
  international maritime power.

Grasping the opportunity of the first
enlargement, the Commission brought a test case in
1973 before the European Court of Justice to clear
up the old controversy, namely, whether Article 48
of the Treaty on the free movement of labour applied
to seamen. In its landmark judgment in the so-
called "French Seamen's case", the Court endorsed
the Commission's view that the general rules of the
Treaty do apply to shipping. The judgment was
important not only for its legal implications but
also for its political implications because it
incorporated maritime transport in the process of
European integration. Although a Court's judgment
cannot be a substitute for a common policy - it
cannot be an "ersatz" of a common policy in the
absence of acts of secondary law or of provisions of
the Treaties - nevertheless the above judgment
triggered actions; it had practical implications
within 48 hours. The judgment was delivered on 4
April 1974 and two days later the final act of the
U.N. Conference on Trade and Development (UNCTAD IV
Session) was initialled in Geneva. During the
course of the Conference, the Commission had not
appeared as representing the Community and had not
negotiated on behalf of the Member States. The
European Court's judgment, however, was such that
the Community had no alternative but to seek a
common position two days before signature of the
final act on the Code. That was the effect of the
judgment upon Articles 113 and 116 of the EEC
Treaty, which were considered to be enlisted among
the general rules of the Treaty that applied to
shipping. Instead of that, and in spite of the
Commission's efforts to establish a common view "a
la recherche du temps perdu", three Member States
(France, Germany and Belgium) signed the Code. With
regard to the voting: France, Germany and Belgium

voted in favour; the United Kingdom and Denmark voted against; Italy, the Netherlands and Greece abstained; Ireland and Luxembourg did not participate in the Conference. Thereupon, the Commission delivered a reasoned opinion to the effect that the three so-called Codist States had contravened the EEC Treaty. The Commission, however, instead of initiating proceedings before the Court, came to an unpublished gentlemen's agreement with the Member States. The result was a standstill compromise on both sides: on the one hand, the Commission would not bring the matter to the Court, on the other hand the Member States were under an obligation not to proceed with the ratification of the Code until April 1979, which was the earliest date for a conference to review it. The common understanding and the hope of both sides were that before then a solution would be found. A compromise of the conflicting views concerning ratification by the Member States of the UNCTAD Code was in fact reached in May 1979 when Regulation 954/79 was enacted.

Although adoption of the main bulk of legislative instruments of this period started in 1977, we consider 1973 as the turning point in the historical process leading, in light of the implications of the judgment in the French seamen's case, to a common shipping policy.

THE LEGAL BASIS OF COMMUNITY MEASURES ON SHIPPING

Community measures for shipping derive from two sources: first, the application of the general rules of the Treaty of Rome and, second, specific acts dealing with shipping and issued under Article 84, paragraph 2 of the EEC Treaty. As far as the first source is concerned the Court judgment in the "French seamen" case was crucial. In that case,[10] the Court decided that Article 48 EEC was directly applicable in the internal legislation of the Member States. France had therefore violated the Treaty by maintaning in its legislation certain provisions whereby employment on French vessels was reserved up to a certain proportion to French nationals. Moreover, in handing down its decision[11] the Court delivered an obiter dictum which had a profound effect on shipping policy within the Community. The Court said that the fundamental and general rules of

the EEC Treaty applied to shipping as well as to any
other means of transport. The Court, however, did
not specify which were these fundamental and general
rules of the EEC Treaty. This omission in the
verdict of the legal oracle of the Community left a
great deal of uncertainty in the Member States.[12]
The Legal Service of the Commission interpreted the
judgment as meaning that the general rules include
provisions dealing with the free movement of goods,
persons, services and capital, free competition and
taxation, the economic policy and institutions of
the Community. The same issue was debated more
recently before the European Court in the so-called
"Nouvelles Frontieres" case[13] where the French
Government argued a restrictive thesis whereby the
judgment in the French Seamen's case concerned only
the application of the second part of the Treaty and
not of the third - which referred to the various
common policies. This thesis was unequivocally
rejected by the Court which upheld an extensive
interpretation[14] of the notion of "general rules" of
the Treaty and lifted the legal smokescreen behind
which some Member States tried to hide.

Community initiatives taken in the period 1973-
1985 may be broadly classified under the following
categories:

1) Consultation procedure.
2) Measures relating to the UNCTAD Liner Code.
3) Measures relating to state trading country
   competition.
4) Measures relating to safety of navigation and
   pollution prevention at sea.
5) Miscellaneous measures with a bearing on
   shipping.

On 24.10.80 the Commission submitted to the
Council a

"Draft for a Council Resolution concerning
priorities and the timetable for decisions to be
taken by the Council in the transport sector during
the period up to the end of 1983 (COM/80 (582
final)[15]".

The draft provided in the Annex for the following
priority actions by the Council in the area of sea
transport: system for monitoring the activities of

certain third countries in sea transport, verifying fulfilment of international safety standards by ships in ports of Community countries, bringing Community interests to bear in relations between the Member States and third countries in the area of sea transport, Community aspects of State aids for shipping, implementing provisions regarding the application of the competition rules to sea transport, social regulations in sea transport.[16]

The Council of Transport Ministers on March 26th, 1981[17] in its resolution on the list of priorities in the transport sector for the period up to the end of 1983 did not widen the scope of its activities for shipping any further than the above areas. It is characteristic of the European Parliament and the Economic and Social Committee that having debated the above list, deplored the absence of decisions and urged the Council of Ministers "to go beyond the lethargy of plain statements of intent"!

1) Decision setting up a consultation procedure on relations between Member States and third countries in shipping matters and on action relating to such matters in international Organisations (77/587/EEC).

On September 13, 1977 the Council took its first decision[18] pursuant to Article 84 paragraph 2 concerning the introduction of a consultation procedure in shipping matters. The procedure is designed to facilitate confidential discussion by the Member States and third countries. This procedure has been the vehicle which allowed the prior preparation of the stance to be taken by the Member States in international organisations dealing with shipping matters.

In December 1977 shipping questions were dealt with for the first time in the regular high level discussions between the Commission and the U.S. and Japanese authorities. Since that time the consultation procedure has provided the framework for regular EEC Commission participation in the ongoing dialogue between the United States and the countries of the Consultative Shipping Group, the so-called CSG/US dialogue.

**2) Measures relating to the UNCTAD Liner Code-
Council Regulation (EEC) No. 954/79 of 15 May 1979[19]
concerning the ratification by the Member States, or
their accession to, the United Nations Convention on
a Code of Conduct for Liner Conferences.**

The most important Community act in shipping,
until 1985, adopted under Article 84 paragraph 2 was
Regulation 954/79 of 15 May 1979 known as the
"Brussels Package" concerning the ratification by
Member States of, or their accession to the United
Nations Convention on a Code of Conduct for the
Liner Conferences. The history of the Code is a
long one.[20] The Code was originally designed to meet
the aspirations of developing countries under
pressure from them to increase their transport
capacities by carrying part of their exports on
board vessels flying their national flag. The Code
distributes maritime transport according to the
famous 40-40-20 formula, i.e., 40% of the sea
transport is carried by liner vessels of the
exporter country, 40% by liners of the importer
country and 20% is left to third flag carriers
(crosstraders). It was believed that the cargo
sharing formula would help the shipping companies of
the developing countries by strengthening their
negotiating position in the conferences and would
also be a deterrent for bilateral cargo sharing
agreements and eastern block competition. The Code
provides that in order to enter into force it has to
be ratified by 24 countries representing 25% of the
world liner tonnage. So far, it has been ratified
by 71 countries well exceeding the required world
liner tonnage. The Community was instrumental in
bringing the Code into effect on October 6, 1983.
The Community managed to reach a compromise of the
divergent views among the Member States after
painstaking negotiations which lasted four years.
The common stance on the Code was necessary for the
following reasons: certain provisions of the Code
are incompatible with the provisions of the EEC
Treaty on the right of establishment (Articles 52-58
of the EEC Treaty), competition (Articles 85 and 86
of the EEC Treaty) the non-discrimination clause of
Article 7 and Articles 113 and 116. Moreover, a
common stance was necessary in view of the UNCTAD V
Session where the Member States had to present a
united front and in view of the renegotiation of the
Lome I Convention with the ACP countries as well as

in the framework of the North-South dialogue.
Negotiations were particularly difficult because
certain Member States (like France and Belgium) with
large trade and small fleets felt that the Code
would help them increase their carrying capacity,
whilst others (like the United Kingdom) heavily
involved in the conferences as well as in
crosstrading were strongly opposed to the idea of
cargo sharing under the Code. According to the
Commission's view the Brussels Package not only took
account of the wishes of the developing countries
for access to liner conferences and cargo sharing
but also maintained commercial principles for cargo
sharing between OECD countries and complied with the
basic principles of the EEC Treaty. Under
Regulation 954/79 the Member States are obliged to
ratify the Code subject to the following
reservations:

a) The Code in its entirety will apply to the
   trades between the developing and developed
   countries.

b) Certain provisions of the Code - specially the
   cargo sharing formula - will not apply in the
   trades between EC countries and on a reciprocal
   basis between EC and OECD countries.

c) The share allocated under the Code to the EC
   lines will be redistributed among them on the
   basis of commercial criteria, in particular: the
   volume of cargo carried by the conference and
   generated by the Member States whose trade is
   served or shipped through their ports, past
   performance of the shipping lines in the trade
   covered by the Conference and the needs of
   shippers (again this principle may be extended
   to other OECD countries on the basis of
   reciprocity).

The Regulation also provides that Member States'
definition of "national shipping line" may include
any shipping line established in a Member State in
accordance with the provisions of the EEC Treaty.

The Code, subject to the reservations set by the
EEC Regulation has been ratified by Denmark,
Germany, France, the Netherlands, the United Kingdom
and Belgium. In spite of its political

significance, the Code, is not a panacea. It has
not in practice proved to be a workable instrument
because of its cumbersome mechanism and the
vagueness of its provisions. The fact that several
countries have ratified it subject to differing
reservations has rendered its application and
interpretation even more difficult.

It is noteworthy that several developing
countries give an extensive interpretation to the
Code as applying not only to liner conference trades
of contracting parties but also to all their liner
trades or, more commonly, as applying its cargo
sharing formula on all their liner and bulk trades.
This interpretation has been persistently rejected
by developed Group B countries which correctly
maintain that the Code by its very title confines
its application to liner conference trades of its
contracting parties. This point has been among the
focal issues of the review conference of the Code
convened in November 1988 when the five year period
since its entry into force expired. The EEC Member
States played a key role during this Review
Conference since together with the Scandinavian
countries they are the only industrialised countries
which have adhered to the Code apart from the Group
of 77.

The Brussels package has not so much attracted
criticism from the developing world as from
socialist countries of Group D which maintain that
the extensive reservations of the Regulation are
contrary to the spirit of the Code and undermine the
principle of universality. To this, Group B
countries respond that reservations deposited
formally by Group D countries with their
ratification exclude from application of the Code
all Government cargoes, thus leaving untouched a
large portion of their trades as well.

Finally, the terms of EEC Member States
ratification laws have been the subject of lengthy
discussions in the series of Round Table meetings
held between OECD Government experts. In 16 Round
Tables that have taken place so far most aspects of
the Code have been scrutinized.

3) Measures relating to state trading countries competition.

Community action in this field was triggered by a Communication of the Commission to the Council (June 1976),[21] asking for countermeasures to be taken against the eastern bloc and, subsequently, (October 1977) proposing a series of alternative solutions. Meanwhile, the Prescott[22] and Seefeld[23] reports on problems in sea transport and relations with the state trading countries submitted to the European Parliament (March 1977) as well as the Parliament's Resolution on it recommended to the Commission and the Council the need for appropriate measures. The Economic and Social Committee in its report on transport problems in East West relations[24] made a detailed examination of shipping problems in relation to the Eastern bloc countries and called on Community institutions to prepare an appropriate legal basis for countermeasures against the threat of serious dislocation in the transport market. All Community institutions agreed on the need to take measures because on the one hand, the Member States realized that bilateral agreements could not cope with the problem, and on the other, were reluctant for political reasons unilaterally to apply restrictive measures possible under their national foreign trade legislation. Therefore, the only effective action was action at the European level under the Community umbrella. Nevertheless, negotiations with the COMECON countries were not precluded. This idea was also taken up by the European Parliament.[25]

The problem mainly concerns liner vessels and partly cruising vessels. State trading countries' vessels, if not accepted for admission to a conference on terms agreeable to them, establish liners which operate as outsiders and compete with the conference by undercutting freight rates offered by their western counterparts. The shipping industries of the eastern countries perform four major functions:[26]

a)   the transport function of national foreign trade to safeguard the economic independence of their country,

b) the profit function to contribute to the growth
    of national income,

c) the military strategic function by treating the
    shipping industry as a potential transport
    component of national defence and,

d) the currency function, i.e., the maximisation of
    foreign currency earnings either in the form of
    foreign currency revenues from the export of
    services or by economising on the use of foreign
    currencies by replacing foreign services with
    domestic ones.

    Since the 1970's the currency function has come
to the fore and to this end COMECON fleets use
several devices. Tariff rates offered are not based
on a calculation of their own costs but cut rates
are offered regardless of the relationship between
costs and earnings. This is obviously possible
because of the state trading character of the
COMECON countries. Their vessels operate with no
commercial criteria, a situation which western
companies cannot meet.[27] Seamen's wages are
relatively low compared to western levels and
national recruits often carry out their military
service on board merchant vessels. Moreover, there
are no insurance premiums or bank costs to be paid
and owing to state aids, shipping countries buy fuel
oil at very low rates. These tactics are coupled
with the insertion of shipping clauses in contracts
whereby COMECON exports are on cif terms and imports
on fob terms so that the COMECON states can choose
the flag of the ships. Finally, western shipping
countries are not allowed to have their own agencies
in the COMECON States: everything must be channelled
through the state transport agencies.

    Because of these tactics, COMECON countries
accumulate hard currencies to pay for imports of
western commodities and technology and they also
undermine the activities of western conference lines
in the trades involved. COMECON countries at
present cover 25% of transport between Northern
Europe and the Mediterranean as well as in the North
Atlantic. Obviously, the low tariffs operate in
favour of western shippers. This is so, however,
only in the short run, because in the longer term
shippers may themselves become vulnerable if these

companies achieve a dominant position in particular trades, allowing them to impose freight rates and to determine the quality of services.

The Community has adopted a flexible strategy in this field on a step by step basis, starting with a harmless monitoring system with countervailing measures to be taken at a later stage. Until 1985, a set of decisions was issued on the collection of information concerning the activities of carriers participating in cargo liner traffic in certain trades.

More particularly, the Council adopted on September 19, 1978 the Decision concerning the activities of certain third countries in the field of cargo shipping (78/774/EEC)[28] based on Article 84 paragraph 2 of the EEC Treaty. This decision required all Member States to set up a system for gathering information on the activities of the fleets of countries whose practices were detrimental to the maritime interests of Member States.

On 19 December 1978 the Council adopted the Decision on the collection of information concerning the activities of carriers participating in cargo liner traffic in certain areas of operation (79/4/EEC).[29] Under this decision, which was also based on Article 84 paragraph 2 of the EEC Treaty, the system for collecting information was expanded to cover the activities of carriers participating in liner trades between the Community and East Africa and Central America.

In December 1980 the Council extended the Decision 79/4/EEC for two years by adopting:

Council Decision of 4 December 1980 amending and supplementing Decision 79/4/EEC on the collection of information concerning the activities of carriers participating in cargo liner traffic in certain areas of operation (80/1181/EEC).[30] The Council also decided to expand this system to cover traffic between the Community and the Far East.

The basic Decision 79/4/EEC was subsequently amended/extended by Council Decisions 81/189/EEC,[31] 82/870/EEC[32] and 84/656/EEC.[33] The latter Decision continued to be in force until 31 December 1986.

According to the above decisions, Member States were under the obligation to collect information about the activities of liner vessels, irrespective of flag, concerning the nature and value of cargo, the level of freight, the ports of loading and unloading, the shipping company, the flag and, subsequently, report to the Commission for assessment of the data. Although the monitoring decisions were not per se sufficient, they reflected the political will of EC Governments not to permit what they considered as unfair practices encroaching upon the freedom of the seas to continue unabated.

A further step in this direction was taken with the adoption of the Council Decision of 26 October 1983 concerning counter-measures in the field of international merchant shipping (83/573/ EEC).[34]

Under this Decision, Member States that have adopted or intend to adopt countermeasures in the field of international merchant shipping are to consult the other Member States and the Commission. Within the framework of this consultation Member States are to endeavour to concert any countermeasures they may take. Without prejudice to the freedom of the Member States to apply national countermeasures unilaterally, the Council may decide on the joint application by Member States of appropriate countermeasures forming part of their national legislation. This Decision supplements the provisions of Decision 78/774/EEC concerning the activities of certain third countries in the field of cargo shipping.

4) **Measures relating to Pollution Prevention at Sea**

Acts in this field are the Community response to a number of tanker accidents causing pollution in Community waters, such as the Amoco Cadiz disaster, and focussing public attention on marine environment issues. Although the main role in this field is played by the Intergovernmental Maritime Organisation (IMO)[35] a United Nations agency, the EC decided to contribute in several ways: by acting as a pressure group in IMO, by urging Member States to ratify and enforce the IMO Conventions and by taking action on matters which are not being dealt with by IMO.

On 26 June 1978 the Council adopted the

Recommendation on the ratification by the Member
States of Conventions on safety in shipping
(78/584/EEC).[36]

This recommendation urges Member States to ratify
the following leading Conventions in this field: the
SOLAS 1974 Convention (International Convention on
the Safety of Life at Sea), the MARPOL 1973
Convention (International Convention for the
Prevention of Pollution by Ships) together with
their 1978 Protocols, and Convention No 147 of 1976
of the International Labour Organisation (ILO)
concerning minimum standards on board merchant
ships. At the same time the Council also adopted a
declaration on the need for better enforcement of
international measures to prevent marine pollution
by ships and to ensure the safety of ships and the
competence of crews. It is noteworthy that under the
terms of MARPOL Convention, Member States are under
the obligation to create reception facilities in
ports for oil residues, as a means to facilitating
the process towards cleaner seas. Nevertheless,
despite the widespread acceptance of MARPOL
Convention, enforcement of this particular provision
is still lagging behind in EC harbours.

Other measures in the area of shipping safety
followed in 1978:

Council Recommendation of 21 December 1978 on the
ratification of the 1978 International Convention on
Standards of Training, Certification and
Watchkeeping for Seafarers (79/114/EEC).[37]

Council Directive of 21 December 1978 concerning
pilotage of vessels by deep-sea pilots in the North
Sea and the English Channel (79/115/EEC).[38]

Council Directive of 21 December 1978 concerning
minimum requirements for certain tankers entering or
leaving Community ports (79/116/EEC).[39]

The above mentioned three Council instruments
were based on Article 84(2) of the EEC Treaty. In
the first instrument the Member States were
recommended to sign the 1978 IMO Convention by 1

April 1979 and to ratify it not later than 31 December 1980. The first of the two Directives sought to improve the qualification standards of deep-sea pilots and encourage the use of these pilots on vessels flying flags of the Community States or other countries. The Second Directive laid down minimum requirements for certain tankers whereby port authorities must be notified about their deficiencies and technical standards as per a tanker check list.

On 23 November 1978 the Council had adopted a statement on the Memorandum of Understanding of 2 March 1978 between certain North Sea maritime authorities on the maintenance of standards on board merchant vessels.[40]

Also on 26 June 1978 the Council adopted a

Resolution setting up an action programme of the European Communities on the control and reduction of pollution caused by hydrocarbons discharged at sea[41] (legal basis: "the Treaty").

Mention should also be made of the proposal for a Council Decision (based on Article 84(2) of the EEC Treaty) rendering mandatory the procedures for ship inspection forming the subject of resolutions of the Inter-Governmental Maritime Consultative Organisation (IMO)[42] which the Commission submitted on 13 November 1978. This proposal was endorsed by both the European Parliament and the Economic and Social Committee but it has not been adopted by the Council.

December 1979 saw the issue of the

Council Directive of 6 December 1979 amending Directive 79/11/ EEC concerning minimum requirements for certain tankers entering or leaving Community ports (79/1034 EEC).[43]

This Directive supplemented Directive 79/116/EEC with provisions on the carriage of liquefied gases (requiring a certificate of fitness under the IMO Code for the construction and equipment of vessels carrying liquefied gases in bulk).

On 2 July 1980 the Commission submitted to the Council a

Proposal for a Council Directive concerning the enforcement, in respect of shipping using Community ports, of international standards for shipping safety and pollution prevention.[44]

The purpose of this draft was to harmonise ship inspections and port controls at Community level and to introduce Community rules for the frequency and criteria of such inspections. Under its terms Member States would be required to identify substandard vessels visiting their ports and compel them to put themselves in order before leaving, thus making the responsibility for inspection of the port state parallel to the responsibility of the flag state. Both the European Parliament and the Economic and Social Committee delivered opinions on the above proposal which was also based on Article 84 paragraph 2 of the EEC Treaty but was never formally adopted.

This proposal should be seen in light of parallel moves taking place in a wider European forum. In December 1980 a Ministerial conference was convened in Paris to discuss port state control. This led to a further ministerial conference on 26 January 1982, at which the maritime authorities of 14 European countries (including the nine seafaring Member States) signed a memorandum of understanding on port state control, and the ministers issued a final communique in which full support was promised. This memorandum of understanding is based largely on the proposal the Commission submitted in 1980. A Committee comprising representatives of the 14 signatory States and the Commission was set up to administer the memorandum of understanding.

The Commission did not withdraw its proposal but did not insist either on its being discussed before the results of the first year of application of the memorandum of understanding were available. Ever since the Commission has reverted on this subject but not convincingly although several annual reports have been delivered. The basic reason for such non translation of the MOU into Community law may be attributed to the reluctance of several EC Governments to transfer competence of ship inspections to the Community. Any transfer of sovereignty from the national authorities to the Community faces a considerable degree of opposition. In this particular instance, fears are linked with the unwillingness to create a Community Coast Guard patrolling EC coasts and divested with draconian powers of enforcement reminiscent of the US Coast Guard.

In the memorandum of understanding each member country undertook to ratify swiftly the relevant leading international instruments (IMO and ILO Conventions): SOLAS 1974 and protocol of 1978, MARPOL 1973/1978, ILO Convention No. 147, Convention on training, certification and watchkeeping 1978, Convention on the prevention of collisions 1972, Convention on load lines 1966. Considerable progress has been made since January 1982. According to the third annual report, the third year of operation of the memorandum of understanding (MOU) may be characterized as the year of international acceptance and increased public interest in port state control. Although the targeted inspection rate of 25%, was not achieved, 23% of vessels visiting the MOU area had been inspected in 1986 and a new conference at ministerial level was held in Paris on 23 April 1987.

Further measures in this field include the following:

Council Decision of 13 December 1982 adopting a concerted action project for the European Economic Community in the field of shore-based navigation aid systems (82/887/EEC).[45]

Commission Opinion of 1 July 1982 addressed to the Greek Government regarding the implementation of the Council Directive of 21 December 1978 concerning minimum requirements for certain tankers entering or leaving Community ports, and of the Council Directive of 6 December 1979 amending the above mentioned Directive (82/452/EEC).[46]

Council Decision of 28 March 1983 on the conclusion of a Community COST concertation agreement on a concerted action project in the field of shore-based marine navigation aid systems (COST project 301) (83/124/EEC).[47]

Community COST concertation agreement on a concerted
action project in the field of shore-based
navigation aid systems (COST project 301).[48]

Council Recommendation of 25 July 1983 on the
ratification of, or accession to, the 1979
International Convention on Maritime Search and
Rescue (SAR) (83/419/EEC).[49]

Proposal for a Council Decision amending the Council
Decision 82/887/EEC adopting a concerted action
project for the EEC in the field of shore-based
navigation aid systems.[50] It is noteworthy that all
decisions concerning the shore-based navigation aid
systems were not based on Article 84 paragraph 2 of
the EEC Treaty but on Article 235.

Finally, mention should also be made of the
Council Recommendation of 15 May 1979 on the
ratification of the International Convention for
Safe Containers (79/487/EEC),[51] which is based on
both Articles 75 and 84 paragraph 2 of the EEC
Treaty. On 18 July 1980 the Commission submitted to
the Council the proposal for a Council Directive on
the harmonised application of the International
Convention for Safe Containers (CSC) in the EEC.[52]

In 1977, the Commission also issued the
following Decision:

Commission Decision of 29 July 1977 establishing the
list of maritime shipping lanes for the application
of Council Directive 76/135/EEC (77/527/EEC).[53]

On the whole, the corpus of Community rules in
this field indicates the Community's deep concern in
creating a zone around the EC coastline free from
substandard vessels considered[54] to be the main
source of marine accidents and of extensive marine
pollution.

5) **Miscellaneous measures with a bearing on
   shipping**

In addition to the above instruments, which have
been produced with direct reference to shipping (art
84 para. 2 EEC Treaty), there exist certain other
measures which also have a bearing on shipping,
namely, trade and cooperation agreements between the

EC and third countries, on sea ports, on shipbuilding. These measures do not make reference to art 84 para. 2 of the EEC Treaty but occasionally to other legal bases.

a)   Cooperation Agreements

The legal basis empowering the EEC to cooperate with international organizations and to look into bilateral relations with third countries is found in article 228 of the EEC Treaty. The extent of the Community's competence for foreign relations was clarified in the famous court case of 1971 the so-called ERTA case n° 22/70. The Community has foreign competence in so far as an agreement would affect a piece of Community law. The foreign competence issue was further developed in the advice of the Court n° 1/76 dating back to 1977, in which the Court stated that if it is necessary for the realisation of the common transport policy to negotiate with third countries even before secondary law has been established the Community can engage in those negotiations. In this context, the Commission is active together with the Member States in OECD, UNCTAD, IMO and ILO, and also maintains bilateral contacts in shipping matters more particularly with the Scandinavian countries.[55]

Sea transport is mentioned in several agreements between the Community and third countries. These agreements are the Lome Conventions and the Economic Cooperation Agreements with Brazil (1980), the Andean Pact countries (1983) and China (1985).

The Lome II Convention between the EC-ACP (November 1979) contained in Annex XIX a joint declaration on shipping whereby "the Community recognises the aspirations of ACP States to have a greater share in the carriage of bulk cargoes"! This statement, which indirectly accepted cargo sharing, was in clear contradiction with the policy vis-a-vis UNCTAD, where at the UNCTAD V Session the EC Member States clearly rejected the cargo sharing demand of the developing countries and declared their firm belief in the principle of free and fair competition in the bulk trades. This contradiction may be attributed to the fact that the Commission was subject to conflicting pressures: first, the economic rationale of having an efficient and

competitive   transport   sector   to   support   the
Community's seaborne trade;   and second, the need to
satisfy the aspirations of third world countries for
fast   economic   development.   These   two conflicting
pressures resulted in contradictory   policies   being
pursued   by   the EC Commission in various aspects of
the sea transport sector.

The   acceptance   of   interventionism   in   the
maritime relations between the EC and the ACP
countries, has been modified considerably in the
current Lome III Convention (1984).   The relevant
title there (Title   V-Articles   86-90)   involves   an
acceptance by the parties concerned of a more
liberal regime in maritime transport.

Article 86 of the Convention contains a
declaration   that   the   objective   of   cooperation
between the EC and the ACP countries in the field of
shipping "shall be to ensure harmonious development
of   efficient   and   reliable   shipping   services   on
economically satisfactory terms by facilitating   the
active participation of all parties according to the
principle of   unrestricted access to the trade of a
commercial basis".

There is still in the new Convention a statement
acknowledging the aspirations of the ACP states   for
greater   participation in shipping and in particular
bulk cargo shipping but this statement is linked   to
the   ideas   of efficiency in the shipment of cargoes
and   of   the   preservation   of   competitive   access
(Article 88).

This   overall shift in proclaimed intentions may
be   attributed   to   a   hardening   of   EC   attitudes
concerning   protectionism   in   maritime transport by
third countries as a   result   of   pressures   by   the
governments of Member States (which strongly opposed
cargo   sharing   in   the bulk trades under UNCTAD) as
well   as   by   interested   pressure   groups   (CAACE,
UNICE).

The   reference to shipping in the context of the
trade   and   economic   cooperation   agreements   with
Brazil[56]   and the Andean Pact[57] countries,   does not
go beyond an exchange of letters of intent that   the
problems   arising   in maritime relations between the
EC and the countries concerned will be examined in a

cooperative spirit. Therefore, this reference is of little practical use.

The cooperation agreement with China[58] constitutes a general framework within which special agreements on specific economic sectors, such as shipping, are to be concluded. The EC Commission is in the process of preparing a draft text for such an agreement in consultation with interested economic groups within the Community.

Under this heading falls also the

Council Decision of 10 December 1984 authorising the automatic renewal or continuance in force of certain friendship, trade and navigation treaties and similar agreements concluded between Member States and third countries (84/640/EEC).[59] (Legal basis: Article 113; validity until 31 December 1986).

On the whole it can be said that from the plethora of trade or economic cooperation agreements concluded by the EC and third countries, those with shipping clauses are very few. Moreover, because they represent a blend of both liberalism and interventionism, these agreements are without any "real teeth" in preserving a competitive environment in the relevant trades.

b) Sea ports

The question of a Community sea ports policy was first raised in the European Parliament in the Reports by Mr Kapteyn, Mr Seifriz and Mr Seefeld.[60] The first Commission initiative was taken in 1972.[61] Between 1972 and 1980 the Commission held meetings with representatives of the major European ports, at which two internal Commission documents were presented.[62] In July 1981 the Commission submitted to the EP a report[63] on its work in connection with a Community sea ports policy. On 11 March 1983 the EP adopted the Carossino Report[64] on the role of ports in the common transport policy and a ten-point Resolution.

c) Shipbuilding

Although shipbuilding forms a separate industrial activity its fortunes are inextricably linked with those of shipping. Hence, any considerations concerning the formation of a shipping policy cannot ignore shipbuilding matters and vice versa.

The Community shipbuilding industry has been affected severely, like shipbuilding activity in other countries, by the prolonged slump in the freight markets which started in 1975 and resulted in a significant drop in the intake of new orders and completions of new vessels. Between 1976 and 1979, according to figures produced by Lloyd's, vessel completions by Community shipyards fell by 42%, whilst the corresponding decrease world-wide was 37%.

The difference between those two percentages indicates that the impact of the crisis upon Community shipyards was heavier than elsewhere as a result of a number of competitive disadvantages they have been suffering such as small scale production, currency depreciation, high operating costs etc.[65]

As a consequence of these developments employment at Community shipyards is estimated to have fallen between 1975 and 1979 by 36%.[66]

The crisis affecting shipyards has compelled the governments of EC Member States to intervene heavily and grant special financial assistance so as to maintain their position by accepting orders at a loss.

The Commission's intervention with respect to the problems of shipbuilding has three dimensions: (a) it attempts to harmonise government subsidies to the shipbuilding sector within the Community, (b) it has proposed a number of measures at Community level to encourage the shipbuilding industry to undertake the necessary structural changes in order to become competitive in the world market, whilst at the same time boosting demand in order to alleviate the social consequences of the crisis and (c) it has taken action at the international level to induce other countries, especially Japan and South Korea, to try to reduce shipbuilding overcapacity.

The Community has so far issued six[67] directives on aids to shipbuilding, the sixth entered into force on 1.1.87, which have defined the aids that could be considered compatible with the rules on competition under Article 92 paragraph 3 of the EEC Treaty and have exercised a discipline in the grant of such aids by the governments of Member States so as to prevent distortions of competition between shipyards within the Common Market.

Moreover, following the Council Resolution of 19th September 1978[68] which recognised the need to make qualitative and quantitative adjustments to the shipbuilding sector, the Commission proposed a scheme[69] to promote the scrapping and building of new vessels at Community yards. The scheme was aiming at providing work for Community shipyards, absorbing some of the fleet overcapacities and modernising the Community fleet. However, owing to difficulties in sharing the costs of its financing, the scheme was not adopted by the Council

With regard to the export credits to shipbuilding as of Jyly 31st, 1981 all EC Member States invariably apply the terms of the 1979 OECD Understanding according to which the duration is set at 8 1/2 years, 20% down payment and interest rate of 8%.

As for home credits for shipbuilding, the Commission has investigated the relevant merits of the two forms of official aid currently in use in the Member States: direct aid for shipyards and credit facilities for shipowners for putting orders to Community shipyards. The Commission considers - as a more effective alternative to other aid systems- the adoption of the system of credit facilities which is devised to meet with sectoral policy guidelines.

APPLICATION OF GENERAL RULES OF THE EEC TREATY TO MARITIME TRANSPORT

1) Social Matters

The application of Articles 48-51 EEC and the deriving secondary law (i.e. the acquis communautaire on social matters) in shipping can be subsumed into the following:

Free movement of Community seamen between vessels under flags of the Member States, employment on board these vessels on the same footing as nationals of the flag state, preference in employment of Community seamen vis-a-vis seamen of third states, aggregation of periods completed under the legislations of several Member States for the acquisition, retention or recovery of entitlement to pensions and other social security benefits.[70]

The application of the general rules in the social sphere to seamen is not wholesale in that there are several exceptions: for instance, the exemption of seamen from the scope of application of the noise directive concerning workers[71]; the transitional period 1/1/1981 - 21/12/1987 of non application of the social rules to Greek workers and seamen (cf. Article 45 of the Greek Treaty of Accession); the transitional period 1/1/1986 - 31/12/1992 of non application of the social rules to Spanish and Portuguese workers and seamen (cf. Article 56 of Spanish Treaty of Accession/Article 216 of Portuguese Treaty of Accession).

In this context, it is noteworthy that the free movement of labour according to the prevailing view in the Member States does not apply to captains due to the dual nature of their functions: private and public. The latter function justifies their exclusion on the basis of Article 48, paragraph 4 EEC according to which employment in the public service is excluded from the application of the free movement of labour. Alternatively, their exclusion could be justified on the basis of Article 48, paragraph 3 EEC referring to "public policy, public security". Such a view has been tacitly accepted by the Commission but does not extend to other officers. The same exception applies to naval (military) vessels where the public service provision in article 48 par.4 would permit a Member State to limit crews and officers of these vessels to its nationals only.[72]

Following a French declaration at the Council of Transport Ministers[73] asking for Community action with regard to minimum standards of ships for the excercise of the seamen's profession and of protection in case of dismissal, the Commission had undertaken a number of studies in this field; namely the so-called Hollesen study,[74] a comparative study with regard to the provisions of national collective agreements on seafarer's pay, working hours, off-duty periods and labour costs on board EC vessels and another study, with regard to the situation of unemployment of seafarers in the EC.

The Hollesen study revealed as was to be expected the existence of significant differences among the fleets of the member countries concerning pay and working conditions for seafarers. Some figures concerning net income have been extracted from the report and are presented on Table 4.1, for four categories of seafarers, chief officer, chief engineer, boatswain and seaman. The information presented on Table 4.1 refers to net income for a single person on a large dry cargo ship, under each of those positions.

Net income estimates have been obtained after deducing from earnings the statutory deductions for income tax, social security contributions by seafarers, and contributions to seafarers' unions. It is worth noting that the differences among fleets concerning net pay are not consistent for all categories of employment, eg. whilst the French chief officer's net pay was higher than that of the Greek Chief Officer, the net pay of a French boatswain appeared to be less than that of his Greek colleague.

This phenomenon can be attributed to the particular conditions prevailing in the individual national labour markets for each category of seafarers as well as the general institutional framework of each economy.

Despite the differences in pay and working conditions, the right of free movement of Community seamen among vessels under the flags of the Member States has not produced any significant real movements between the fleets since that right was consecrated by the European Court. This can be attributed to a number of impediments such as the lack of action concerning the mutual recognition of the national certificates of seafarers at Community level, the lack of knowledge by seafarers of other Member State languages, and the opposition of national trade unions to the employment of seafarers from other countries.

Such impediments make it extremely difficult for the forces of economic integration to produce a unified labour market for seafarers within the Community. In fact, bearing in mind the progress achieved so far with respect to the removal of the impediments to the unification of other labour markets for which efforts had started much earlier, it is quite reasonable to speculate that progress towards a unified labour market for seafarers within the Community will be very slow indeed.

In our assessment, however, even in the absence of the above obstacles there would be no significant mobility of seafarers from one Member State to another.

Table 4.1

Net Income per Annum for a Single Man on Board a Large Dry Cargo in 1978 in EUA

Category

Country	Chief Officer	Chief Engineer	Boats-wain	Able Seaman
Belgium	14.613	17.269	8.730	7.712
Denmark	14.675	14.003	11.368	11.435
France	13.253	14.701	7.804	6.172
FRG	12.553	13.623	10.420	9.378
Greece	12.205	10.681	8.160	6.025
Italy	9.562	10.497	6.873	5.850
The Netherlands	12.830	14.004	8.109	6.839
United Kingdom	6.978	7.835	6.768	5.718

Source: Commission of the European Communities,
       "Hollesen Report"

2) Right of Establishment

The application of Articles 52-58 of the EEC Treaty on sea transport means that national provisions restricting the right of establishment of shipping companies from a Member State to a Member State are inapplicable vis-a-vis nationals or companies of other Member States or rather that they should be applied without discrimination on the grounds of nationality and such infringements may be brought before national courts. The main problem in this field hinges on the subject of registration[75] under the national flag. For the time being, national legislation of all Member States reserves in varying degrees the right of registration of vessels to nationals or national companies. Table 4.2 illustrates national legislation of EEC Member States relating to ownership of ships as a criterion for nationality.[76] Member States favour the view that there is no relation between establishment and registration, since the latter is an act of national sovereignty escaping from the demands of Community law. On the contrary, the Commission's view is that registration is a corollary of establishment and that, in any event, all financial advantages deriving from the flag should be granted to EC nationals without discrimination. Thus, the Commission maintains that a Member State which requires all or a proportion of the shareholders and/or directors of a company owning ships of its nationality to possess its nationality is in breach of Community law. Equally, requiring individuals owning ships having a particular Member State's nationality to be of the same nationality is contrary to the freedom of establishment. To be compatible with Community law, such legislation would have to be amended to allow ships having the nationality of a particular Member State to be owned not only by nationals of that State but also by nationals of other EC Member States established in that State. If the view of the Commission is correct, then the legislation of virtually all Member States is contrary to Community law. The problem has wider implications because the flag is linked in certain Member States with a series of economic advantages. This is the case with respect to coastal shipping, the so-called "cabotage".[77] The Commission in a report[78] on the economic implications of coastal shipping in the Community

concluded that the economic consequences from the
lifting of the privilege are minimal. It is
noteworthy that a case[79] on this matter was brought
before the Court concerning an action of the
Commission versus France but, thereafter, was
settled.

As contrasted with the right of establishment,
the combined application of Community Law
provisions[80] meant that freedom to provide services
did not apply to sea transport so long as a
unanimous decision by the Council was not issued in
this direction under Article 84 paragraph 2.
Therefore, until 1.1.87 when Regulation 4055/86
entered into force we were facing the paradox in
this field in that the major issue - establishment -
was allowed and the minor issue - services - was
prohibited.

Table 4.2
EEC Member States' Legislation relating to the
ownership of ships as a criterion for nationality

Member States	Requirement for Ships Owned by Individuals	Requirement for Ships Owned by Companies
Belgium	At least 50% of ship must be owned by Belgian nationals	At least 50% of ship must be owned by a company incorporated in Belgium
Denmark	Must have Danish nationality	Must be incorporated in Denmark. Two-thirds of directors must be Danish nationals domiciled in Denmark.
France	At least 50% of ship must be owned by French nationals	All of ship must be owned by a company incorporated in France and whose directors are French nationals.
FRG	Must have German nationality	Partnerships must have a place of business in Germany and a majority of partners must be German nationals. Companies must have a principal place of business in Germany and a majority of directors must be German nationals
Greece	Must have Greek nationality	Company need not be incorporated in Greece, but if a foreign company more than 50% of company must belong to Greek nationals.
Ireland	Must have Irish nationality	Company must be incorporated and have its principal place of business in Ireland.
Italy	Must either have Italian nationality or have been resident in Italy for five or more years and been given permission	Must either be incorporated in Italy and a majority of directors must be Italian nationals or, if a foreign company, must have a representative in Italy of Italian nationality.
Netherlands	Must have Dutch nationality. No such requirement for fishing vessels, but vessels must operate from Netherlands.	Company must be incorporated and have its seat in Netherlands and either two-thirds of shares must be owned by Dutch nationals and majority of directors Dutch and domiciled in the Netherlands. Fishing vessels as for individuals.
Portugal	Must have Portuguese nationality	Company must be incorporated and have its principal place of business in Portugal.

Table 4.2 Continued

Member States	Requirement for Ships Owned by Individuals	Requirement for Ships Owned by Companies
Spain	Must be Spanish nationals resident in Spain or non-nationals resident in Spain provided appropriate authorisation obtained	Company must be incorporated in Spain If a subsidiary of a foreign company, foreign shareholding must not exceed 40%.
United Kingdom	Must be British subject	Company must be incorporated and have its principal place of business in the UK or some other part of Her Majesty's dominions. The Merchant Shipping Bill limits latter to dependent territories and Crown dependencies. In case of fishing vessels the Bill provides 75% of shareholders and directors must be British citizens resident and domiciled in the UK.

Information taken from L.Hagberg (ed.), Handbook on Maritime Law, Vol.III (1983) and Robin Churchill "EEC Law and the Nationality of Ships and Crews", in "EEC Shipping Law" Conference 4-5/2/88, Rotterdam, European Study Conferences Ltd.

3) Competition Rules

It is characteristic that special rules of competition were gradually issued concerning the whole range of economic activities covered by the Community Treaties, with the exception of sea and air transport. However, by virtue of the judgment in the French seamen's case, the competition provisions of the EEC Treaty are applicable to sea transport. The applicability of competition rules of the Treaty to maritime transport was reiterated expressis verbis by the European Court of Justice more recently in the so-called Nouvelles Frontieres case.[81], where it was stated that Articles 85-90 of the EEC Treaty are applicable to the transport sector and more particularly to the air transport sector. The Court based its reasoning, inter alia, to the fact that whenever the Treaty wished to exempt certain activities from the application of competition rules, it provided for a clear cut derogation to this effect, as is the case of agricultural products by virtue of Article 42 of the Treaty. Impetus was given by the very words of the preamble of Regulation 954/79 on the accession of the Member States to the UNCTAD Code of Conduct for

Liner Conferences whereby "...the Commission will
forward to the Council a proposal for a Regulation
concerning the application of those rules to sea
transport...".

On 16 October 1981 the Commission presented the
Council with the

Proposal for a Council Regulation (EEC) laying down
detailed rules for the application of Articles 85
and 86 of the Treaty to maritime transport.[82]

The set of rules elaborated by the Commission
soon became the subject of controversy among Member
States, the European Parliament[83], the Economic and
Social Committee[84], shipowners and shippers.

The draft Regulation, which concerned sea
transport generally, propounded the conditions under
which liner conferences - which are basically
cartels - could be granted exemption from Articles
85-86 of the EEC Treaty. The basic bones of
contention concerned the conditions for such
exemption and the balance to be struck between
shipowners' interests and shippers' interests, the
treatment of the bulk sector, (namely, the claim for
non-application of the regulation on the bulk sector
due to the highly competitive environment in which
it operates), and finally the cumbersome procedural
rules of control and investigation established under
the Regulation. The end result after extensive
deliberations was the non-adoption of this
Regulation as presented at the time which, however,
served as a forerunner of the amended Competition
Regulation 4056/86 adopted under the common shipping
policy package.

ASSESSMENT OF COMMUNITY INITIATIVES (1958-1985)

An assessment of Community initiatives between
1958-1985 can be made from two points of view: a)
the external front as distinguished from the
internal front; and b) the mosaic approach as
distinguished from the global approach.

a) Development of Community initiatives in shipping
    can be pursued on two fronts: the external and
    the internal. The former is much more important
    than the latter because shipping as a trunk
    industry is much more important for extra-

Community trade. Measures adopted until 1985 indicated that the Community was occupied with the external side,[85] i.e. it endeavoured to help the shipping sector of the Member States to cope with the problems of international transport. On the other hand, no concrete efforts were made to adopt uniform rules to regulate the activities of the vessel, the seaman and the shipping company.

b) With regard to the shaping of common shipping initiatives, shipping policy enthusiasts fell into two camps divided on their general approach to the subject.[86] There were the fundamentalists, led by France, who favour a global approach, believing that there is a need to establish a set of general precepts to underline such a policy and that these should provide the skeleton around which a policy on a particular subject should be built. This was the continental and most ambitious approach, and presupposed a great deal in terms of common philosophy on the part of the Member States. The second group, led by the U.K, favoured what had been widely termed the "mosaic" approach, a policy " a petits pas". Adherents of this doctrine felt that vital issues of common concern, such as the Code of Conduct for Liner Conferences, eastern bloc competition, substandard vessels and so on should be tackled one by one. They preferred concrete proposals for solving individual problems which could be dealt with more easily under a joint approach. Common agreement on any of these issues would provide the first brick in an expanding policy mosaic. The origins of these differences between the two approaches can be found in the different emphasis given to the national shipping sector in the context of each national economy. Eg. France looked at the national shipping sector in terms of its importance as a trunk industry; and a significant customer of the national shipbuilding industry, i.e., shipping as subservient to trade and shipbuilding. On the other hand, the U.K. attached much more importance to having a healthy competitive fleet which could generate employment for national seafarers and contribute to the balance of payments of the country. The difference here was between shipper countries and carrier countries. The latter were naturally concerned about the ability of their fleets to offer their services in the cross-trades between third countries and, consequently, wanted to see specific Community action against protectionist measures practiced by other countries, whilst at the same time feared that any process of regulating sea transport within the Community would threaten the international competitive position of their maritime sector. The practice of the Council in its adoption of some 20 legal instruments on shipping until 1985 demonstrated that the Community turned to practical realities and adopted the mosaic or piece-meal approach. It refrained from putting forward an overall arrangement for sea transport. That approach was also in line with the views of CAACE[87] which saw the need for the EC to act as a compact group of countries on specific international shipping policy issues in order to safeguard its shipping interests, but viewed with alarm attempts to regulate shipping within the EC which would deprive it of its commercial freedom.

Under the mosaic approach supported by the Commission any idea of dirigisme in shipping was discarded: measures were to be taken when necessary. Therefore, the idea of setting up a Federal Maritime Commission with wide - ranging powers at Community level seemed more than remote and very rightly so, since the FMC interventionist stance has been constantly the subject of attack from shipping and political ranks in the U.S. and abroad[88].

This piecemeal approach to shaping a common EC shipping policy was further enhanced by the accession of Greece[89] which with a fleet founded and operating on free enterprise principles, is opposed to state intervention in the operations of shipping policies.

Thus, it appears that the two biggest maritime Member States were in accord on the shape that a Community shipping policy should take.

From the assessment of the above positions it was reasonable at the time to infer that the Community reaction to the external pressures on its fleets, such as the Eastern Bloc competition and flag discrimination practices by third countries would not lead to the adoption of extensive internal harmonisation measures which would lead to regulation of the sea transport sector. It is against such a background that the Commission proposals were produced in 1985.

NOTES

1   For the amended Article 84 par.2 by the European Single Act, Article 16 par.5, cf Chapter 8.

2   DOC. VII/S/05230 final of 12 November 1960.
3   DOC. VII/COM (61)50 final of 10 April 1961.
4   DOC. VII/COM (62)88 final of 23 May 1962.
5   DOC. VII/COM (62) 103 final of 16 July 1962 and DOC. VII/COM (62) 261 final of 27 September 1962.

6   O.J. No. 124 of 28 November 1962, p.275.
7   O.J. No. L. 175 of 23 July 1968, p.1.

8   Eighth General Report of the Commission of the EEC on the activities of the Community (1 April 1964 - 31 March 1965) p. 234/235, point 239.

8   Fourth General Report on the activities of the EEC 1970, p.253, point 302.

10 CJEC Judgment of 4 April 1974, case 167/73 Commission v. France

11 The same principle was upheld by the Court later in judgment of 12 October 1978, case 156/77, ie, the ruling indirectly confirmed that the rules on competition formed part of the general rules.

12 Cf A. Bredimas: "Maritime Transport before the Court of Justice of the European Communities", Epitheorissis Emborikou Dikaiou, Athens, 1977, p. 328 (in Greek).

13 No. 209-213/84 Judgment 30/4/86 on "fixing of air tariffs".

14 Cf Anna Bredima "Methods of Interpretation and Community Law", European Studies in Law n° 6, North-Holland Publishing Co., Amsterdam, 1978.

15 OJ No. C. 294 of 13 November 1980, p.6.

16 Cf on 28 November 1977 the Commission submitted to the Council a programme of priority action in the transport sector up to 1980. The Commission regarded the following as priority matters: problems concerning the organisation of liner shipping; the Code of Conduct and flag discrimination; definition of competition rules for sea transport; sub-standard vessels and mutual recognition of seafarers' certificates. Eleventh General Report of the activities of the EC 1977, p. 211, point 380 and p. 125 points 15-17.

17 OJ No. C. 177 p. 1 of 11 July 1981.
18 OJ No. L. 239 of 17 September 1977, p. 23.
19 OJ No. L. 121 of 17 May 1979, p. 1.

20 L. Schmidt - O. Seiler: The UNCTAD Code of Conduct for Liner Conferences, Hamburg, 1979; ACB McIntosh: "Anti-trust implications of liner conferences. Alternatives to the regulation of liner trades with emphasis on the European approach" Lloyd's Maritime and Commercial Law Quarterly, May 1980, pp. 139-154.

21 Communication on relations with third countries in the sea transport sector EC Bull. 6-1976, point 2274, COM (76) 341 final of 30 June 1976, cf also Council Resolution on a Community solution to the problems of sea transport (4/11/75). Tenth General Report on the Activities of the European Communities 1976, p. 257, point 451.

22 EP Resolution of 10 February 1977, OJ No. C. 57 of 7 March 1977, p. 5.

23 EP Resolution of 20 April 1977, OJ No. C. 118 of 16 May 1977, p.4.

Chapter 8
THE 1986 PACKAGE OF MEASURES ADOPTED

Table 2.11
Age Distribution of Principal Fleet by Number of Ships

EEC Countries

EEC Countries	UNDER 5 YEARS 1982	1986	1987	5-10 YEARS 1982	1986	1987	10-15 YEARS 1982	1986	1987	15-20 YEARS 1982	1986	1987	20+ 1982	1986	1987	UNDER 10 YEARS 1982	1986	1987	CHANGE IN PERCENTAGE 1987/1982	1986/1982
BELGIUM	21	21	NA	22	20	NA	16	15	NA	14	12	NA	27	32	NA	43.4	41	NA	NA	-2.39
DENMARK	13	16	16	30	15	13	16	16	22	15	17	15	26	31	34	43	31	29	-14	-12
FRANCE	9	11	11	25	15	14	17	21	24	19	17	13	30	36	38	34	26	25	-9	-8
FRG	21	24	NA	21	22	NA	19	12	NA	16	12	NA	23	30	NA	42	46	NA	NA	4
GREECE	6	11	8	13	21	10	21	38	21	18	19	18	42	11	43	19	32	18	-1	-13
HOLLAND	26	24	NA	28	27	NA	19	22	NA	14	12	NA	13	15	NA	54	51	NA	NA	-3
IRELAND	NA	NA	NA	NA	NA	NA	NA	NA	NA	NA	NA	NA	NA	NA	NA	NA	NA	NA	NA	NA
ITALY	10	7	7	13	13	14	18	19	43	16	20	18	43	41	18	23	20	21	-2	-3
PORTUGAL	11	NA	NA	11	NA	NA	21	NA	NA	21	NA	NA	36	NA	NA	22	NA	NA	NA	NA
SPAIN	12	7	6	27	14	12	17	25	25	18	17	15	26	37	42	39	21	21	NA	-18
UNIT. KINGDOM	13	11	10	24	15	15	18	20	19	15	16	16	30	38	40	37	26	25	12	11

NON EEC Countries

NON EEC Countries	UNDER 5 YEARS 1982	1986	1987	5-10 YEARS 1982	1986	1987	10-15 YEARS 1982	1986	1987	15-20 YEARS 1982	1986	1987	20+ 1982	1986	1987	UNDER 10 YEARS 1982	1986	1987	CHANGE IN PERCENTAGE 1987/1982	1986/1982
BAHAMAS	NA	14	12	NA	23	27	NA	28	32	NA	15	15	NA	20	14	NA	37	39	NA	NA
BRAZIL	24	16	16	23	24	25	20	20	20	6	8	11	31	31	28	47	41	41	-6	-6
CHINA	16	13	11	23	17	18	13	22	17	15	16	41	33	32	13	39	30	29	-10	-9
TAIWAN	16	3	5	16	17	18	45	24	17	37	35	41	2	11	13	32	28	29	-3	-4
CYPRUS	3	5	22	6	12	12	20	27	32	11	8	17	55	25	16	9	13	17	8	-1
HONG-KONG	24	33	28	29	19	24	19	29	30	20	19	30	17	11	12	53	52	46	-7	8
INDIA	17	24	21	23	31	17	20	22	21	11	19	21	21	9	19	40	43	45	5	-1
JAPAN	28	21	8	26	15	32	33	20	21	11	26	19	5	7	38	54	52	53	-1	-3
S. KOREA	14	17	16	15	27	12	24	38	41	8	15	17	14	31	8	29	23	22	-7	-6
LIBERIA	17	23	9	39	27	24	25	23	NA	7	12	NA	7	3	4	56	44	38	-18	-12
N. ZEALAND	30	11	19	24	17	NA	21	17	16	17	17	16	17	15	NA	54	50	24	-17	-4
NORWAY	17	20	10	24	17	15	20	20	22	17	18	17	30	38	44	41	28	36	6	-13
PANAMA	12	23	17	18	12	17	20	15	15	18	25	24	34	25	25	30	37	26	7	7
PHILIPPINES	9	12	NA	10	21	16	21	30	31	12	15	24	40	36	35	19	24	40	-5	5
SINGAPORE	18	11	20	27	18	23	15	15	NA	11	18	21	23	8	NA	45	44	NA	NA	NA
SWEDEN	18	11	25	20	19	NA	20	21	NA	9	15	NA	32	41	NA	38	29	NA	NA	NA
TURKEY	15	15	13	25	15	15	16	19	20	21	23	21	35	30	31	40	32	28	-1	-1
U.S.S.R.	12	NA	NA	17	31	29	20	17	20	14	14	13	30	28	33	29	30	NA	-13	-8
U.S.A.	25	8	5	22	31	29	15	17	20	14	14	13	28	30	33	47	39	34	-13	-8

Source: Lloyd's Register of Shipping: Statistical Tables

24 Economic and Social Committee of the European Communities: "EEC's Transport Problems with East European Countries", Opinion, Brussels, 1977 and OJ No. C. 59 of 8 March 1978, p. 10 and 12 point 15.

25 OJ No. C. 163 of 15 June 1978, p. 49 (Rapporteur Mr. Schmid), OJ No. C. 140 of 5 June 197, p. 171 (Rapporteur Mr. Jung), OJ No. C. 238 of 13 September 1982, p. 96.

26 K. Kwasniewsky: "Shipping Policy of the Comecon Countries" Marine Policy, 1977.

27 Economic and Social Committee of the European Communities "EEC's Transport Problems with East European Countries" Opinion Brussels 1977.

28 OJ No. L. 258 of 21 September 1978, p. 38.
29 OJ No. L. 5 of 9 January 1979, p. 31.
30 OJ No. L. 350 of 23 December 1980, p. 44.
31 OJ No. L. 88 of 2 April 1981, p. 32.
32 OJ No. L. 368 of 28 December 1982, p. 42.
33 OJ No. L. 341 of 29 December 1984, p. 92.
34 OJ No. L. 332 of 28 November 1983, p. 37.

35 The IMO was called IMCO at the time (Intergovernmental Maritime Consultative Organisation).

36 OJ No. L. 194 of 19 July 1978, p. 17 cf also Commission Communication to the Council on marine pollution arising from the carriage of oil OJ No. C. 269 of 13 November 1978, p. 31.

37 OJ No. L. 33/31.
38 OJ No. L. 33/32.
39 OJ No. L. 33/32.
40 EC Bull 11-1978, point 2.1.91
41 OJ No. C. 162 of 8 July 1978, p. 1.
42 OJ No. C. 284 of 28 November 1978, p. 3.
43 OJ No. L. 315 of 11 December 1979, p. 16.
44 OJ No. C. 192 of 30 July 1980, p. 8.
45 OJ No. L. 378 of 31 December 1982, p. 32
46 OJ No. L. 206 of 14 July 1982, p. 46.
47 OJ No. L. 84 of 30 March 1983, p. 9.
48 Idem.
49 OJ No. L. 237 of 26 August 1983, p. 34.
50 OJ No. C. 182 of 20 July 1985.

51 OJ No. L. 125 of 22 May 1979, p. 18.
52 OJ No. C. 228 of 8 August 1980, p. 43.
53 OJ No. L. 209 of 17 August 1977, p. 29.

54 Lord Bruce of Donington : Report to the European
    Parliament on 1) the best   means   of   preventing
    accidents   to   shipping and consequential marine
    and coastal pollution, 2) shipping regulations,
    EP Doc. 555/78, 15/1/79.

55 Cf.   J.Erdmenger   in   "EEC   Shipping   Law",
    Conference 4-5/2/88, Rotterdam, European Study
    Conferences Ltd.

56 October 1, 1980.
57 December 17, 1983.
58 May 21, 1985
59 OJ No. L. 339 of 27 December 1984, p. 10.

60 Cf Doc.   EP 106 of 11 December 1961,   Doc EP 148
    of 24 November 1967,   Doc EP 10/72 of   12   April
    1972.

61 Doc 16/VII/71 of 24 March 1970.
62 Doc. cb/77-863 and VII/440/80.
63 Doc. EP 73. 762.

64 Doc. EP 47.110 and OJ No. C. 96 of 11 April
    1983, p. 116.

65 Commission   of   the   European   Communities,
    "Shipbuilding   -   Reorganisation   Programme".
    Bulletin of the European Communities, Supplement
    7/77.

66 Commission of the European Communities, "Report
    on the State of the Shipbuilding Industry in the
    Community", Com (80)448 final.

67 78/388 EEC OJ No.L.98 of 11 April 1978, p.   19.
    81/363/EEC OJ No.L.137 of 23 May 1981, p.   39.
    82/880/EEC OJ No.L.371 of 30 December 1982,p.46.
    85/2/EEC OJ no.L.2 of 3 January 1985, p.13.
    87/167/EEC OJ no. L.69/55 12 March 1987.

68 OJ No. C. 229 of 27 September 1978, p. 1. This
    resolution related the size of the shipbuilding
    industry to the size of the Community's maritime
    trade   and   its "economic, social and strategic
    importance".

69 Commission of the European Communities, "Communication from the Commission to the Council on a Scheme to Promote the Scrapping and Building of Ocean - Going Ships" "Bulletin of the European Communities", Supplement, 7/79.

70 For a detailed analysis of the issue of nationality of crews cf Robin Churchill "EEC Law and the Nationality of Ships and Crews" in "EEC Shipping Law", Conference 4-5/2/88, Rotterdam, European Study Conferences Ltd.

71 Application of the principle of free movement of workers has given rise to problems in two areas: fishing vessels and pilots. There are currently three cases before the European Court concerning fishing vessels: Case 223/86, Pesca Valentia Ltd v. Minister for Fisheries and Forestry, Ireland; Case 3/87, R. v. Ministry of Agriculture, Fisheries and Food ex p.Agegate Ltd; Case 216/87, R. v. Ministry of Agriculture, Fisheries and Food ex p. Jaderow Ltd.

72 cf. Directive 86/188/EEC 12/5/86, OJ L 137/28, 24/5/86.

73 February 20th, 1979 - under Documents MAR 10, MAR 11, MAR 12.

74 Commission of the European Communities, Survey on Working Hours and Wages in Sea Transport in 1979 in the Member States of the European Communities, June 1980.

75 M. Dubois: "Le principe de la liberte d'etablissement et de Prestations de services en matiere de Transports Maritimes", Colloque 10-12/10-79, Institut Mediterraneen des Transports Maritimes, Marseille.

76 cf. Robin Churchill "EEC Law and the Nationality of Ships and Crews" in "EEC Shipping Law", Conference 4-5/2/88, Rotterdam, European Study Conferences Ltd.

77 Robin Churchill, ibid, argues as follows: where a shipowner having the nationality of Member State B and established in that State, wishes to

transport goods in a ship flying the flag of
State B between two ports in Member State A,
which reserves such cabotage to ships having its
nationality, the exclusion of the shipowner is
not contrary to Community law. Freedom of
establishment is not at issue, but the right to
provide services. There is, however, no
automatic freedom to provide services in
transport. Thus, reserving cabotage to the
national flag as per the above case, is not
contrary to Community Law.

78 "The Economic Implications of the Reservation of
    Coastal Shipping to National Flag Ships within
    the Community and of the Abandonment of such
    Reservation", August 1979.

79 Infringement case B/70/78 Commission v. France.
    The case was discontinued following exchange of
    letters between the Commission and France and
    subsequent changes of French Ministerial
    decisions.

80 Although Articles 59-66 EEC are included in the
    fundamental rules of the Treaty that could apply
    to shipping, under Article 61, freedom to
    provide services in the transport sector is
    governed by the provisions of Title IV on common
    transport policy among which Article 84 para 2
    is enlisted. Thus it is left to the Council
    acting on the various legal bases to be found in
    the chapter of the Treaty on Transport to make
    suitable provision as regards the freedom to
    provide transport services. In case 13/83
    (European Parliament v. Commission), the Court
    found that the Council was at fault for not
    having adopted provisions applying this freedom
    to inland transport, whilst it made no express
    finding as regards air and sea transport. It
    may be inferred from this that the Council is
    under no duty to elaborate such provisions for
    air and sea transport. cf George Close "Free
    Access to Cargoes and Freedom to Operate" in
    "EEC Shipping Law", Conference 4-5/2/88,
    Rotterdam, European Study Conferences Ltd.

81 No. 209-213/84, on "fixing of air
    tariffs"/judgment 30/4/86.

82 OJ No. C. 282 of 5 November 1981, p. 4 and No.
    C. 339 of 29 December 1981, p. 4.

83 Resolution adopted on 24/5/84 and Nyborg Interim
    Report of 21/5/84, Doc-1-249/84/B, PE 78-
    589/fin.

84 Opinion of 27 January 1983 (Rapporteurs R.
    Bonety, A. Bredima) OJ No. C. 77 of 21 March
    1983, p. 13.

85 The reason obviously being that 90% of the extra
    Community trade is carried by sea as contrasted
    to 25% of the intra-Community trade.

86 R. Burke: "Towards a Shipping Policy for the
    EEC", Seatrade Conference, Brussels, 11/9/78.
    R. Burke: "Shipping Policy a view of Western
    Europe", Stockholm School of Economics, 22/6/79.

87 CAACE Annual Report 1978, Brussels, May 1979.

88 See also Seatrade Publication Ltd Seatrade U.S.
    Yearbook, 1979.

89 A. Bredimas "The Common Shipping Policy of the
    EEC", Common Market Law Review 1981, p. 9-32, S.
    Plyntzanopoulos: "The Greek Merchant Marine
    after accession to the EEC", Greek Association
    of Maritime Law, Athens 1980 (in Greek). J.G.
    Tzoannos "Greek Merchant Marine and EEC
    implications from accession", Institute of
    Economic and Industrial Research, Athens 1977
    (in Greek)

CHAPTER 5

1985 COMMISSION MEMORANDUM AND PROPOSALS
FOR A COMMON MARITIME POLICY

INTRODUCTION

It is evident from the preceding analysis that the case law of the European Court of Justice and the Community measures adopted in the period between 1958-1985 were far from constituting a common maritime policy. Since developments were equally slow in land and air transport, the European Parliament under the influence (in fact it was the wrath) of the then Chairman of its Transport Committee, Mr. Horst Seefeld, introduced before the European Court of Justice in 1983 a recourse for inaction against the Commission and the Council for non respect of the general purposes of the EEC Treaty in the transport sector. The Court[1] ruled that the Commission was under the obligation to elaborate proposals in the transport sector. Here again, a pronouncement of the Court triggered action and the Commission volens nolens formally submitted policy papers in February 1983 (on inland transport), in March 1984 (on civil aviation) and in March 1985 (on maritime transport).

The paper, entitled, "Communication and Proposals by the Commission to the Council on Progress towards a Common Transport Policy-Maritime Transport"[2], was officially released on 14 March 1985. At this juncture it is worthwhile stating a bit of history concerning elaboration of the Commission paper. The paper was officially approved by the Commission in collegium in December 1984 under the Greek Transport Commissioner, Mr. G. Contogeorgis. Thereafter, in January '85 the Transport portfolio was entrusted to the British Commissioner, Mr. S. Clinton Davis. From the outset, Mr. Clinton Davis made it publicly known that he had certain misgivings about the Memorandum and that he would wish it to be more pronounced over labour issues, flags of convenience and, thus, in its overall approach less liberal. Taking advantage of the fact that in the "interregnum" between the two Commissioners - over Christmas 1985 - the versions in all languages were not ready, the new Commissioner proceeded with some amendments in the text of the Memorandum, not in the legislative proposals. These amendments were basically the following:

The wording of the Memorandum concerning open registries has been toned down without its being coupled, however, with a change in the overall policy on open registries. Thus, there are changes to the effect that open registry shipping is considered as having "undesirable effects" and in some respects may "not be in conformity with international conventions" and that measures should be taken to eliminate "unacceptable practices".

In the paragraphs concerning manpower and social aspects there is a series of presentational changes designed to adjust the tone of the section and to stress that social and employment issues are closely linked to international policy. More particularly, attention is drawn to the adverse consequences for the EEC of a reduction in the number of available seafarers. Moreover, an official dialogue between the social partners should be established to promote a greater consensus on general problems in shipping. The new text also calls for a detailed study on the problems of non domiciled seafarers to be undertaken in this area, whilst the previous text gave a degree of acceptance to EEC owners employing non-EEC nationals. There are also some other changes, such as adding to the list of major long-term factors affecting the structure of Community shipping the following factors: major takeovers, diversification by shipping companies into non-maritime activities and increased influence of financial institutions as beneficial owners of ships. Finally, reference is made to the need for concerted action on hydrography.

It is this amended version that was adopted by the Commission on the 14 March 1985. Nevertheless, although it was initially accepted by the Commission in December 1984 and subsequently as amended in March 1985, the basic structure of the document and the basic data upon which it was based was that gathered in 1983 or even 1982. This is a drawback when assessing the proposals because we are dealing with a constantly changing perspective as far as shipping is concerned. The Commission believes that the time has come "to develop a more coherent overall framework for a Community shipping policy" and that this overall concept of shipping policy "should be read in conjunction with the policy papers on inland transport and civil aviation because "taken together they meet the Parliament's request for a comprehensive approach to the common transport policy". The policy paper, however, should also be read against the background of the sharp decline of the Community fleet and of the prolonged shipping crisis. These were in fact as acknowledged in the first few lines of the Commission's proposal the main causes which necessitated a common policy.

GIST OF THE COMMISSION MEMORANDUM

The Memorandum analyses, on the one hand, the importance of maritime transport for the Community as follows:

The European Community is the leading trading area in the world. Its trade with third countries in 1982 represented 21% by value of world imports and 20% of world exports. The share of the USA, the second most important trading area, amounted to 16% of world imports and 10% of world exports. Maritime transport is far and away the most important carrier of this trade. About 95% of the total quantity of EC trade with third countries and about 30% of intra-Community traffic is carried by sea. In 1982 the fleets belonging to EC Member States earned net incomes of approximately U.S.$ 9.1 thousand million, of which approximately 50% derived from cross trades varied from approximately 90% in the case of Denmark and Greece to approximately 35% in the case of France. These figures show in the Commission's view, how dependent the EC is on world trade and how dependent its maritime shipping interests are in turn on the international maritime shipping markets.

Thereafter, the Memorandum proceeds to an analysis of the development of the Community fleet in the course of recent years, this part constituting the reasoning for the Commission proposals. The Commission recognizes that between 1975-1983, the Community share of world tonnage has fallen from 29% to 23,3% in 1983. There has, thus, been a marked decline in the share of world tonnage represented by the merchant fleets operating under the flags of Community countries. This development is contrasted with the growth of the fleets of developing countries and to a lesser extent of open registry fleets and COMECON fleets. Nevertheless, since 1975 the absolute size of merchant fleets under Member States' flags has decreased only slightly. The Memorandum also notes that the effects of the recession may be seen in the age profile of Member States' fleets which are now marginally older than the world average.

The Memorandum acknowledges as well that the proportion of world trade carried by the Community fleet in 1983 was still about 40%. This is the reason why the Commission believes that the relative decline of the Community fleet has not reached the critical point that would necessitate a stark choice between "maintaining the fleet at the expense of the taxpayer" or of "letting the fleet go".

The Commission identifies the long term causes of the relative decline of the Community fleet as follows:

1) The slump in world demand has imposed financial strains on Community shipowners which have caused them to sell off ships to buyers in third countries.

2) The comparative advantage of European shipping is being eroded. Technological innovation (eg. container ships), greater specialisation (eg. liquefied gas carriers), higher quality services are becoming increasingly costly, and this has stimulated "flagging out", ie, registering ships under non-EEC flags; this kind of measure allows Community firms to retain economic control of the ships while avoiding what they see as the competitive disadvantage of operating under Community flags.

3) In the liner trades the situation has become worse as a result of competition from state trading countries and cargo reservation by developing countries.

4) There has been a marked shift in trade patterns over the last decade, particularly in the oil

trades, where a large number of oil tankers have become redundant.

5) These structural weaknesses have been exacerbated by the prolonged world recession in which world trade has stagnated while the size of the world fleet has grown, leading to a massive excess of supply over demand for shipping services.

In considering what policy to adopt in face of the decline of Community fleets, the Commission argues that a protectionist policy would almost certainly encourage further protectionism in the USA and most other countries and cross trading opportunities would be lost, whilst in the direct trades little or nothing would be gained. In view of the Community's dependence on world trade and the dependence of its shipping interests on international shipping markets, the Commission is of the opinion that the maintenance of a multilateral market-economy oriented maritime shipping policy is still in the interests of the EC shipping industry and that of shippers. The Commission holds this view despite the fact that as a result of the continuing recession in world trade, reductions in comparative cost advantages and increasing protectionism on the part of third countries, EC vessels have a declining share of the world fleet. Such a policy is, in the Commission's view, the best way of achieving the objectives of the Treaty. This liberal, free trade approach becomes the key element that permeates the Memorandum and the legislative proposals. The Commission remarks that it is, however, now more necessary than ever for the Community and the Member States to take action against the growing danger to EC interests posed by practices and protectionist measures employed by non-EC countries which make it more difficult, if not impossible, to maintain a market economy system. One of the priorities of the Memorandum is, therefore, to set out proposed countermeasures by means of which the Commission hopes it will be possible to negotiate an effective solution to the problem.

The Memorandum expresses willingness on the part of the Commission to intensify its cooperation in shipping matters with the ACP countries, through the

Lome III Convention, but expects them to refrain from acts restricting access to sea transport.

In pursuing a non protectionist policy, Community action should be guided by a number of basic principles:

1) International agreement is preferable to unilateral Community action.

2) The predominant issues in shipping concern trade with third countries.

3) Common action towards third countries should be matched by equality of treatment of Community shipowners by Member States.

4) The Community should seek to improve the competitiveness of Community shipping and in this way the better employment opportunities for seafarers.

5) The Community should support international measures to improve maritime safety.

The Memorandum equally contains more detailed analyses, sector by sector.

In the social field, in 1983 some 250.000 to 300.000 people were registered as ratings in the Community countries. Due to the increasing size of the vessels and the overall reduction of the fleet, the number of seafarers declined by one third between 1960 and 1980. Non-EEC seafarers represented 15% to 20% of the manpower of the Community fleet, percentage varying considerably among Member States. There are also differences in the wages paid to seafarers and in the social security systems. The Commission does not propose any harmonisation measures but limits itself to the elaboration of a study in the context of an ad hoc Consultative Committee on maritime matters giving emphasis to a favourable direct tax system for Community seafarers and to mutual recognition of diplomas, licences and certificates of competency.

In the technical field, the Commission proposes studies to improve the competitiveness of the European fleet as well as for the safety of navigation and pollution prevention to which all it attaches a great importance. In this regard, the Commission wishes to reinforce the system of port control established by the 1982 European Memorandum (MOU) by writing the MOU into Community law. Moreover, it proposes a Directive establishing a Community wide list of approved ship equipment in order to facilitate the transfer of ships between Member States. It also invites:

- consideration of the need for a network of shore-based navigation aids to improve maritime safety in the Community's coastal waters, followed by the establishment of such a network if it proves advisable;
- the establishment of common standards for the training of Vessel Traffic Management Services (VTS) staff (captains and crews).

More specifically with regard to the liner sector, the Commission continues to subscribe to the view that the liner conference system is beneficial to world seaborne trade in providing stability of freight rates and regularity of service. Nevertheless, the Commission views with concern the increasing trend to excluding non conference competition (eg. outsiders) from trades in which closed conferences operate. Accordingly, the Commission proposes modifying its original draft competition regulation with a view to tightening up conditions of liner conference exemption from the application of the competition rules of the EEC Treaty. In the same sector, the Commission recommends ratification of the UNCTAD Liner Code under the reservations of the Brussels Package (Regulation 954/79) and the declaration on outsiders elaborated in the Round Table of April 1984.

With respect to the bulk sector, the Commission concludes that world shipping operates by and large in a competitive environment. There is, therefore, no need to apply the competition rules of the Treaty and maintenance of the status quo for the Community -apart from specific action proposed in the legislative annexes- is the best possible policy for the Community. The Commission also surveys developments in open registry shipping and here states that the real problem does not lie in the distinction between open registries and other flags but rather with substandard vessels to be found under any flag. It considers that EC beneficial ownership of shipping is not negligible as a complement of the fleets under the registry of Member States. Thus, it enables Community shipowners to average their costs between high cost operations under the national flag and lower cost open registry operations.

The Commission subscribes to the distinction made by OECD countries - in the context of prolonged discussions in the UNCTAD forum - between open registries and substandard vessels. It believes that economic advantages accrue to the Community by the operation of these fleets, which is by and large beneficial, namely, keeping low transport costs to the benefit of the consumer. On the other hand, the Commission affirms that there is a need to tighten the administrative link between flag state and ship in order to enable more transparency and accountability of the owership and the improvement of ship safety and social standards by implementation and control of relevant international conventions. The Commission Memorandum, thus, dismisses claims of the so-called economic genuine link between flag state and ship, which may be subsumed into a nationality requirement of the flag state in the manning, management and ownership of the vessel.

As regards sea ports, the Commission asserts that they should be considered against the background of the establishment of a common transport policy covering maritime shipping and inland transport. In its Communication the Commission, therefore, draws attention to the proposal which it recently submitted to the Council on the elimination of distortions in competition between sea ports owing to different regulations laid down by the various Member States with regard to hinterland traffic. The Commission has let it be known that it will be taking a fresh look at State aids to sea ports and intends to tackle this issue on the basis of Articles 92 and 93 of the Treaty.

The Commission also intends to intensify its cooperation with sea ports in the field of information technology (exchange of information).

Finally, the Commission intends to put forward proposals by 1986 at the latest, with regard to research programmes in the field of maritime transport (maritime systems, transport needs, new means of transport, ship-harbour interfaces, ship safety and environmental protection, ship economy and competitiveness). The Commission also wishes to exercise more effective control over the transport of EC food aid to developing countries and maritime fraud.

SYNOPSIS OF THE COMMISSION PROPOSALS

The above analyses in the Memorandum are further substantiated by a list of statistical tables contained in Annex I, which, because drafted rapidly in the last months of 1984, do not take into consideration statistics for 1983. In view of the rapidity of developments in world maritime transport since then, relatively outdated statistics are obviously a handicap. Thereafter, comes Annex II containing the six legislative proposals on a common maritime policy as follows:

1) Draft Council Regulation concerning coordinated action to safeguard free access to cargoes in ocean trades (II-1).

2) Draft Council Regulation applying the principle of freedom to provide services to maritime transport (II-2).

3) Draft Council Decision amending Council Decision No. 77/587/EEC of 13/9/77 setting up a consultation procedure on relations between Member States and third countries in shipping matters and on action relating to such matters in international organisations (II-3).

4) Draft Council Directive concerning a common interpretation of the concept of "national shipping line" (II-4).

5) Amendments to the Proposal for a Council Regulation (EEC) laying down Detailed Rules for the application of Articles 85 and 86 of the Treaty to Maritime Transport (II-5).

6) Draft Council Regulation on unfair pricing practices in maritime transport (liner trade) (II-6).

1) Draft Council Regulation concerning coordinated action to safeguard free access to cargoes in ocean trades.

The first proposal concerns a draft regulation based on Art. 84 paragraph 2 of the EEC Treaty to coordinate action between Member States and the Commisssion against third countries in the liner or bulk trades so as to safeguard free access to cargoes in the ocean trades by shipping companies of the EC or the OECD.

The purpose is to reinforce the position of Member States in resisting protectionist measures taken by third countries. Coordinated action is to proceed in two stages:
a) diplomatic measures, and if these fail,
b) counter-measures directed at the shipping companies of the offending country.

The counter-measures may consist of a partial or total restriction of access to cargoes (quotas), permits or financial charges.

There is immunity, however, from EC counter-measures if the third country restricts access according to the provisions of the UN Code.

EEC Member States officials together with officials of other OECD countries participate in the so-called Consultative Shipping Group (CSG) which has been holding for a number of years (since 1981) meetings with the United States in the context of the CSG/US dialogue with a view to signing an agreement concerning mutual resistance to protectionist practices by third countries. One of the purposes of Annex II-1 was in fact to enable the Community to honour its commitment vis-a-vis the United States in view of the mutual agreement signed on April 28, 1986 by providing with a legislative instrument for the mechanism of coordinated resistance against protectionism.

2) Draft Council Regulation applying the principle of freedom to provide services in sea transport.

The second proposal (Annex II-2) involves a draft Regulation for the application of the principle of freedom to provide services to sea transport, based again on Article 84 paragraph 2 of the EEC Treaty.

The Regulation will abolish restrictions in the provision of such services by persons (legal or natural) established in a member state other than that of the person for whom the services are intended in (a) the trades between any two Member States, (b) the coastal trades of a Member State (cabotage) including its overseas territories, (c) the trades between a Member State and third countries (cross-trading) and (d) the supply of off-shore installations.

In the case of cabotage the abolition will take place within a transitional period of ten years from the date the Regulation comes into force (or longer in particularly difficult cases in specific regions), while in the cases of bilateral cargo sharing agreements between a member country and a third country or off-shore supply services, the transitional period for the abolition is five years. During these transitional periods no member state will be permitted to make existing provisions restricting access to cargoes less favourable to persons established in other member states.

Annex II-2 has the purpose of applying to maritime transport one of the fundamental principles of Community law, namely, the removal of any national obstacle in the activities of a national of another Member State, that is, equality of treatment of Community shipowners by Member States.

Annex II-2 was designed to encourage free trade in shipping operations within the EEC, whilst Annex II-1 was designed to counter protectionism practised by non-EEC countries.

3) Draft Council Decision amending Decision 77/587/EEC setting up a consultation procedure on relations between Member States and third countries in shipping matters and on action relating to such matters in international organisations.

The third proposal (Annex II-3) based on Article 84 paragraph 2 of the EEC Treaty concerns a draft Decision which amends the existing one (Decision 77/587/EEC) setting up a consultation procedure among member countries on their maritime relations with third countries or on their action relating to maritime affairs in international organisations.

The aim here is to make the consultation procedure more meaningful by obliging a Member State that is negotiating shipping agreements with third countries to consult other Member States ex ante (prior) to the conclusion of the bilateral or multilateral agreements so that these agreements respect the measures adopted jointly in pursuance of Community maritime policy in light of the principles of the EEC Treaty. Indirectly, this decision also aims at discouraging the conclusion of such agreements by individual Member States.

4) Draft Council Directive concerning a common interpretation of the concept of "national shipping line".

The fourth proposal (Annex II-4) based on Article 84 paragraph 2 of the EEC Treaty concerns a draft Directive on the definition of "national shipping line" for the purposes of implementing the UN Code of Conduct of Liner Conferences as modified by the Brussels Package (954/79).

In adopting Regulation 954/79 concerning ratification of the UNCTAD Liner Code, the Council envisaged the possibility of a joint interpretation of the concept of national shipping line which confers, in Code based trades, important rights on liner shipping companies. The Commission's draft Directive suggests a set of criteria for such a definition designed to avoid any discrimination between shipping lines in the Member States and, subject to reciprocity, shipping lines of other OECD countries, without denying each Member State the flexibility to take into account its particular national circumstances. The directive is also aimed at preventing the abuse of the criterion of the national shipping line by companies belonging to nationals of third countries by imposing additional criteria to those imposed by the Regulation 954/79.

The criteria proposed by the draft Directive are the following according to Article 1 para 2:

a) The head-office of management and the effective control must be situated in a Member State.

b) The executive board must consist of persons the majority of whom are nationals of EEC Member States.

c) The company shares must be controlled effectively through a majority shareholding by nationals of EEC Member States who have their domicile or registered office, in one of the EEC Member States.

Moreover, the draft provides for the criterion of ships flying the flag of a Member State which may be added in certain circumstances.

5) Amendments to the proposal for the Council Regulation laying down detailed rules for the application of Articles 85 and 86 of the Treaty to maritime transport.

The fifth proposal (Annex II-5) based on both Articles 84 paragraph 2 and 87 of the EEC Treaty contains amendments to the 1981 draft Regulation laying down rules for the application of the competition rules to liner trades. Tramp vessel services are expressis verbis not covered by the scope of the Regulation.

Whilst acknowledging the stabilizing role of liner conferences, guaranteeing regular and reliable services to transport users, the Commission, in laying dowing the conditions for the exemption of the conferences from the competition rules, seems concerned about the increasing trend towards exclusion of outsider competition from trades in which closed conferences operate.

The new version results from extensive discussions in the Community institutions over the original 1981 draft. Thus, on the one hand it validates the positions of liner conferences (associations of shipping lines) under Community law by exempting them en bloc from the EEC Treaty's ban on restrictive agreements. The exemption, on the other hand, would be subject to certain conditions:

1) conferences must not discriminate between ports or shippers on non justifiable economic grounds,
2) they should consult shippers on matters on common interest,
3) their "loyalty agreements" with their customers should fulfil reasonable criteria,
4) they should publish tariffs,
5) they should not act predatorily towards competitors.

Breach of these conditions would result in sanctions, which could include withdrawal of the block exemption, though this could be replaced by an individual exemption on terms to be decided by the Commission.

6) Draft Council Regulation on unfair pricing practices in maritime transport.

The final proposal (Annex II-6) concerns a draft Regulation to deal with unfair pricing practices in cargo liner shipping practiced by shipowners established in a third country and it is based on article 84 paragraph 2 of the EEC Treaty.

"Unfair pricing practices" are taken to mean the continuous charging of a freight rate on a particular shipping route which is lower than the lowest rate charged during at least one year on the same route and for the same commodity by an established and "representative" outsider.

The draft Regulation envisages detailed procedures for the lodging of complaints, the examination of the injury on Community shipowners and the imposition of redressive duties (levies) on the offenders.

In the Commission's view, the proposal on the application of the competition articles of the Treaty to liner shipping needed to be complemented by this proposal ensuring that Community liner shipping can compete with third countries liner shipping companies on the basis of fair and commercial principles. The Commission, therefore, proposes to be empowered to act against unfair

practices where they cause or threaten to cause
material injury to Community liner companies or
where they enjoy unfair competitive advantages (eg.
through state ownership, cargo reservation
agreements, or operation under the flag of a state
outside IMO and ILO Conventions). In fact, the
draft Regulation is an anti-dumping Regulation for
the liner shipping sector.

NOTES

1   European Parliament v. Council, Case 13/83,
    22/5/85, O.J C 144, 13/6/85.

2   Doc. COM (85) 90 final. Cf also Bulletin of the
    European Communities, Supplement 5/85 and O.J
    C212 of 23 August 1985 pp. 2-21 (proposals only).

CHAPTER 6

ATTITUDES VIS-A-VIS COMMON SHIPPING POLICY PROPOSALS BY VARIOUS INTEREST GROUPS

The release of the Commission's Memorandum - the gestation of which was public and common knowledge to interested parties which were frequently consulted in the course of its preparation in Brussels - triggered debates at several levels: in the various Community institutions involved in the EC legislative process, ie, Council, EP, ESC; within the Member States between the government and private interest groups focussing evidently on the national interest of each one of them; and within interest groups at Community level, such as the ESC, CAACE, ITF, Shipbuilders.

It is interesting to register the various points of view on the various aspects of the Memorandum and its proposals against the melting pot of all these views that the Commission's paper purports to have taken into consideration.

EUROPEAN SHIPPERS COUNCILS

In late December 1985, the European Shippers Council (ESC)[1] produced a document with their detailed views on the EC Commission's Maritime Transport Memorandum. The same views were widely publicized in the press and the ESC participated in numerous occasions at hearings or gatherings to put forward their views, such as the EP Hearing on February 26, 1986 and in oral testimony before the U.K. House of Lords on November 7, 1985 and February 12, 1986.

The ESC view is that the main task of the Community maritime policy should be to secure healthy competition both within the EC and in trade with third countries. The ESC therefore welcome the rejection by the Commission of a protectionist policy as well as the criticism of bilateral cargo allocation. Their views are based on the fundamental principle that maritime policy should be directed at equipping the fleet to meet the needs of the Community's industries in international trade. A basic shortcoming of the Memorandum is the fact

that shipping markets are examined in isolation
without due regard to developments in international
trade markets. The question centres on the
Community fleet's ability to compete with maximum
efficiency. The ESC are more confident than the
Commission regarding the general health of the
Community fleet: in the shippers' view, the EEC
fleet is relatively strong in the main growth areas
(cellular containers) with a reasonable share of
world trade and is sensibly reducing tonnage in the
tanker and bulk trades. The Commission, however,
fails to pay due regard to market developments in
international trade and misinterprets the reasons
for structural changes in the Community fleet. This
is reflected in the nature of some of the draft
proposals.

The ESC expresses concern that some proposals
might already be overtaken by economic events and
points to consequences of failing to prepare for
changes in liner shipping that will affect the
structure of the conference system. The Memorandum
is based on the assumptions that the conference
system as it existed for many years is generally
beneficial and that it will continue in existence
for years to come unchanged but it does not offer an
analysis of the pros and cons of the system. In the
view of ESC neither of these assumptions is valid.
On the one hand, ESC face in recent years rate
instability attributed to conference practices. On
the other hand, the trend towards high technology
fleets will increase the quality gap among groups of
shipping lines within conference and will result in
competition among them. ESC therefore see a danger
that legislation will enshrine obsolete practices
concerning the liner conference system and will lack
the flexibility to accommodate and encourage future
beneficial commercial developments.

By and large, shippers do not consider as
important Annex II-4 (national shipping line) and
see no need for a regulation on unfair pricing
practices (Annex II-6). Shippers agree that the
remaining proposals are interdependent and should be
treated as a single policy package. Nevertheless,
ESC consider that priority should be further given
to Annexes II-1 (access to cargo), Annex II-2
(freedom to provide services) and Annex II-3
(consultation procedure). Thereafter, the

competition Regulation (Annex II-5) will be seen in its proper perspective in that there are significant omissions from the draft regulation. Specifically, there are no clear references to shippers' associations, to service agreements and to the inherent risks of large consortia and international shipping companies achieving a dominant position in specific markets.

With regard to the legislative proposals, we highlight some of the basic comments put forward by ESC:

Annex II-1

The immunity for action (article 1) taken in accordance with the UNCTAD Code is extremely dangerous because third countries, in particular less developed countries, usually claim the UNCTAD Code as the legal basis of practices which often exceed its provisions.

Annex II-2

The Draft Regulation will create a more competitive maritime market within the EC in that any Community shipping line would be able to provide services from any EC port. In order to minimise turn-round time, conferences continue to reduce the number of ports of call, thus increasing the need for feeder services; this development makes this draft Regulation even more important. It will also widen the choice of services available to shippers who will welcome the resulting elimination of existing bilateral cargo sharing agreements. The period for gradual abolition is excessive; total abolition should be achieved before the programmed implementation of the policy package.

Annex II-5

The ESC consider that the conference system as such is in contradiction with Article 85 of the EEC Treaty and in many cases with Article 86. The present Regulation should be a means by which the present imbalance of advantages between shipowners and shippers is corrected through the elimination of a number of serious faults in the present system. As it was found necessary for the EC Member States

to disregard several fundamental provisions of the
Code in the interest of shipowners (eg. cargo
sharing), this disregard will also be necessary on
other issues (eg. loyalty) in the interest of
Community shippers.[2]

Article 5 paragraph 1

The definition of "transport user" under Article
1 paragraph 3(c) would seem to exclude Shippers'
Councils in Europe; therefore, it will be necessary
to add "and/or their organisations" after "transport
users".

Aritcle 5 paragraph 2

The legal fairness of a loyalty contract will be
unchallengeable if this article becomes law in the
Community. Loyalty is a major tool by which the
conference maintains its large market share and
limits the possibility of competition by compelling
the shipper to commit all his cargo to the
conference. The ESC believe that old style loyalty
should now be replaced by a new relationship between
shippers and conference lines taking into
consideration the advent of service contracts. Such
contracts have been to the benefit of large shippers
who are required to supply a specific volume of
goods over a specific period of time at an
individually agreed rate. The Regulation should,
therefore, provide for service contracts. It should
also provide improved protection for small shippers
who may not have sufficient traffic to negotiate
service contracts. Such protection could be
provided by introducing the concept of shippers
associations which combine cargoes of various
shippers and negotiate collective contracts. The
shippers associations should be granted exemption
(under Article 85 paragraph 3 of the Treaty) in
Article 6.

Instead of prescribing in great detail how the
antiquated loyalty system should operate, the
regulation should set out a number of general
criteria to be fulfilled in the contractual
relationsip between shippers and conference lines.
The general criteria form a four-tier system:

1) rights and obligations under a contract should be fairly divided between the parties.
2) No contract may be required by a conference to cover the totality of any shipper's cargo.
3) Any contract must be for a specified duration. Notice of termination should be given not more than three months.
4) Shippers should have a choice of signing a contract either with the conference or with an individual line since service standards vary between conference lines and price is based on them.

Article 7 paragraph 2(c)

ESC believe that if effective competition is eliminated, the block exemption should be withdrawn and any new special exemption should be conditional upon the reappearance of effective competition.

Annex II-6

This proposal is clearly out of line with the declared goals of the Memorandum, namely, rejection of a protectionist policy. This proposal would actually introduce a protectionist policy and is, therefore, opposed by European Shippers. If the proposal were to be adopted it would result in a general increase in the level of freight rates quoted by independent lines to be "on the safe side"; it would result in a reduction in the number of independent lines since more lines would seek conference membership and in an alignment of the competitive pattern in a given trade on that dictated by the conference cartel. A further negative effect is that the EC would lose credibility in international discussions on maritime policy and it would no longer be possible for the EC to combat flag discrimination. With regard to the specific problem of alleged unfair competition from Eastern bloc fleets, Member States agreed in 1983 under the terms of a Decision to consult on and coordinate any measures to be taken. So, existing instruments are sufficient rather than creating new ones of such sweeping scope. The competition rules of the EEC Treaty have as their purpose to protect normal market competition against cartels. The purpose of the present proposal seems to be the contrary. Finally, the Memorandum offers no documentation of the presence of unfair pricing practices and, thus, does not substantiate the need for the legislation being proposed.[3]

Articles 1 and 2

By limiting the application of a redressive duty to "foreign shipowners", the EC would discriminate unfairly in favour of a number of Community shipowners who are to be found in one or all of the categories set out in Article 3 paragraph 2:

- some Community shipping lines are government controlled
- some EC Member States have bilateral cargo sharing agreements
- some EC Member States have not ratified all the Conventions referred to in the Annex.

The Commission proposes to use as a standard of assessment the lowest freight rates charged by an established and representative independent shipowner. This means that ultimately the rate policy of the Conference is taken as the standard.

On the whole, despite particular criticisms, the Memorandum was supported by the ESC.

COMITE DES ASSOCIATIONS D'ARMATEURS DES COMMUNAUTES EUROPEENNES (CAACE)

CAACE[4] as early as October 1983 forwarded in a submission to the Commission a list of priorities for measures to be taken by the EC. Rather than advocating a comprehensive and cohesive long term shipping policy, CAACE -recognizing the difficulties in structuring and implementing such a policy- proposed that the Community pursue a realistic and pragmatic approach in the following fields: entry into force of the UNCTAD Liner Code and tackling the problems arising in the context of the CSG/US dialogue, the definition of a national shipping line, consultation with non OECD countries as to their terms of application of the Code; countermeasures vis-a-vis non' commercial competition, measures in the social field as well as in the anti-pollution, safety of navigation field. The overriding consideration still was that shipowners did not like "to find themselves in a situation whereby, through over-regulation or administrative measures, they were being put in a straight jacket". This first move still indicated preference for a mosaic approach that prevailed in the seventies but at the same time indicated awareness of the need for urgent measures to be adopted in a number of fields.

The shift in CAACE policy in favour of a global approach is clearcut and pronounced in the Memorandum containing CAACE views on the Commission's policy paper released in April 1985. CAACE welcomes the Commission's policy paper introducing a comprehensive shipping policy. The present critical situation of the Community fleet demands clear political action and the paper represents an important starting point in this political process and a valuable basis for a policy to defend and promote the EC fleet. CAACE stresses the importance of shipping to the EC as an earner of foreign exchange, as an employer at sea and ashore, as a provider of transport services for external trade to and from the Community and for its strategic value. CAACE shipowners - as home traders but also cross traders - believe whole - heartedly in a liberal policy and in resisting protectionism in shipping under any name. It must, however, be said that the commercial and political realities of today's world are unfortunately eroding the free market approach. In the liner trades, the choice is not necessarily a stark one between a free market and a protectionist path. CAACE sees the need for a balanced and pragmatic approach through a free trade policy aimed at improving the competitiveness of the EC shipping industry in the international markets and selective/defensive actions where political or economic distortions exist, coupled with the opening up of a genuine common market in shipping as between Member States. The CAACE Memorandum attributes the drastic decline of the relative importance of the Community fleet to the following reasons: the world trade recession, overtonnaging, the growth of protectionist practices by third countries and the unfair pricing behaviour of subsidised or state controlled carriers.

The CAACE paper characterizes the Commission's Memorandum as a useful endeavour to try to translate the principles of the EEC Treaty into shipping terms and stresses that while no individual Member State can hope effectively to tackle these problems, together there is a real opportunity for the health of the industry to be restored. The paper endorses the concept of a "package" of four regulations to be given priority in terms of adoption but recognizes that all six proposals will not solve all the difficulties and should be followed by further positive measures to enhance the competitiveness of the EC fleets.

Nevertheless, the "package" of four proposals should be adopted as soon as possible. Without urgent action, CAACE can only foresee a further decline in the fortunes of the industry.

With regard to the issue of countermeasures, CAACE endorses the Commission's stance and - whilst an advocate of free and fair competition in both liner and non - liner trades - justifies it in view of the problems of unfair pricing practices encountered in the liner sector.

CAACE further welcomes the Commission's concern about prompt finalization of the CSG/US dialogue and proposes extension of the principles to emanate from the dialogue to non-liner trades, the cruising market and cross trades.

The external common policy, as envisaged by CAACE, needs to be complemented by achievement of the internal market, so that the liberalisation process should be coupled with a certain harmonisation in order to remove distortions in competitive capabilities.

On the more specific issues of the Commission Memorandum, which are not covered in the Annexes, CAACE comments as follows:

- There should be greater coordination of national assistance to shipping companies within the EC and the EEC should resist undesirable national shipbuilding subsidies worldwide where they contribute to the overtonnaging crisis. Recourse to scrapping at Community or national level rather than to second hand market is also necessary.

- With regard to social aspects, CAACE fully endorses the Commission's views and more particularly the statement in the Memorandum that it is impossible to insulate employment problems from the full international dimensions of shipping. Similarly, CAACE fully espouses the Commission's views on bulk markets and open registries, safety of navigation, pollution prevention and maritime fraud.

Concerning the Annexes to the Memorandum, we highlight some of the basic comments advanced by CAACE:

Annex II-1

The beneficiaries of this Annex[5] (the same applying to Annex II-2) should be - apart from companies established in an EC Member States - alternatively "vessels flying the flag of a Member State".

The countermeasures proposed are more liner oriented and therefore in devising them, the particular nature of the bulk sector should also be taken into consideration.

Non discriminatory shipping clauses should be incorporated in EC trade agreements with third countries.

Annex II-2

Whilst supporting early enactment of this proposal, CAACE recognizes that in certain circumstances transitional periods[6] may be necessary because of the sensitivities of the sectors involved. Namely, the social/political dimension in the serving of islands should be fully recognised and dealt with in the context of cabotage provisions. In order to encourage the principle of freedom to provide services to become a reality, CAACE believes that the differences in Member States laws affecting the basic costs of EC shipowners should be considered, namely, taxes, manning scales and the implementation of international standards.

Annex II-3

CAACE sees merit in advance consultations but fears that the process could be abused in order to delay unduly the ability of Member States to conclude agreements with third countries.

Annex II-4

CAACE in dismissing the proposal adds that it comes too late and that the most suitable way forward is for individual countries to develop their own definition of a national line.

Annex II-5

CAACE seems most disappointed with this proposal, which it considers as a reiteration of a paper produced by the Commission in October 1983 amending the original 1981 proposal. The present draft seems to disregard two concerns advanced by CAACE vis-a-vis the previous drafts:

First, it is not completely aligned with provisions of the UNCTAD Liner Code and second, a breach of any requirement could lead to annulment of a conference agreement with retrospective effect.

In Article 1 paragraph 2 an all embracing definition of bulk transport is put forward incorporating criteria of the nature of cargo carried (cargoes without mark or count and cargoes dry, wet or others) as well as of the nature of freight fixing (against rates of freight established in free competition in accordance with conditions of supply and demand).

Article 1 paragraph 3(c)

The definitions of "shipper" and "shipper organisations" as set out in the Liner Code should be retained but the definition of "transport user" to be deleted.

Moreover, the question of consortia[7] or joint ventures should be dealt with by the Regulation.

Article 3

Passenger liner conferences should also be specifically exempted.

Article 4

CAACE is opposed to the retention of any "conditions" as opposed to "obligations" because of the retrospective effect of annulment of the agreeement in case of breach of the former.

Article 5 paragraph 2

CAACE[8] proposes alignment of this article concerning loyalty agreements with the provisions of the Liner Code. It opposes, inter alia, provisions which set forth the maximum notice period of 6 months, the maximum penalties, the spread between immediate and deferred rebates.

Article 7 paragraph 1 and 2

CAACE[9] believes that the maximum sanction for breach of an obligation should be fines and is opposed to the possibility of withdrawal of the block exemption.

Finally, CAACE believes that the declaration concerning Article 86 attached to the Commission's 1981 draft should also be published. This declaration emphasizes the particularities of the shipping sector in assessment of abuse of dominant position under Article 86.

Annex II-6

CAACE[10] considers this draft as an essential element of the new maritime policy. It endorses the draft regulation subject to certain improvements as follows:

- The regulation is of too narrow a scope. In addition to state controlled lines, those which benefit from internal cargo reservation laws and those whose ships do not fulfil the main ILO and IMO Conventions, foreign liner companies which receive a high level of subsidy should be covered.

- With regard to the definition of unfair pricing
  practice, the rate charged by a single commercial
  outsider is too restrictive if used as the only
  yardstick when assessing whether a freight rate
  is unfair. CAACE suggest applying a concept of a
  weighted average more or less along the general
  lines of Regulation 2176/84, properly adjusted.

- In many situations, a sanction other than a duty
  might be appropriate (eg. quotas on sailings,
  carryings or earnings).

By and large, CAACE believes that the merit of
the mechanism of this proposal lies essentially in
its very existence and the threat it represents to
possible offenders. The mere fact of initiating
"unfair trading" proceeding will serve as a
deterrent for any company which may be tempted to
engage in such practices.

The above views can be summarised into a clearly
and broadly supportive attitude by Community
shipowners vis-a-vis the Commission Memorandum and
proposals subject to particular comments. CAACE had
the opportunity to submit these views and make oral
presentations to the EP Hearing on February 26, 1986
and to the U.K. House of Lords on 15 January 1986.

INTERNATIONAL TRANSPORT WORKERS' FEDERATION (ITF)

European seamen were also actively involved in
the debate over the shaping of EC shipping policy. A
report of ITF[11], representing the great majority of
the seafarers' Unions in the Community, was released
by the end of 1985. ITF submitted this report
containing the views of European seafarers to the EP
special hearing on February 26, 1986 and to the U.K.
House of Lords where ITF appeared for oral evidence
on December 4, 1985.

The ITF report reviews the structure of the
merchant fleets of the Member States and emphasizes
the importance of shipping to the economy of the
Community the contribution of which it characterises
as "enormous". Thereafter, follows a long string of
criticisms of the Commission Memorandum as follows:

"Unfortunately, these poposals are inadequate, largely because the Commission has not provided an adequate analysis of the current and likely future problems facing the fleets of Member States". This failure to examine EC shipping in the wider economic, political and social context is a major criticism of the Commission's statement and must be connected with the desire of Commissioners to produce "something on shipping" before they completed their terms of office at the end of 1984. Although there were some amendments to the paper by the new Transport Commissioner, removing some of the excesses of the original document, the basic philosophy of the paper remains the same.

The EC is now "burdened with a short sighted view of shipping and regulations which will give no real improvement and hope for the future. Unless, there is a major reappraisal of the Commission's statement and policy, the prospects are for ever-decreasing fleets for Member States with consequential adverse effects for related industries".

The report argues that the decline of the Community fleet is not ascribed to the right reasons by the Commission: for instance, the loss of comparative advantage of the EC fleet and higher crew costs for Community vessels which are both being quoted by the Commission. The report further argues that a favourable direct tax regime for seafarers should be promoted -as the Commission proposes - but flagging out (as a means of EC shipowners' retaining control of vessels) should not be permitted. The alternatives facing EC shipping companies are not simply either to retain vessels under the national flag or to use a flag of convenience, as the Commission suggests. Clearly, flagging out is not the simple solution which the Commission presents. It is not enough to state that there has been loss of comparative advantage, when measures can be taken to offset the advantages which competitors have from paying meagre wages, providing poor social security and expecting low standards of living from their seafarers as well as from providing state aids (subsidies), fiscal privileges and cargo reservation.

The report then, analyses the features prevailing in each particular shipping sector (dry cargo vessels, tankers, cruise shipping) and then to domestic and intra-Community shipping.

With regard to the issue of beneficiaries of the common shipping policy, the report seems to be against the criterion of the nationality of the operator under any flag and under any nationality of crew propounded by the Commission. It, thus, implies the use of Member State registered vessels using Community crews as the proper criterion for the beneficiaries of the policy.

Following an analysis of employment problems in the Community fleet, the report reaches its most important chapter entitled "Future developments" where a conceptual approach to common policy issues is put forward as an alternative to the basic approach of the Commission.

Basing the future prosperity of the EC fleets on a new era of "free trade" and a reversal in the trend towards cargo sharing seems ill-advised. The "free trade" approach was embodied in the Treaty of Rome drawn up some 30 years ago, in a period of rebuilding of Europe after World War II when colonial and post colonial ties by European countries were still strong. "However, with "free trade" in shipping having failed the developing nations and having been rejected by socialist countries, the survival of EC fleets should not be tied to an ideological commitment to any particular economic system. This does not mean that "protectionism" should be embraced wholesale, rather practical intervention should be undertaken".

The report reaches its culmination in advancing a plan[12] of ten points to guide future EC policy in shipping as follows:

1) Instead of opposing cargo sharing arrangements, the Commission should tackle the question of how management of cargo movements can be developed in an orderly way.

2) The relationships among shipping, shipbuilding and other industries (such as steel) should be examined and an integrated approach adopted.

3) A European scrap and build policy should be introduced with the aim of getting rid of substandard ships and building new ships in European shipyards.

4) The capital side of shipping should be examined to see how the financing of EC shipping could meet the competitive advantages offered in non-Community shipyards and to non-Community shipowners, (eg. Far Eastern shipyards and shipowners).

5) The fiscal regimes of flags of convenience countries should be considered with a view to eliminating the unfair advantages which arise from the way in which capital and profits are treated.

6) The social aspects of seafarer employment should be examined with reference to hours of work and the pressure to reduce crews. Regulations on minimum rest periods, leave and time off should be introduced.

7) The research on crewing and technology which is being carried out by Member States should be coordinated with specific attention to the training required.

8) Actual living and working conditions on board ship and terms and conditions of employment should be harmonised as far as possible, taking account of the general variation in pay and conditions which exist between Member States.

9) Port state control should be quickly developed to ensure that similar standards operate in all EC ports and to avoid competition between them. Particular attention needs to be paid to implementation of ILO Conventions 87 and 98. The publication of deficiencies by flag is necessary.

10) The extension of the concept of port state control to provide coastal state control should be a priority, with a complementary instrument being introduced so that vessels passing through

EC waters are subject to the same standards as vessels entering ports.

The 10-point plan can be subsumed into a shipping policy to encourage international trade and improve collective standards of living. It must be based on trade management, take account of inter-related industries and deal with social issues.

The paper concludes by casting all blame for flagging out of EC fleets to flags of convenience in the following terms:

"Shipping has wider economic benefits to provide than can come from further flight of the EC's merchant fleets to flags of convenience, which as recently reported[13] have produced a net social disbenefit to the world at large, rather than marginal benefits in the form of lower freight rates".

By and large, both on basic policy issues and on detailed points, the ITF report has no words of sympathy for the Commission Memorandum and Annexes which are completely dismissed on all counts.

COUNCIL OF EUROPEAN AND JAPANESE NATIONAL SHIPOWNERS' ASSOCIATIONS (CENSA)

European Shipowners have been particularly concerned about the future directions of the common shipping policy of the EC, not only in the strictly Community forum of shipowners, ie, CAACE but also in the larger forum where shipowners from non-EC European countries and Japan are represented, ie, CENSA[14]. The latter has closely followed developments and its position is clearly articulated in a Memorandum addressed to the U.K. House of Lords and in oral evidence given on January 15, 1986.

The non-EC European countries and Japan are interested in many aspects of the policy to emanate from the EC because, apart from the international repercussions of such a policy by the major trading bloc in the world, these countries work closely with the EC countries in the context of the Consultative Shipping Group for the CSG/US dialogue. Several aspects of the dialogue are dependent upon the outcome of EC shipping policy discussions. Moreover, these countries also work together with the EC countries in the context of successive Round Tables to determine a harmonised approach to the ratification of the UNCTAD Liner Code. Likewise, these countries together with EC countries, were involved in general shipping policy discussions in the context of the OECD.

Like CAACE, CENSA[15] broadly supports the Commission's Memorandum and Annexes and the general policy options contained therein. Nevertheless, CENSA seems concerned about several aspects of the Memorandum and Annexes as follows:

Basically, CENSA applauds the Commission's exemplary advocacy of an open market philosophy. The proposed regulations on coordinated action, freedom to provide services and unfair pricing practices could benefit CENSA shipowners as a whole and not just those within the EC.

The causes of the decline of the EC fleet as identified by the Commission are not disputed; they are germane to the decline of fleets of other CENSA countries. Nevertheless, the Annexes deal only with the problems of protectionism and non-commercial competition, whilst the major problem facing shipowners in all sectors of the industry is gross overcapacity. Instead, no attempt has been made to address the overall problem of supply/demand disequilibrum, at least by promoting scrapping. The example upon which it might be possible to build is the current Japanese scheme that establishes cash-grants that enable shipowners to apply for release from encumbrances and obligations to mortgagors in order to dispose of an unwanted ship by scrapping. Since the problem is a global one, CENSA suggests an initiative to be developed inside a wider grouping such as the OECD. As regards the fourth cause of decline identified by the Commission, the loss of comparative advantage, according to CENSA this loss cannot be restored solely by measures aimed at defending the open market. Positive measures are also needed to enable European shipowners to compete on the same level as their rivals from other parts of the word.

It would be helpful if the EC could consider a study on the steps necessary to restore competitive advantage in fiscal regimes, manning levels, implementation of IMO/ILO standards and funding of research.

With regard to the legislative proposals, CENSA comments as follows:

Annex II-1

CENSA supports the concept embodied in the draft regulation and in particular the possibility of extension to other OECD countries. However, the procedures for coordinated resistance have two shortcomings: they lack a degree of automaticity and they lack provision for expeditious consultation.

Annex II-2

CENSA sees this regulation as the cornerstone of the package of regulations since it sets out the principle of elimination in due course of barriers to entry by any EEC carrier into any EC internal or external trade. In light of the sensitivities and difficulties in setting such a principle into practice, a time scale is needed. CENSA hopes that the expeditious liberalisation of the EC internal shipping market will form the foundation of an effective external policy, thus giving a basis for the principle to be extended further.

Annexes II-3 and II-4

CENSA believes that these two proposals should be given a lower priority than the other four proposals. It supports basically Annex II-3 and believes that the necessity for introducing Annex II-4 has been overtaken.

Annex II-5

CENSA, whilst acknowledging the political need for such a regulation to be included in the priority package of proposals, is on the whole disappointed with the Commission's draft proposal for the same reasons as CAACE. The detailed comments concerning this draft are virtually identical to those advanced by CAACE.

Annex II-6

The proposal is most welcome by CENSA but needs to be extended to unfair pricing practices in the cruise ship market. The most serious concern about this proposal is that the "yardstick" contemplated to establish unfair competition is unrealistic. CENSA argumentation on this proposal is again the same as the argumentation of CAACE.

The preceding analysis reveals clearly that the common shipping policy Memorandum failed to win unanimity on the part of the various interest groups at European level, eg, carriers, seamen, shippers, in that diametrically opposed views were put forward. However, carriers and shippers seemed to be smiling more than seamen.

NOTES

1   The European Shippers' Councils constitute a federation of the National Shippers' Councils in the following countries: Austria, Belgium, Denmark, Finland, France, United Kingdom, Greece, Israel, Italy, Netherlands, Norway, Portugal, Spain, Sweden, Switzerland, West Germany. ESC represent exporters and importers who use maritime transport.

2   Following adoption of Regulation 4056/86 it was remarked that "had the EEC followed the United States example and introduced a condition whereby in certain cases individual lines in a conference had the right of independent action, many shipper aspirations would have been achieved". Jack Welsh "Shipper Reaction to the 1986 EEC Shipping Regulations", in "The EEC and Shipping", Institute of Maritime Law, Conference 11/2/88, London.

3   Following adoption of Regulation 4057/86 it was observed by shippers that "the shippers' overall view is that complaints and investigations of unfair pricing are more akin to politico/economic evaluation than legal judgments". Jack Welsh, op.cit.

4   CAACE is the association representing the national shipowner associations of the EC Member States (apart from Luxembourg) and over the fifth of the world's fleet.

5   It is noteworthy that the Union of Greek Shipowners (UGS) disassociates itself from the concept of countermeasures as propounded in both Annexes II-1 and II-2 as being protectionist measures. UGS could accept the principle of countermeasures in Annex II-1 if adopted simultaneously with Annex II-2 providing for a clear cut interdiction of all bilateral agreements on cargo sharing.

6   The General Council of British Shipping (GCBS) is convinced that arrangements in respect of all sea transport services referred in Article 2 have to be agreed upon before the regulation can be introduced, whilst accepting a degree of flexibility in relation to transitional periods.

7   UGS disassociates its position from CAACE comments concerning loyalty agreements. This association is against 100% loyalty ties and favours only a certain percentage of a shipper's cargo (preferably 70%) being subject to loyalty. UGS is also against the possibility of deferred rebates. The notice period of termination of a loyalty contract should be fixed at 3 months. By and large, the views of UGS coincide with the views of the European Shippers' Councils on this issue.

8   UGS believes that withdrawal of the block exemption should not be precluded if circumstances justify it and fines should not always be the maximum sanction (Article 7 paragraph 1). Acts of conferences restricting the operation of outsiders should be penalised like acts of third countries leading to the same result. There should be access to conferences if

the trade is closed either because of acts of third countries or acts of conferences. The abuse of dominant position by acts of conferences should be punished.

9 UGS consider consortia as being cartels in the sense that through appropriate agreements, consortia succeed in restricting free competition. Hence, the Commission should not, by generalising and over-simplifying the matter, grant an a priori exemption to consortia.

10 UGS disassociates itself from CAACE comments on this proposal. UGS is in principle against the redressive duties mechanism of this draft regulation because they are considered to be a protectionist instrument.

11 The ITF represents seamen's (officers and lower crew-ratings) associations in all countries around the world.

12 It is worthwhile comparing these points with EP first draft opinion by rapporteur, Mr. K. Stewart.

13 "Flags of Convenience" B.N. Metaxas, Gower Press, 1985.

14 CENSA represents national shipowner associations from: the United Kingdom, France, Germany, Italy, Greece, Belgium, Ireland, Norway, Sweden, Finland, Denmark, Japan, Portugal, Spain.

15 UGS disassociates itself from CENSA comments on the same issues as under the CAACE Memorandum.

CHAPTER 7

POSITIONS BY COMMUNITY INSTITUTIONS

TRANSPORT COUNCIL DELIBERATIONS 1985-1986

In order to facilitate an agreement, the Commission and the Committee of Permanent Representatives of the Council (COREPER) focussed discussions on the most essential proposals, leaving the others in abeyance. This move was judged necessary in order to speed up things in view of the well known cumbersome mechanisms and procedures that prevail in order to adopt significant legislative pieces of the Community. This was so all the more in light of the third enlargement of the Community from 10 to 12 Member States which rendered the reaching of decisions an even more difficult and slow process.

Thus, at the Council meeting of 24 June 1985 it was stressed that a careful examination of all aspects (internal and external) of the Commissions's Communication should be conducted as soon as possible. It was also agreed that the Council would examine the six proposals contained in the Communication giving priority to the proposals on co-ordinated action to safeguard free access to cargoes in ocean trades (II-1), on freedom to provide sea transport services (II-2), on detailed rules for the application of Article 85 and 86 of the Treaty to maritime transport (II-5) and on unfair pricing practices in maritime transport (II-6).

So, the idea of a "package" of 4 regulations emerged and the numerous meetings at expert level (Transport Group) in the Council, thereafter, concentrated on the examination of this package and left aside Annexes II-3 and II-4. This move proved correct in that the package of four Regulations which emerged from the Council on 16 December 1986 became the subject of intensive negotiations, strenuous efforts by the Presidency and consultations which, however, by Community standards did not last very long.

The first Transport Council to examine the Commission proposals was held on 24 June 1985 under the Italian Presidency. Thereafter, the package of 4 proposals was examined at the Council of 11/11/85 under the Dutch Presidency. Whilst discussions at expert level and Coreper had cleared the ground considerably in all drafts and definitely in Annexes II-1, II-5 and II-6, it was a French torpedo that rendered decisions impossible. On 20/11/85 France submitted a Working paper[1] concerning the creation of a Community wide cabotage with regard to Annex II-2. Moreover, France asked that realignment measures between Member States be adopted on social, technical and fiscal issues concurrently with the adoption of the package. Such novel ideas did not gain enough support to be accepted but were sufficient to halt the movement forward of the package.

The following Transport Council, held on 15 March 1986, did not do much but witness a consensus in broad lines vis-a-vis Annexes II-1, II-5 and II-6 despite the remaining thorns on some points of the drafts. Nevertheless, there was a wide divergence of opinions vis-a-vis Annex II-2 and, more particularly, the issue of cabotage. The scheduled Transport Council for May 8, 1986, was cancelled and shipping matters were again discussed under the Dutch Presidency on June 19, 1986.

Despite the strenuous efforts of the Dutch - who chaired the Transport Council on shipping for an entire year (in lieu of Luxembourg)- it again proved impossible to resolve differences on the cabotage issue. In an attempt to break the deadlock Germany[2] proposed a draft on cabotage which provided that cabotage restrictions be lifted in transportation between a list of Community ports specifically mentioned in Annex. This draft was coupled with a lifting of cabotage for vessels between 500-6.499 grt plying in the above trades.

To add to the difficulties, Spain - as a newcomer to the Community - came forward with new ideas, namely, questioning the veracity of the agreement reached before its accession by the 10 partners as to the issue of "beneficiaries" of the Common Shipping Policy. In fact, Spain submitted a draft on this issue whereby the common shipping policy should apply to companies established in an EEC Member State owning ships under a Community flag. This position torpedoed the agreement on the two alternative criteria to apply on the issue of beneficiaries. This position was diametrically opposed to that of Greece and of the U.K., both interested in having a choice between two alternatives: the former interested in vessels flying the flag of a Member State, the latter in companies incorporated in a Member State. The issue of a "Community Company" owning vessels under a Community flag was added to the remaining difficulties on the chess board.

The Dutch Presidency - whose efforts must not be under-estimated - concluded a year of discussions on June 19, 1986 with a sad remark to those countries impeding the process. The Transport Council of 30 June 1986 made a passing reference to shipping issues and urged Member States to proceed to the adoption of the package. In this state of play, the United Kingdom took the chair and as the second maritime power of the Community - even if on the decline - attempted to break the deadlock. The "device" used was splitting Annex II-2 into two separate regulations, the first, dealing with freedom to provide services in maritime transport between Member States and third countries; the second within Member States (ie, cabotage). This device enabled national delegations entrenched so far in their positions to clear the ground further on Annexes II-1, II-5, II-6 and the so called "1/2 regulation" on freedom to provide services between Member States and third countries, leaving the stumbling block of cabotage more or less untouchable due to the prevailing divergence of opinions. In September 24-25, 1986, the Transport Group of the Council registered this movement but it was impossible to detect any breakthrough on the deadlock over adoption of the whole package of 4 Regulations that was being clouded basically by the issues of cabotage and the beneficiaries.

In preparation for the Transport Council of December 15-16, 1986 high level Government officials took part in two meetings in autumn of that year, on October 3 and November 26. It is remarkable that the second one ended with gloomy prospects for the outcome of the December Transport Council. There

was a hardening of positions on all sides, Portugal
joining Spain, France, Italy over the remaining
issues of Annex II-2 as well as addition on the
table of a draft declaration on convergence of
operating conditions to be adopted with the package.
This declaration dealt with the issue of
competitiveness of Community fleets and with further
measures required to be adopted in the future by the
Community for this purpose. The declaration
concerned the second stage of common shipping policy
proposals and laid down its foundations by broadly
delineating the ways and means to achieve this
competitiveness. The draft declaration attempted to
introduce harmonisation of operating conditions of
vessels between Member States but presented it in
terms of alignment of provisions or reduction of
disparities between Member States on social, fiscal
and technical issues and invited the Commission to
proceed with detailed studies on these matters as a
first step to the adoption of the measures. The
declaration also referred to the achievement of this
process in the context of completion of the internal
market by 1992.

It is in this state of play that the December
16, 1986 achievement came as a surprise to all.
Nevertheless, it justified the great expectations of
the British to add a feather in their cap under
their Presidency.

Before proceeding to the outcome of the December
1986 Transport Council, we should look more closely
at the two issues which proved to be the stumbling
blocks of the negotiations, namely, the issues of
"beneficiaries" and of cabotage.

a)   **The issue of beneficiaries**

One of the gordian knots of negotiations in
Council soon emerged at the issue of "beneficiaries"
of the common maritime policy. This is a horizontal
problem, ie, it permeates debates on virtually most
of the proposals, namely, II-1, II-2, II-3 and II-6.
The problem has legal and economic implications and
it turns on the official interpretation of the texts
of the above proposals of the notion of "national"
of the EC in the sense of the "beneficiary" of the
shipping policy.

Article 56 of the EEC Treaty refers to the freedom to provide services in respect of nationals of Member States who are established in a State of the Community other than that of the person for whom the services are intended. Such nationals according to the Treaty are natural persons or legal entities within the meaning of Article 58 of the Treaty. Thus, the whole corpus of Community law turns on the issue of nationality of persons but it does not confer by fictio iuris upon goods the notion of rights and obligations arising from the nationality. In light of the above, there is no provision for the nationality of vessels in the corpus of primary and secondary Community Law.

On the other hand, the notion of nationality of vessels is one of the basic principles of international law[3] - enshrined in a number of leading Conventions - and of national laws of several countries. In international Law reference is made in unequivocal terms to the principle that "vessels have the nationality of the country whose flag they are entitled to fly". Such reference is found in the following, inter alia, Conventions: UN Convention on the Law of High Seas 1958 (Article 6), UN Convention of the Law of the Sea 1984 (Article 92), UN Convention on Conditions of Ship Registration 1986 (Article 8).[4] Moreover, nationality of vessels is a well enshrined principle in the laws of some sixty countries (developed and developing) according to a comparative legal examination on the grant of nationality conducted by the UNCTAD Secretariat.[5] Thus, both international and national law recognize that the ship may be the subject of rights and obligations and by fictio iuris it is a person having the nationality of the country granting her flag.

By contrast, there are no specific provisions of Community law dealing directly with the conditions upon which nationality will be granted to ships, a matter which still remains the function of the Member States.[6]

The legal gap in Community law may be explained by the fact that at the time of conclusion of the EEC Treaty, the founding fathers of the Community did not have maritime transport in mind. This judgement is corroborated by the fact that according to the provisions of Article 84 paragraph 2 EEC, maritime transport was confined to a watertight compartment. This state of things prevailed throughout the years because no practical problem had arisen but very soon became one of the focal points of the common shipping policy discussions in 1985. The solution of the problem had economic parameters due to the sui generis position of the Greek fleet.

According to Greek law[7] it is possible to register under the Greek flag vessels that do not belong to Greek companies (in the sense of companies incorporated in Greece) but to foreign companies which, however, should be majority (over 51%) owned by Greek nationals. This possibility, which introduced the so-called dual system of the law on registration, has been widely used in practice so that the overwhelming majority of the Greek flag fleet is owned by companies incorporated off shore (eg. Liberia, Panama) but belong over 51% to Greek nationals. In light of the above, a legal controversy of major financial implications soon emerged among the Member States. Did the Community wish to adopt a common shipping policy that would not apply to the biggest fleet of its Member States - amounting to 1/3 of the whole Community fleet - and to the fleet of the fourth maritime power in the world? That was the question put by Greece which - corroborating its position in light of international law and national law precepts - declared that the solution to this problem was a condicio sine qua non for further participation by this country in shipping policy discussions. It is noteworthy that national seamen's Unions in EEC Member States concurred in supporting inclusion of the flag criterion. Moreover, positive consideration to the issue was given both by the European Parliament and the Economic and Social Committee in their respective opinions on the common shipping policy.

On the other hand, most of the other EC Member States were in a situation where either vessels registered in one Member State belonged to companies incorporated and established in the same country or, at least, such companies incorporated and established in a Member State owned vessels registered in non EC Member States. In the latter case, there was no problem since there was still

possibility of compliance with the criterion of
national in the sense of a company incorporated and
established in the EEC. The criterion of "company"
perfectly suited countries like the United Kingdom,
where massive deflagging from its flag had occurred
in recent years, but where these third country flag
vessels remained under the ownership of companies
incorporated and established in the United Kingdom.
Despite heated debates over the merits of the
different legal regimes on this issue, practical
realities prevailed. Therefore, finally by agreement
between Greece and the other Member States, it was
accepted by the end of 1985 that the Greek situation
would be accommodated in the texts of the
legislative proposals in question by providing an
alternative to the existing criterion of company,
namely, the registration of the vessel (the flag).
In this state of play, Spain[8] in mid 1986 - as a
newcomer to the Community and to the negotiations -
put a reservation on the compromise formula by
stating that, in their view, the beneficiaries of
the common shipping policy should only be "Community
companies" in the sense of companies established and
incorporated in a Member State of the EC majority
owned by nationals of the EC Member State and owning
vessels registered in a Member State. The debate
was reopened once again and a certain part of the
delay in formally adopting the package of
regulations may be attributed to the solution of
this problem. The Spanish position created problems
not only for Greece which could be accommodated only
by the provision of alternative criteria (company or
flag) but also for the United Kingdom which would
also not be covered by the definition of Community
company propounded by Spain because, in several
instances, it could not meet the second additional
criterion of the flag of a Member State, at least so
far as the bulk of its fleet that had deflagged to
non EC countries. The solution was provided by the
Transport Council of December 16, 1986 where Spain
lifted its reservation leaving the two alternative
criteria as agreed earlier on.

b) The issue of cabotage

    Another stumbling block in the negotiations
proved to be the issue of cabotage, that is, the
privilege granted by certain Member States only to
vessels flying their flag to carry goods and

passengers between their national ports (including trade between the mainland and offshore islands). Cabotage may be attributed to historical and geographical reasons. For instance, the existence of extremely long coastline as with Italy, or of an archipelago with scattered islands as with Greece, explains why plying between national ports was allowed only to national flag vessels in these countries. On the other hand, the geographical formation of the Belgian coastline explains why cabotage does not exist in Belgium, since virtually all transportation between Belgian ports is by land. Cabotage thus exists in the following countries: France, Italy, Greece, Spain, Portugal and Germany. In legal terms, this is undisputedly an issue of flag discrimination.

Since cabotage covers not only the ordinary volume of goods and passengers servicing islands and remote geographical locations[9] but also the highly profitable business of cruising, it is evident why this issue soon became one of the focal points of negotiations. Member States were soon divided into two blocks:

On the one hand, the countries of Southern front -France, Italy, Greece, Spain and Portugal- insisting on maintenance of cabotage while on the other, the Northern front countries -the United Kingdom, the Netherlands, Belgium, Ireland, Germany and Denmark[10]- insisted on lifting it as soon as possible. There was clearly a division between Mediterranean and Northern countries on the issue. The United Kingdom, a champion of the anti-cabotage campaign, threatened on several occasions whilst negotiations continued to impose cabotage unilaterally around its coast or, alternatively, to proceed to the European Court of Justice for a final pronouncement on the controversy.

The whole issue was even more complicated because within the group of countries that favoured maintenance of cabotage, the reasoning advanced by some differed substantially from that of the others. Thus, Greece put forward reasons of national security and the strategic location of its islands in close proximity to its perennial enemy, Turkey. For Greece, these reasons militated in favour of maintenance of cabotage. On the other hand, in a

Working Paper submitted after the November 11, 1985
Council, France proposed the creation of a Community
maritime space where national restrictions between
Member States would be abolished in favour of
Community flags, not only for the trades actually
reserved by national laws but equally for all
internal maritime transports which actually are
free. This position, which would have aligned the
whole of Europe with the American system of the
Jones Act, did not gain much support from other
delegations on the grounds that by giving an example
of interventionism within its own frontiers, the
Community would justify the protectionism of other
countries. Such a move would contradict the general
principles of maritime liberalism that is underlying
the European edifice. Moreover, Spain, Italy and
Portugal subordinated the lifting of cabotage
restrictions to the harmonisation among Member
States of social costs and employment conditions of
seamen.

Discussions in Council proved that most
delegations were ready to accept the maintenance of
cabotage restrictions with regard to the ordinary
servicing of islands and remote geographical
locations which are financially insignificant but
usually are vested with the character of public
service and, in some instances, justified for
reasons of national defence. With respect to
lifting cabotage restrictions on cruise ships, views
differed widely. In light of the above, no solution
was possible on this part of the initial Annex II-2,
which after June 1986 had taken the form of a
separate regulation concerning freedom to provide
services within Member States. In adopting a
package of 4 regulations, the December 16, 1986
Council instructed the Coreper to clear more the
ground on the cabotage regulation with a view to its
adoption at a later stage in 1987.

THE ECONOMIC AND SOCIAL COMMITTEE

The Economic and Social Committee (ESC), by its
very nature and by its tripartite constitution
encompassing representatives of shipowners,seamen,
shippers and shipbuilders, proved a very useful
forum for contributing to the debate over the
Commission's Memorandum. The ESC delivered two
opinions, one, on 27 November 1985 on the priority

package of four annexes; and the other, of 21 May 1986, on the remaining two annexes and on the Memorandum. The ESC also adopted a detailed report on the above. Rapporteurs were: Mr. K. Mols Sorensen (from the Federation of Merchant Navy Officers, Denmark) and Dr. A. Bredima (from the Union of Greek Shipowners, Greece). Despite differences of opinion expressed in the debate, a very broad consensus was developed in support of both opinions. The first was adopted unanimously and the second with just one negative vote out of 189.

The ESC stressed that Annexes II-1 and II-2 should be adopted simultaneously and implemented at the earliest possible time. It recognised the need for a Regulation such as Annex II-5, which applied the competition articles of the Treaty to maritime transport, and it welcomed the draft Regulation in Annex II-6 on unfair pricing practices. Moreover, the ESC fully endorsed the principle of ex ante consultation in Annex II-3 but dismissed Annex II-4 on grounds that it comes too late, is unclear and requires further reexamination by the Commission.

Within this general attitude of support for the Commission's proposals, the ESC made a number of detailed suggestions for amendments. The main ones were:

1)   Annex II-1 should alternatively apply to vessels flying the flag of Member States (the same comment applied also to Annexes II-2, II-3 and II-6); it should include action against OECD countries which restrict Community shipping; it should encourage the insertion of non discriminatory shipping clauses in trade or other agreements between the Community and third countries and it should contain commercial countermeasures against offending countries exports apart from purely maritime countermeasures.

2)   Annex II-2 should exclude from Community coastal trade ships flying the flags of countries which restrict the access of Community vessels to their coastal trades.

3)   Annex II-3 should apply the ex ante consultation procedure not only to future maritime agreements

but also to trade or other agreements having repercussions in the maritime field.

4) Annex II-5 should treat passenger or combined passenger/freight conferences in the same way as freight conferences; it should exclude tramp vessel services or bulk transport to be defined basically according to the criterion of transportation under contract "against rates of freight which are established in free competition in accordance with conditions of supply and demand"; it should also clarify how exempted agreements will be monitored and should clarify the criteria of application of abuse of dominant position (Art. 86 of the EEC Treaty) in maritime transport.

5) Annex II-6 should be extended to other shipping services besides liner shipping; it should improve the definition of unfair practices and the definition of Community shipowners; it should allow complaints from seafarers as well as from shipowners; it should cover foreign shipowners who compete unfairly because of high subsidies, including credit and fiscal privileges and those who avoid social and economic responsibilities as well as those who operate under flags of countries which do not ratify and/or implement certain IMO and ILO Conventions. Finally, it should provide for greater flexibility regarding sanctions besides duties (eg. quotas on sailings).

The Memorandum was also the subject of heated debates which, however, ultimately yielded to realism and reason. Thus, the ESC generally welcomes the Memorandum but expresses a number of critical comments:

i) The Commission's analysis is confined to a static review of the situation, failing to appreciate fully its seriousness and also failing either to assess the most recent trends and the outlook for various sectors or to consider the effects of the fundamental change taking place in the level and pattern of world trade.

ii) It endorses the Commission's stance in favour of the liberal approach but notes that the latter is unfortunately being eroded by the commercial and political realities of today's world. In view of these factors, it urges the Commission to adopt a pragmatic approach, intervening when necessary in certain trades and sectors.

iii) It urges the Commission to consider measures encouraging the scrapping of vessels as a means of reducing overtonnaging.

iv) With regard to state aid, it believes the EC should resist any undesirable national shipbuilding subsidies world-wide where they contribute to the overtonnaging crisis. It also requires the elaboration by the Commission of a more complete study covering not only investment subsidies but levels of direct and indirect subsidy and protective legislation given to shipowners both within and outside the EC.

v) With regard to social aspects, the ESC has a lot to say: it recognizes that the best way to secure employment for seafarers is to secure the future of Member State fleets and expresses anxiety over the reduction in number of skilled or semi-skilled seafarers within the Community. It also welcomes the Commission's support for favourable direct tax regimes for Community seafarers but expresses scepticism with respect to the freedom of movement of seamen in the Community fleet -which is to be facilitated by a mutual recognition of their diplomas- by reason of national defence considerations prevailing in certain Member States.

vi) Following a heated debate about open registries, the ESC finally endorsed the view that flags of convenience are not necessarily synonymous with substandard operations and that all vessels regardless of flag should be made subject to more stringent port state control. In this respect, whilst the ESC believes the Commission has given insufficient attention to the economic impact of flags of convenience on Member State economies, it concludes only that the administrative link between flag state and vessel should be tightened.

By and large, the two opinions of ESC can be characterized by a sense of realism and the need for a sensible consensus on speedy measures to save the declining Community fleet. The driving force which permeates these opinions is all the more impressive when seen against the wide spectrum of differences expressed in the debates -reflected in the report of the ESC- as well as given the extremely limited time allotted for elaborating the opinions in order to meet constraints requested by the Council.

THE EUROPEAN PARLIAMENT

Unfortunately, the same spirit of cooperation did not prevail in the parallel workings of the EP. The appointment of rapporteur became a subject of controversy which finally was solved by the appointment of Mr. Ken Stewart (U.K, Socialist). Thereafter, the EP decided that the time limits requested by the Council could not be met and unilaterally decided that, instead of delivering an opinion on the priority package by December 1985, its opinion on the Memorandum and six annexes would be delivered by June 1986. The Transport Committee deliberations in June 1986 revealed a wide gap of opinion between the views of the rapporteur, supported by the Socialist Party, and the rest of the Committee. The draft opinion presented by the rapporteur, K. Stewart, is interesting to examine against the background of a special hearing conducted on February 26-27, 1986 to facilitate the rapporteur's work. At the Hearing, all sides of the industry at European level were represented -UNICE, CAACE, the European Shippers Councils and the ITF- as well as representatives of ILO and IMO and other Organisations. The result of these well substantiated presentations covering a wide spectrum of interests was that the draft opinion as presented to the Transport Committee was a completely one sided document totally disregarding the need for a balanced approach. We highlight some of the basic themes of the explanatory statement (March 3, 1986) which could have been drafted in the UNCTAD Secretariat headquarters during a period, the years 1980-1984, when a confrontational mood prevailed there. Whilst the Explanatory Statement agrees with

the Commission's analysis on the importance of
shipping to EC and on the serious problems it faces,
the Statement remarks that "the diagnosis is correct
but the cure proposed by the Commission is wrong".
The rapporteur argues that the pursuit of free
market policies in shipping would no longer serve
the social and economic interests of the EC and,
therefore, offers an alternative appoach. The
rapporteur proceeds to a long economic analysis of
the concept of "perfect competition" in maritime
transport to conclude that the free trade approach
is unequal and that cargo management is realistic.
Furthermore, rejection of the free trade approach is
based on an analysis of the flag of convenience
phenomenon which is characterised as an "economic
symptom" of free trade. The analysis clearly
espouses the UNCTAD Secretariat cause vis-a-vis
phasing out of open registries which are to blame
for deflagging from the EC fleet, for record levels
of unemployment among seamen, for dehumanising
employment conditions. The alternative approach is
based on the following premises: it recognises that
the world is characterised by varying degrees of
protection; that the free market policy that
underlies the Treaty of Rome has not been applied in
several instances and that the Brussels Package does
not preclude the development of cargo sharing
arrangements among members. This alternative
policy[11] recognises, inter alia, that:

- the free trade approach has failed developing
  countries, has been rejected by COMECON countries
  and might not in an interdependent world serve
  the future needs of the EC,
- management of cargo movements can be developed in
  an orderly way,
- the problem of preventing "flagging out" should
  be an EC priority and dealing with unfair
  advantages offered by flags of convenience is
  essential to ensuring the future of EC shipping.

The debate in the Transport Committee on 20-
22/5/86 proved an unbridgeable gap between the
opinions of the rapporteur and a substantial part of
the EP. The rapporteur, therefore, resigned and the
Chairman of the Transport Committee, Mr. G.
Anastassopoulos, was entrusted with the "tache
ingrate" to produce a new draft opinion taking into
consideration some 320 amendments submitted during

the debate. The new text was examined by the Transport Committee on July 16, 1986 and some subsequent 134 amendments were introduced. It was ultimately adopted on September 11, 1986 with 191 votes in favour, 3 against and 15 abstentions (out of 209) and with 8 additional amendments being accepted. The reason we refer to all the stages of the deliberations is to explain and justify the final result of the September 1986 Plenary. The report consists of, inter alia, a Motion for Resolution, a text of amendments (adopted) concerning the six legislative Annexes and a minority opinion.

The New Motion for Resolution is canvassed along the following lines: It acknowledges the importance of maritime transport to the EC and attributes the decline of the Community fleet to the same reasons as those of the Commission. It welcomes the Memorandum of the Commission as a first step towards a comprehensive shipping policy. Community shipping policy should have the following characteristics:

- elimination of overtonnaging,
- special attention to be paid to developing countries and their right to a fair share of world cargoes should be recognized,
- a coordinated package of measures should be adopted to counteract and reduce flagging out,
- the terms of employment of seafarers should be based on the principle of harmonisation,
- incentives for EC shipowners to place orders with EC shipyards,
- there is a need for coordination within the EC: among Member States, shipowners, shipyards
- The EP supports the freedom to provide services on the basis of fair competition, reciprocity, effective regulations in the social and technical fields.

The basic philosophy must be grounded on the following principles: safeguard for the principle of free and fair competition, the free movement of goods and services, non discrimination in flag policy.

A "pragmatic approach" is proposed, one based on a policy of management of cargo movements "consistent with the Brussels Package", a scrap and build policy, a policy of seafarer training.

The Motion attaches great importance to the development of an EC port policy and to enforcement of safety at sea/pollution prevention. The latter objective requires translation of the European Memorandum of Understanding on Port State Control into a Community Directive and implementation of ILO Conventions 87 and 98.

The Motion refers to the social aspects of shipping and requires measures on minimum crew levels, maximum hours of work per week and a policy on training, and invites the Commission to examine the effects of employment of non-EC crews on EC ships.

With regard to flags of convenience, the Motion "regrets the fact that the third memorandum has adopted the shipowners' view that flags of convenience are an economic necessity, while, in reality, they are a means of exploitation not consistent with the Treaty's obligations to enhance the working conditions and the standard of living for seafarers". Still on the same issue, the Motion "voices deep concern with the unsatisfactory aspects of the Convention on the conditions for registering ships for it neither defines what satisfactory part of the crew shall be nationals of the flag state and whether this is mandatory nor does it specify the legal provisions for the participation of nationals of the flag state in the ownership of vessels so that the state in question could exercise effectively its jurisdiction and control".

More specifically, with regard to the various annexes the Motion for Resolution provides:

Annex II-1

The EP supports this Regulation, which is consistent with the approach pursued by Member States in other fora and urges that "a flexible approach should be chosen geared towards support for Community shipping and trade". With regard to beneficiaries, the EP recognises that "ships have the nationality of the state whose flag they are entitled to fly" and urges that the flag criterion be an integral part of this Annex.

Annex II-2

Whilst the EP agrees that the freedom to provide services must in future be applied to maritime transport, it considers important that Member States be able, for reasons of national security, to restrict their coastal trade to ships flying their own flag. Member states should be allowed to maintain restrictions in the case of cabotage providing transport between the continent and islands and between islands themselves; these restrictions are to be removed gradually on the basis of reciprocity.

Annex II-4

The EP considers it essential to include among the criteria for definition of "national line" those of flag nationality and crew nationality.

Annex II-5

The EP calls on the Commission to submit a proposal for a regulation which regulates group exemption for consortia and joint ventures.

Annex II-6

The EP notes a number of shortcomings in this draft. It fails to promote competitiveness although it risks retaliatory measures from third countries. The EP requests new definitions for "unfair pricing practices", "Community shipowner" to satisfy the criteria of effective management control, Community flag and employment of EC nationals, "injury" and "foreign shipowners".

The Motion for Resolution is a difficult text to judge and assess, although it contains valuable statements, they are subsequentloy negated by opposing statements (probably the effect of amendments). For instance, whilst on the one hand the Motion asserts that "the basic philosophy of this Memorandum must be safeguarding the principle of free and fair competition and non-discrimination in flag policy", on the other, it proposes "a pragmatic approach based on policy of management of cargo movements"! How, with such conflicting statements, is one going to reconcile texts and find a general line of thought? The text also makes inaccurate statements on certain issues. For instance, Amendment No. 27 (adopted) on Article 3 of Annex II-5 defines "intermodal transport" as "maritime transport including transport to and from ports", whilst it is the transportation of goods simultaneously by more than one way of transport.

Moreover, with regard to flags of convenience, the EP seems totally entrenched in ITF/UNCTAD Secretariat philosophy and clearly at odds with the policies proclaimed by Member States on this issue.

How is the Council expected to be advised by such contradictory and self-defeating statements on basic issues, such as the main approach to be adopted: liberalism or protectionism? Whilst the document was disclaimed by seamen's Unions, it was bitterly criticized by CAACE as "a hotchpotch of conflicting statements" and that " at best it should be forgotten".

Finally, the Minority opinion reproduces the themes encountered in the first rapporteur's explanatory statement: the basic philosophy underlying the Memorandum and the motion for resolution adopted by EP is "inappropriate, contradictory and logically flawed". The philosophy is inappropriate because "it does not recognize the profound underrelationship of shipping with its user industries, shipbuilding, ports etc and it proposes countermeasures in Annex II-2, liberalisation without harmonisation in Annex II-2, and protective duties in Annex II-6 which would lead to retaliation from third countries". The philosophy is contradictory because "it adheres to the doctrine of free trade for its first and second proposals whilst it institutionalises the cartel type conferences in its fifth proposal and over protects shipowners in the sixth proposal". It is logically flawed because "it pursues the free market approach in imperfectly competitive markets".

NOTES

1 According to the working paper submitted by
  France to the Council, existing restrictions on
  freedom to provide services cease to exist as
  from 1/1/87 with regard to vessels registered in
  a Member State, nationals of Member States and
  shipping companies established in a Member State
  other than that for which the services are
  intended. Cabotage restrictions are open to the
  above beneficiaries as from 1/1/88, ie, the paper
  provides for the creation of a Community wide
  cabotage. A Member State may continue to
  maintain restrictions (other than cabotage) for a
  period of five years in its trades with another
  Member State and for ten years in its trades
  between the ports of that Member State. A
  safeguarding clause may be used by a Member State
  experiencing particularly difficult economic
  situations of its fleet or special situations of
  certain regions. Moreover, the working paper
  provides for the creation of a Consultative
  Committee on alignment of operating conditions of
  vessels (technical, financial) which is entrusted
  with the task of submitting proposals on the
  above subject to be decided by the Council (cf
  Doc. MAR/85/36 (20/11/85).

2 According to the working paper presented by
  Germany to the Council, existing cabotage
  restrictions would cease to exist as from 1/1/88
  with regard to transportation by ships registered
  in a Member State and of a tonnage between eg.
  500-6499 grt in a specific list of Member States
  ports including: all ports in the Baltic, the
  North Sea, the British Isles, the Channel and the
  French coasts as well as continental ports in
  Spain, Portugal, Italy and Greece. The German
  approach was based on the idea of a limited
  positive list of cabotage elements that would be
  liberalised (cf Doc. MAR/86/9 Annex 3/4/86).

3 The concept of nationality of ships was not fully
  developed until the end of the 18th century when
  a growing practice emerged in bilateral treaties
  of commerce and navigation that a ship's
  nationality was to be decided in accordance with
  the laws of the state under whose flag the ship
  was operated.

4 See also the Muscat Dhows case (1905) where the
  Permanent   Court   of   Arbitration   said that
  "generally speaking it belongs to every sovereign
  to decide to whom he will accord the right to fly
  his flag and to prescribe the rules covering such
  grants" (1908)2. A.J.I.L. 921.

5 With respect to the legal background to the
  question of nationality of ships cf: UNCTAD/Trade
  and Development Board/Committee on Shipping/8th
  Session, Geneva 12/4/77, Reference TD/B/C.4/168,
  10 March 77, pp 3,6,7. See also: B.A. Boczek,
  Flags of Convenience: An International Legal
  Study, Cambridge, Mass., Harvard University
  Press, 1962, p. 92 who observes that "the
  subjection of the high seas to juridical order is
  organized and effected by means of a permanent
  legal relation between ships flying a particular
  flag and the state whose flag they fly. This
  permanent legal relation is traditionally called
  the nationality of ships".

6 For a detailed analysis of the implications of
  this issue cf Robin Churchill "EEC Law and the
  Nationality of Ships and Crews" in "EEC Shipping
  Law", Conference 4-5/2/88, Rotterdam, European
  Study Conferences Ltd. Churchill argues that
  despite the absence of specific provisions of
  Community law, the general body of Community law
  applies and restricts the discretion Member
  States have to legislate as follows:
  1. It is contrary to Community law for a Member
     State to require ships having its nationality
     to be owned by individuals having its
     nationality or by companies whose shareholders
     and directors have its nationality. In each
     case ownership must be widened to include not
     only nationals but any other EEC national
     established in the Member State in question.
  2. A Member State cannot require as a condition
     of a ship having its nationality that the ship
     be built in that Member State.
  3. A Member State cannot require the crews of its
     ships to have its nationality but must allow
     any suitably qualified Community seafarer to
     serve on its ships. Churchill concludes that
     despite   the   considerable   divergence   among
     Member State laws on the nationality of ships,

there seems no point in harmonisation's sake and, in any event, he sees no real justification for it or benefit to be gained.

7 Article 13 of legislative decree No. 2687/1953.

8 The reservation introduced by Spain follows: For the purposes of this Regulation (ANNEX II-2) a Community shipping company shall mean any shipping company set up in accordance with the laws of a Member State which has its head office in, and is effectively controlled from a Member State and majority ownership of which is in the hands of nationals of the Member States. The Community shipping companies for the above purposes must own vessels flying the flag of a Member State.

9 In a study conducted by the Commission in August 1979, entitled "The economic implications of the reservation of coastal shipping to national flag ships within the Community and of the abandonment of such reservation", it was found that the economic consequences from liberalisation of cabotage in the Community were insignificant. The study did not cover the cruise sector.

10 Only minimal restrictions exist in Denmark. In France, Germany and Italy there is provision for waivers. France recognizes the "petit cabotage", ie, between French ports, and the "grand cabotage", ie, between ports of Metropolitan France and ports in its overseas territories, eg. Guadeloupe, Martinique.

11 It is worthwhile comparing these passages with the Memorandum submitted by ITF to the U.K. House of Lords for verbatim reproductions.

CHAPTER 8

THE 1986 PACKAGE OF MEASURES ADOPTED

The Transport Council of December 16, 1986, under the British Presidency, made considerable headway in progress towards a common shipping policy by adopting the package of four regulations. These were the following:

- Regulation No.4055/86 applying the principle of freedom to provide services to maritime transport between Member States and between Member States and third countries.

- Regulation No.4056/86 laying down detailed rules for the application of Articles 85 and 86 of the Treaty to maritime transport.

- Regulation No. 4057/86 on unfair pricing practices in maritime transport.

- Regulation No.4058/86 concerning coordinated action to safeguard free access to cargoes in ocean trades.

Despite strenuous efforts by the British Chairman, Mr. John Moore, the Council was unable because of differing views on the issue of future treatment of cabotage restrictions to reach a consensus on the draft Regulation applying the principle of freedom to provide services to maritime transport within Member States. Hence, the Council instructed Coreper to intensify its work with the objective of reaching a consensus on this issue as soon as possible in 1987.

The four regulations adopted are coupled with a number of official statements entered in the Council minutes, which were made by the Council itself, by the Commission and by the delegations of the various Member States. Three of these statements are by far more important than the others in that they prescribe work of the Community in the near future, and thus, merit particular attention.

STATEMENT ON COMMUNITY SHIPPING POLICY

This resounding Council statement, in fact, delineates the framework and purposes for future measures to be taken by the EC in the second phase of its common shipping policy. In its statement, the Council declares that "its adoption of the present Regulations marks only a first stage in the elaboration of a Community shipping policy whose aims are to maintain and develop an efficient competitive Community shipping industry to ensure the provision of competitive shipping services for the benefit of Community trade".

The Council recognises that if these aims are to be achieved, efforts will be needed to reduce the disparities in operating conditions and costs between the Community fleets as a whole and their foreign competitors.

In this connection measures are required to promote the Community fleet.

Accordingly, it "welcomes the Commission's programme proposals set out in Annex I to document 8107/86 MAR 48, relating to fiscal, social and technical aspects. The Council invites the Commission to submit appropriate proposals as rapidly as possible, with a view to contributing to the completion of the internal market by 1992".

STATEMENT ON CONSULTATION PROCEDURE

This Commission statement made with regard to Articles 4 paragraph 2 and 6 paragraph 5 of the Regulation 4058/86 "requests the Council to take up as a matter of priority its proposal to amend the consultation procedure established by Council Decision 77/587/EEC".

STATEMENT ON TRAMP SHIPPING AND CONSORTIA

This Council statement was made with regard to Articles 1 and 3 of Regulation 4056/86. According to its terms, the Council invites the Commission "to study the situation regarding competition in the sectors of passenger shipping, tramp shipping, joint ventures, consortia and agreements between transport users to consider whether it is necessary to submit new proposals". The Council notes, however, that where the object and effect of joint ventures and consortia are either to achieve technical improvement or co-operation as provided for in Article 2 of the Regulation or where close-knit consortia only cover minor market shares, the prohibition laid down in Article 85(1) of the Treaty does not apply to such consortia.

The Commission undertakes to submit within one year from the date of adoption of the Regulation a report to the Council, on whether to provide for block exemptions for passenger transport services, joint ventures and consortia,[1] and to submit proposals to that effect if necessary. The Commission will meanwhile examine carefully any request for individual exemption relating to passenger transport services. In doing so, it will examine, inter alia, "the extent to which such agreements are conducive to facilitating services in this area and favour their continuity and their optimum operation".

Preambles to the package of four regulations in their final form were added to the regulations following the Council meeting of December 16. These preambles together with the operative part of the Regulations and the statements to the minutes were officially adopted as an "A"[2] item by the Industry Council on December 22, 1987. Thereafter, the Regulations were published in the Official Journal of the European Communities on December 31, 1986 (L.378)[3].

REGULATION NO. 4055/86 APPLYING THE PRINCIPLE OF FREEDOM TO PROVIDE SERVICES TO MARITIME TRANSPORT BETWEEN MEMBER STATES AND BETWEEN MEMBER STATES AND THIRD COUNTRIES

The preambular paragraphs of this Regulation confirm the anti-protectionist stance of the Community by upholding the principle of free and fair competition and condemning bilateral agreements on cargo sharing between third countries and some Member States. The same paragraphs also make reference to the issue of "beneficiaries" of the Regulation as follows: "whereas the structure of the Community shipping industry is such as to make it appropriate that the provisions of this Regulation

should also apply to nationals of the Member States
established outside the Community and to shipping
companies established outside the Community and
controlled by nationals of a Member State, if their
vessels are registered in that Member State in
accordance with its legislation". This statement
implies that accommodation of the Greek registration
system has necessitated the provision of an
alternative category of beneficiaries of the freedom
to provide services in maritime transport. It
implies acceptance by the Community of the notion of
nationality of ships strengthened with the
additional caveat that the shipowning company
established outside the EEC will be majority owned
by EEC nationals. The legal basis of the Regulation
is art. 84 para 2 EEC.

(a) Scope of Application

The Regulation (Article 1) applies to maritime
transport services between Member States and between
Member States and third countries which are intended
to incorporate the following: a) intra-Community
shipping services, ie, the carriage of passengers or
goods by sea between any port of a Member State and
any port or off-shore installation of another Member
State and b) third-country traffic, ie, the carriage
of passengers or goods by sea between the ports of a
Member State and ports or off-shore installations of
a third country.

(b) Beneficiaries

As explained above, the Regulation (Article 1)
applies the freedom to provide services in maritime
transport to two alternative categories of
beneficiaries: a) nationals (natural persons or
legal entities) of Member States, b) nationals of
Member States established outside the Community and
to shipping companies established outside the
Community and controlled by nationals of a Member
State, if their vessels are registered in that
Member State in accordance with its legislation.

The Regulation also may extend its benefits to
another category of persons subject to Council
decision: the nationals of a third country who
provide maritime transport services and are
established in the Community (Article 7). This

provision is basically intended to be used in order to extend the benefit of the liberalization process to other OECD countries which are not Member States of the EEC. It is remarkable, however, that this provision is unduly vague: it does not specify when, how, under what criteria such a Council decision may be taken. This provision may open the door to misinterpretations and claims by nationals of other countries apart from the above group.

(c) Phasing out of Unilateral National Restrictions

The Regulation differentiates the treatment of restrictions on freedom to provide services in maritime transport according as to whether these restrictions emanate from unilateral national action or bilateral agreements on cargo sharing. Unilateral national restrictions in existence before 1 July 1986 on the carriage of certain goods wholly or partly reserved for vessels flying the national flag shall be phased according to a timetable provided in Article 2:

- carriage between Member States by vessels flying the flag of a Member State: 31 December 1989,
- carriage between Member States and third countries by vessels flying the flag of a Member State: 31 December 1991,
- carriage between Member States and between Member States and third countries in other vessels: 1 January 1993.

These rather long periods, as compared to periods initially provided for the phasing out of such restrictions, are a last moment concession to Portugal, France and Spain[4] (the last being the Member State with the most protective legislation).

(d) Bilateral Agreements on Cargo Sharing

The Regulation differentiates the treatment of restrictions on freedom to provide maritime services depending on whether these emanate from existing or future bilateral agreements on cargo sharing[5]. Cargo sharing arrangements contained in existing bilateral agreements concluded by Member States with third countries as a matter of principle shall be phased out or adjusted (Article 3).

The adjustment (Article 4) of such agreements shall be made in accordance with Community legislation taking into account the following parameters:

- for (liner) trades governed by the UN Code of Conduct for Liner Conferences, agreements shall comply with this Code and with the obligations of Member States under Regulation 954/79,
- for trades not governed by the UN Code of Conduct, agreements shall be adjusted as soon as possible and in any event before 1 January 1993 so as to provide for fair, free and non-discriminatory access by all Community nationals to the cargo shares due to the Member States concerned.

National action in adjustment to the Regulation shall be notified immediately to the Member States and to the Commission and a progress report will be made every six months initially and subsequently every year. Finally, the consultation procedure established under Decision 77/587 will also apply. In extreme cases of difficulty in the adjustment process, the Council shall take appropriate action (Article 4).

The above procedure concerning the treatment of existing restrictions, apart from its importance as a matter of principle, is expected to be of significant importance in practice in view of the number of Member States involved in bilateral agreements and the volumes of trade already involved.

Cargo sharing arrangements in future agreements with third countries are prohibited as a matter of principle (Article 5). Such arrangements may be permitted only in exceptional circumstances where Community liner shipping companies would not otherwise have an effective opportunity to ply for trade to and from the third country concerned. Such occasions may arise in cases of insistence of the third country concerned basically due to the traditional pattern of conducting its foreign shipping and trade relations, for instance, COMECON countries or some other countries due to their sociopolitical system. Whilst the principle of prohibition of such agreements yields vis-a-vis liner trade a per above, this is not the case of bilaterals in the bulk trades, where the Community appears adamant with regard to their condemnation. In such cases, where a third country seeks to impose cargo sharing arrangements on Member States in liquid or dry bulk trades, the Council activates coordinated action under Regulation 4058/86. This differentiation in treatment between liner and bulk trades was a disputable issue till the end of discussions in Council and a bone of contention between, on the one hand, France, Italy, and Spain, which claimed that the treatment finally reserved only to liner trades should be the same destined for all trades (non liner trades) and, on the other hand, Greece and Denmark, which maintained that the derogation to the prohibition of future bilateral agreements should be restricted only to liner trades.

The Regulation provides (Article 6) that future agreements in liner trades may be permitted in compliance with the following caveats. If a Member State's national or shipping companies (ie, the beneficiaries of the Regulation) are experiencing or are threatened by a situation where they do not have an effective opportunity to ply for trade to and from a particular third country, the Member State concerned shall inform the Commission and the other Member States. Thereupon, the Council by qualified majority on a proposal of the Commission, shall decide on the necessary action, which may include the conclusion of a cargo sharing arrangement. In the absence of decision by the Council within six months, the Member State may take the action necessary to preserve an effective opportunity to ply for trade. Such action should provide for fair, free and non-discriminatory access to the relevant cargo shares by nationals or Community shipping companies (the beneficiaries of the Regulation). Finally, the national action shall be notified immediately to the Member States and the Commission and the consultation procedure of Decision 77/587 shall apply (Article 6).

(e) Transitional Provisions - Entry into Force

Furthermore, a non-discriminatory clause is provided in the meantime and so long as the existing restrictions have not been abolished. Thus, Member

States   are   under   the   obligation   to   apply
restrictions   without   distinction   on   grounds   of
nationality or residence to the beneficiaries of the
Regulation.

The Regulation, which entered into force on the
day   following   its   publication   in   the   Official
Journal of the EC, ie, 1/1/87, is subject to review
before 1/1/1995.

A number of criticisms may be levelled against
the mechanism introduced by the Regulation: it   is
doubtful   how successful the provisions on adjusting
existing   bilateral   agreements   containing   cargo
sharing clauses will prove to be; what is meant
precisely by "cargo sharing aggangement" and what
does the phrase "fair,   free and non-discriminatory
access" mean? How well will the   procedure   for   a
Council   decision on new cargo sharing arrangements
for liner shipping work out? Will Member States
always   inform   the   Commission   of   their proposed
arrangements and will the Council be   able   to   act
within   the   6   months   time limit? Finally, it is
doubtful whether   the   provisions   whereby   existing
cargo sharing agreements need not be phased out -
even if they must be adjusted- and permitting the
conclusion of   new   cargo   sharing agreements even
exceptionally are compatible with the OECD   Code   of
Liberalisation of Invisible Transactions.[6]

REGULATION NO.4056/86 LAYING DOWN DETAILED RULES FOR
THE   APPLICATION OF ARTICLES 85 AND 86 OF THE TREATY
TO MARITIME TRANSPORT.

The purpose of this Regulation as set   forth   in
the   preambular   paragraphs   is   to   steer a middle
course   between   two   evils: undue   distortion   of
competition within the common market by a complete
laissez faire attitude and excessive regulation of
the   sector.   Adoption   of   the   competition   rules
originates in the misgivings expressed by developing
countries in the 1970's about the functioning of the
conference system.[7] It is also the result of the
last   preambular paragraph of Regulation 954/79
concerning ratification or accession by EC Member
States   to   the   UN Code of Conduct for liner
conferences where it is stated that:

"Whereas the stabilizing role of conferences in ensuring reliable services to shippers is recognized, but it is nevertheless necessary to avoid possible breaches by conferences of the rules of competition laid down in the Treaty; whereas the Commission will accordingly forward to the Council a proposal for a Regulation concerning the application of those rules to sea transport".

Furthermore, the Regulation attempts to steer a middle course between conflicting interests of liner conferences and shippers. The result of this Regulation is group exemption to liner conferences couched in the widest possible terms, ie, a very generous treatment of liner conferences unprecedented in other fields of competition law of the Community. Finally, whilst its detailed procedural part is a verbatim reproduction of Regulation 1017/68 applicable to inland transport operations, the substantive law of the Regulation takes into consideration the particularities of maritime transport. The legal basis of the Regulation is dual, namely, both articles 87 and 84 para 2 EEC.

(a)   Scope of Application

The Regulation applies to international maritime transport services from or to one or more Community ports, other than tramp vessel services (Article 1 paragraph 2). This non-application to tramp trades is in recognition that this sector broadly operates in a freely competitive environment.[8] The definition of "tramp vessel services" which has been the subject of debates since the first version of the draft Regulation in 1981 ended up including a number of elements which take into consideration both the nature of the cargoes carried (in bulk or in break-bulk) and the way the contract of affreightment is concluded (non-regularly scheduled or non-advertised sailings, freight rates freely negotiated case by case in accordance with the conditions of supply and demand). The former elements were basically propounded by the United Kingdom, the latter by Greece and the Netherlands. The non-application of Regulation 4056/86 to the tramp vessel services does not, of course, preclude the direct application of articles 85-90 of the Treaty to these trades.

There is also provision for the definition of liner conferences as "the group of two or more vessel - operating carriers which provides international liner services for the carriage of cargo on a particular route or routes within specified geographical limits and which has an agreement or arrangement, whatever its nature, within the framework of which they operate under uniform or common freight rates and any other agreed conditions with respect to the provision of liner services".

Furthermore, transport users are defined as being under-takings (eg. shippers, consignees, forwarders etc.) provided they have entered into, or demonstrate an intention to enter into, a contractual or other arrangement with a conference or shipping line for the shipment of goods, or any association of shippers.[9]

(b)   Technical agreements

With regard to technical agreements, there is in article 2 the usual clause concerning the non-applicability of the prohibition of article 85 para 1 of the EEC Treaty if such agreements have as sole object and effect to achieve technical improvements or cooperation by means of:

a)   the introduction or uniform application of standards or types in respect of vessels and other means of transport, equipment, supplies or fixed installations;
b)   the exchange or pooling for the purpose of operating tran-sport services, of vessels, space on vessels or slots and other means of transport, staff, equipment or fixed installations;
c)   the organization and execution of successive or supplementary maritime transport operations and the establishment or application of inclusive rates and conditions for such operations;
d)   the co-ordination of transport timetables for connecting routes;
e)   the consolidation of individual consignments;
f)   the establishment or application of uniform rules concerning the structure and the conditions governing the application of transport tariffs.

(c) Exemptions (Articles 3 and 6)

Two exemptions from the prohibition of Article 85 paragraph 1 of the Treaty are granted under the terms of the Regulation: the first, in Article 3, concerns agreements, decisions and concerted practices of all or part of the members of one or more liner conferences. The second, in Article 6, concerns such agreements between transport users and conferences. It is inferred from the above that agreements between conferences and non-conference lines (ie, outsiders), the so-called tolerated outsider agreements, are not equally exempted. Exemptions, as constituting a deviation from the orthodox application of the rules, can only be restrictively interpreted. We make this inference all the more because of the nature of conferences permissible under the Regulation, namely, the closed conferences. Another reason militating in favour of a restrictive interpretation is that the group exemption granted to liner conferences is the widest possible and without precedent in other fields of competition law of the Community.

Under the terms of Article 3, the exemption of such agreements (subject to the condition of Article 4 of the Regulation) is granted when they have as their objective the fixing of rates and conditions of cariage and one or more of the following objectives: coordination of shipping timetables, sailing dates, dates of calls, determination of frequency of sailings, coordination or allocation of sailings among members of the conference, regulation of the carrying capacity offered by each member, allocation of cargo or revenue among members.

(d) Condition attaching to exemption

The Regulation then draws a distinction between obligations and condition attaching to exemption. The legal effects in case of breach of the former are less onerous than in case of breach of the latter. Thus, according to article 4 the exemption provided for in Articles 3 and 6 is granted subject to the condition that the agreement shall not, within the common market, cause detriment to certain ports, transport users or carriers by applying for the carriage of the same goods and in the area

covered by the agreement, rates and conditions of
carriage which differ according to the country of
origin or destination or port of loading or
discharge, unless such rates or conditions can be
economically justified. In case of breach of the
above condition, the agreement - or part of the
agreement, if it is severable -will automatically be
void pursuant to Article 85 para 2 of the Treaty.
This is the ultimate penalty under the Regulation.
Thus the group exemption of closed conferences from
the interdiction prescribed in Article 85 par.1 is
subject to the condition that the closed conferences
operate in open trades, i.e., that the trade must
remain open to access of non-conference lines.

(e)   Obligations attaching to exemption - loyalty
      arrangements

     As far as the obligations attaching to
exemption - as set out in Article 5 - there is a
list of five obligations, the most important being
the loyalty arrangements. According to Article 5
para 2, the shipping lines members of a conference
shall be entitled to institute and maintain loyalty
arrangements with transport users, the terms of
which shall be a matter for consultation between the
conference and the transport users' organizations.
The loyalty agreements shall be based on the
contract system or any other system which is also
lawful. Thereafter, the provisions relating to
loyalty agreements are taken verbatim from the
relevant provisions of the UNCTAD Liner Code
(Article 7), whereby transport users shall be
offered a choice between immediate rebates and
deferred rebates. Under the former, each of the
parties shall be entitled to terminate the loyalty
agreement at any time without penalty subject to a
period of 6 months' notice (the period will be
reduced to 3 months when the conference rate is the
subject of a dispute). Under the latter, the
loyalty period may not exceed 6 months and again the
period will be reduced to 3 months if the conference
rate is the subject of a dispute. There is also
provision that, following consultation, the
conference shall set out a list of cargo which is
specifically excluded from the scope of the loyalty
agreement with the caveat - inserted at the last
minute in the December 16, 1986 Council following
reservation by Greece - that "100% loyalty

arrangements may be offered but may not be unilaterally imposed". This is a significant improvement in the Regulation compared to its previous versions and may be also attributed to the persistent firing at the loyalty arrangement system by the European Shippers' Councils. Nevertheless, the Council and the Commission did not go as far as regulating the time/volume service contracts[10], which are considered as the latest development in shipment contracts, leaving aside the "antiquated forms" of loyalty agreements. Finally, following consultation, the conference shall set out a list of circumstances in which transport users will be released from their obligation of loyalty.

The other four obligations attaching to the exemption are: consultations between transport users and conferences concerning the rates, conditions and quality of scheduled maritime transport services and which shall take place whenever requested by any of the parties; availability of tariffs to transport users setting out all the conditions concerning loading and discharge and the exact extent of the services covered by the freight charge; notification to the Commission of awards at arbitration and recommendations made by conciliators; services not covered by the freight charges (inland transport operations and quayside services).

(f) Monitoring of exempted agreements

Article 7 entitled "monitoring of exempted agreements" is by far the article containing the crux of the Regulation in that it provides for the consequences in case of breach of an obligation attaching to the group exemption of the conference or in case of effects incompatible with article 85 para 3 of the EEC Treaty.

In case of breach of an obligation (Article 7 para 1), the Commission may proceed to an escalation of acts starting with recommendations to the persons concerned; in the event of failure to observe those - depending upon the gravity of the breach - the Commission may adopt a decision either prohibiting them from carrying out or requiring them to perform specific acts or, whilst withdrawing the benefit of the block exemption, granting them an individual exemption or withdrawing the benefit of the block exemption.

In case of effects incompatible with Article 85 para 3 of the EEC Treaty, due to special circumstances, the Commission, on receipt of a complaint or on its own initiative, shall take a series of measures. The special circumstances are created, inter alia, by acts of conferences or a change in market conditions in a given trade resulting in the absence or elimination of actual or potential competition, such as restrictive practices whereby the trade is not available to competition or acts of conferences which may prevent technical or economic progress or user participation in the benefits;

- prevent the operation of outsiders in a trade,
- impose unfair tariffs on conference members, or
- impose arrangements which otherwise impede technical or economic progress (cargo - sharing limitation on types of vessels).

In the above circumstances, if actual or potential competition is absent or may be eliminated as a result of action by a third country, the Commission shall enter into consultations with the competent authorities of the third country, followed by negotiations in order to remedy the situation. If the special circumstances result in the absence or elimination of actual or potential competition contrary to Article 85 para 3 (a) of the Treaty, the Commission shall withdraw the benefit of the block exemption and it shall rule on whether an individual exemption should be granted to the relevant conference with a view to obtaining access to the market for non-conference lines. The above provision indicates the tacit acceptance of the Council that the trades (ie, the market) must remain open to outsiders, even if the conferences operate under the "closed conference system", which is the case for all European based conferences, as contrasted to the American based conferences that are open. It is noteworthy in this regard that the Greek delegation insisted on inserting a provision whereby in such circumstances the Commission "would positively examine applications for admission to conferences". This provision, whilst endorsed by the Commission, was originally intended to be inserted in the minutes of the Council but in the last phase of negotiations was ultimately dropped.

(g)   Effects incompatible with Article 86 of the Treaty

A Regulation applying Articles 85 and 86 of the Treaty to maritime transport would not justify its existence had there not been provision in its operative part for application of Article 86. This was, however, the case in the earlier versions of the draft regulation, but owing to the persistence of Greece, Article 8 entitled, "effects incompatible with Article 86", was introduced. Article 8 indicates that the abuse of a dominant position within the meaning of Article 86 shall be prohibited, no prior decision to that effect being required. Furthermore, where the Commission finds that the conduct of a conference benefitting from group exemption has effects which are incompatible with Article 86 of the Treaty, it may withdraw the benefit of the block exemption and take all appropriate measures for the termination of the infringement.

Determination of a dominant position in maritime transport depends upon a series of factors including the level of services and not only upon percentages of the trade shared between the conference and the outsiders. Each given trade must be examined per se and there is no hard and fast answer depending only upon the percentage.

(h)   Conflicts of international law

Community law does not operate in a vacuum. The Commission, conscious of the possible frictions in the application of the competition Regulation, provided Article 9 for the solution of conflicts of International Law. Article 9 may prove in practice a very interesting source of litigation in that it attempts to solve such conflicts of international law and disputes over the extra - territoriality in the application of Community Law. Bearing in mind the impressive anti-trust corpus of law in the United States administered by the Federal Maritime Commission, it will be interesting to see how the mechanism provided in Article 9 will delineate the extent of application of Community law vis-a-vis

United States Law and whether it will prove to be an efficient tool for demarcation lines between EEC jurisdiction and other jurisdictions. Under the terms of Article 9, in case the application of the Regulation is liable to enter into conflict with the provisions of or administrative action of certain third countries which would compromise important Community trading and shipping interests, the Commission shall undertake consultations with the competent authorities of the third countries concerned aimed at reconciling the above mentioned interests with respect for Community law. If agreements with third countries need to be negotiated, the Council shall authorize the Commission to conduct such negotiations in consultation with an Advisory Committee (established under the Regulation) and subject to the guidelines provided by the Council. Here again, the decision-making procedure of the Council shall be based on Article 84 para 2 of the Treaty.

(i) Procedural Rules

The procedural part of the Regulation (Articles 10-27) is a verbatim repetition of the relevant provisions in Regulation No. 1017/68 on inland transport operations and at the same time has a strong Federal Maritime Commission flavour. Although identical provisions exist for inland transport and for other types of economic activities under the EEC Treaty, it will be interesting to see if their application to maritime transport will prove difficult, if not impossible. The par excellence international character of shipping activities and operations may prove to be an impediment to the smooth application of the rules as provided for in the procedural part of the Regulation. The nature of shipping operations may render investigations by the Commission difficult and justify criticisms levelled at the entire procedural mechanism as onerous and utopian.

The procedural mechanism is triggered by complaints submitted by Member States, natural or legal persons who claim a legitimate interest or on the initiative of the Commission (Article 10). Where the Commission finds that there has been an infringement of Article 85 para 1 or 86 of the Treaty, it may require the undertakings concerned to

bring the infringement to an end and address
relevant recommendations for its termination. If
the Commission concludes that on the evidence before
it there are no grounds for intervention, it shall
issue a decision rejecting the complaint as
unfounded. If the Commission concludes that the
agreement satisfies the provisions both of Article
85 para 1 and 85 para 3, it shall issue a decision
applying Article 85 para 3 indicating the date from
which it is to take effect. This date may be prior
to that of the decision.

Undertakings seeking application of Article 85
para 3 in respect of agreements falling within the
provisions of Article 85 para 1, to which they are
parties, shall submit applications to the
Commission. If the applications are judged
admissible, the Commission shall as soon as possible
publish in the Official Journal of the European
Communities a summary of the application inviting
interested parties to submit their comments within
thirty days. It is noteworthy that in proceeding to
such publications, the Commission will seek to
protect the business secrets of the undertakings
concerned. The Regulation, however, does not
explain how the formal application is going to be
made. The Commission is preparing a special form
for notifications. The Regulation does not provide
for applications for negative clearance (i.e., a
decision stating that the agreement or practice does
not fall within the competition rules at all).
Until the Commission rectifies this omission, use of
the standard Form A/B which is used for all other
categories of non-maritime agreements should suffice
for the making of such applications.[11]

Within ninety days from publication in the
Official Journal, the agreement shall be deemed
exempt from the prohibition for the time already
elapsed and for a maximum of six years thereafter
(Article 12). This is so unless the Commission
finds to the contrary. In fact, the Commission is
empowered to revoke or amend its decision or
prohibit specified acts by the parties (Article 13).

(j)   Liaison with the authorities of Member States

Although the Commission has the primary responsibility for administering the procedure and the sole power to grant exemptions and to impose obligations, subject to review by the Court of Justice of the European Communities, there is also provision for constant and close liaison with the relevant national authorities of the Member States. The national authorities have unusually wide rights under the Regulation. Thus, according to Article 14, the authorities of the Member States shall retain the power to decide whether any case falls within the provisions of Article 85 para 1 or Article 86, until such time as the Commission has initiated proceedings with a view to formulating a decision. In this regard, one should bear in mind the direct applicability of Articles 85-86 of the Treaty in the national laws of Member States. Apart from an exchange of documents between the Commission and the competent authorities of the Member States, an Advisory Committee on agreements and dominant positions in maritime transport is created under Article 15. The Committee shall be consulted prior to the taking of any decision by the Commission and prior to the adoption of implementing provisions. It shall be composed - as similar Committees for other sectors of economic activities - of national officials competent in the sphere of maritime transport and agreements and dominant positions. Consultation shall take place at a joint meeting convened by the Commission and the relevant report, annexed to the draft decision shall not be made public. It must be reckoned that the relationship between the national and the Community authorities is not entirely clear and will require clarification in the future. It is also important to note the position of national courts. Although they have the legal power to apply Articles 85-86 of the Treaty, they do not have the power to grant an exemption under Article 85 para 3. In such cases, a national court would have no option but to grant an injunction and/or award damages. It is also possible that the Court could stay proceedings to allow the parties the right to apply to the Commission for an exemption.

(k)   Requests for information - Investigation

The   Commission   is   entitled   to   request
information from the competent authorities of the
Member States and from the under-takings concerned.
Moreover, the authorities of the Member States -
assisted by Commission officials, if need be -
undertake the investigations which the Commission
considers   necessary.   Such   investigations   are
conducted upon production of an authorization in
writing issued by the authorities of the Member
State in whose territory they are being made
(Article   17).   The   Commission   may   undertake
investigations by its own authorized officials and,
to this effect, examine books and other business
records,   take copies,   ask for   oral   explanations,
enter   any   premises,   land   and   vehicles   of
undertakings (Article 18).   It is obvious that the
latter provisions have just been extrapolated to the
maritime transport Regulation without any attempt to
take into consideration the particularities of the
sector.

(l)   Fines - Periodic Penalty Payments

The   Commission - subject to the unlimited
jurisdiction (within the meaning of Article 172 of
the EEC Treaty) of the European Court of Justice to
review decisions fixing fines/penalties, cancel,
reduce or increase same - is empowered to impose on
undertakings fines of from 100 to 5.000 ECU, where
intentionally or negligently they supply incorrect,
incomplete or misleading information. The decision
of the Commission is a legally binding instrument
akin to an administrative judgment. Fines may range
from 1000 to 1.000.000 ECU or a sum not exceeding
10% of the turnover of the preceding business year
to each of the undertakings participating in the
infringement, where the latter intentionally or
negligently infringe Article 85 para 1 or Article 86
or do not comply with an obligation imposed by the
Regulation (Article 19)[12]. An undertaking is defined
as the whole corporate group and thus the Commission
is entitled to look to the global turnover of a
whole network of connected companies. Thus, the
Commission has an immense fining capacity.

Periodic penalty payments of from 50-1000 ECU
per day may be imposed by the Commission upon

undertakings in order to compel them to put an end
to the infringements and breaches as per above
(Article 20).

In reaching its decisions under the procedural
mechanism, the Commission shall give the opportunity
to interested parties of being heard whilst all
information acquired by the Commission and the
authorities of the Member States in the course of
investigations shall be covered by the obligation of
professional secrecy.

(m) Entry into force

The Regulation entered into force on July 1,
1987.

COUNCIL REGULATION NO. 4057/86 ON UNFAIR PRICING
PRACTICES IN MARITIME TRANSPORT

This Regulation based on Article 84 para 2 of
the EEC Treaty refers in its very title to unfair
pricing practices "in maritime transport" although
it becomes clear expressis verbis from the terms of
its first preamble to its last Article that it
refers only to liner shipping. Is this an oversight
of the title or does it indicate intention to
proceed, at a later stage if need be, along the same
lines to a Regulation covering non liner shipping?
Whichever was the case, we consider the title of the
Regulation misleading.

The need for the Regulation is justified, inter
alia, on the grounds of evidence procured by the
information system set up by the Decision
78/774/EEC, ie, the monitoring system[13] whereby
according to its findings "there is reason to
believe that the competitive participation of
Community shipowners in international liner shipping
is adversely affected by certain unfair practices of
shipping liners of third countries" (1st recital).

The crux of the Regulation lies in defining what
constitutes an unfair price in the maritime
transport field since such rules are not
internationally agreed[14] (6th recital). The
calculation of what constitutes the "normal freight
rate" below which freight rates are judged unfair
has been under attack by various sides in that here

lies the protectionist character of the whole Regulation seeking to protect Community shipowners in liner shipping vis-a-vis their foreign competitors.

It is also interesting to note that the Regulation in its twelfth recital expressly delineates the extent of its application and interaction vis-a-vis the Competition Regulation; ie, Regulation 4057/86 cannot be invoked and misused in order to avoid application of Regulation 4056/86.

(a)   Objective of the Regulation

The Regulation, as set forth in Article 1, is a procedural regulation "laying down the procedure in order to respond to unfair pricing practices by certain third country shipowners engaged in international cargo liner shipping which cause serious disruption of the freight pattern on a particular route to, from or within the Community and cause or threaten to cause major injury to Community shipowners operating on that route and to Community interests". In such cases, a redressive duty may be applied by the Community (Article 2).

(b) Definitions - Unfair pricing practices

According to Article 3 (b) unfair pricing practices are "the continuous charging on a particular shipping route to, from or within the Community of freight rates for selected or all commodities which are lower than the normal freight rates charged during a period of a least six months, when such lower freight rates are made possible by the fact that the shipowner concerned enjoys non-commercial advantages which are granted by a State which is not a member of the Community". It is noteworthy that the Regulation does not define the non-commercial advantages[15] enjoyed by the foreign shipowner. The original version submitted by the Commission was eloquent in defining in Article 3 such advantages as follows: being owned or controlled directly or indirectly by any State which is not a Member of the Community, and/or being more favourably placed than Community shipowners as to the access to cargo in ocean trades through national legislation, and/or, operating the ships of countries which have not ratified and do not implement a list of leading international Conventions of IMO and ILO (referred to in an Annex). The Regulation only refers to unfair pricing practices made possible by government intervention. Therefore, it is to be compared to the anti-subsidy rules applicable in trade of goods and not to the anti-dumping rules. The Regulation certainly includes subsidies of any nature granted directly to the shipowners. It is questionable whether the concept covers subsidies to shipbuilders from whom the shipowner bought the ship and whether it also refers to freight quota not provided for in accordance with the Liner Code that guarantee a shipping line a competitive advantage enabling shipowners to charge lower freight rates.

(c) Normal Freight Rate

Normal freight rates are determined by taking into account, alternatively, two factors, the comparable rate and the contructed rate as follows in Article 3 (c): the comparable rate actually charged in the ordinary course of shipping business for the like service on the same or comparable route by established and representative companies not enjoying non commercial advantages; or otherwise the constructed rate which is determined by taking the costs of comparable companies not enjoying non commercial advantages plus a reasonable margin of profit. This cost shall be computed on the basis of all costs incurred in the ordinary course of shipping business, both fixed and variable, plus a reasonable amount for overhead expenses.[16]

(d) Community Shipowners

The Regulation for the first time provides a definition of Community shipowners as meaning alternatively "all cargo shipping companies established under the Treaty in a Member State of the Community; nationals of Member States established outside the Community or cargo shipping companies established outside the Community and controlled by nationals of Member States, if their ships are registered in a Member State in accordance with its legislation".

Reference to "Community shipowners" (Article 3) and to persons acting on behalf of the "Community

shipping industry" (Article 5) amounts to the same,
ie, that only shipowners are the beneficiaries of
the Regulation. Shippers or exporters do not come
under the definition of beneficiaries. Such
categories at best can be considered as an
"interested party" and can only submit their views
in a pending procedure.

It is noteworthy that a comparative examination
of the beneficiaries of this regulation as
contrasted to the beneficiaries under Regulation No.
4055/86 or even Regulation No. 4058/86 reveals a
number of differences. Under Regulation No.
4058/86 (Article 1) beneficiaries are "companies
established in a Member State or vessels flying the
flag of a Member State". The second criterion
implies a clear cut acceptance of the notion of
nationality of ships as an alternative to the
nationality of natural persons or legal entities.
According to Article 1 of Regulation No. 4055/86 the
notion of beneficiaries applies to "nationals of
Member States who are established in a Member State
other than that of the person for whom the services
are intended" or "alternatively to nationals of
Member States established outside the Community and
to shipping companies established outside the
Community and controlled by nationals of a Member
State, if their vessels are registered in that
Member State in accordance with its legislation".
The above definition - which is identical to the
definition of Article 3 of the present Regulation
with the exception of the word "that" in lieu of "a"
indicates a qualified acceptance of the notion of
nationality of ships, only in cases where such
vessels are owned by companies established outside
the EEC and controlled by Community nationals.
Thus, the wholesale acceptance of the nationality of
ships under Regulation No. 4058/86 is more
restricted according to the terms of Regulations No.
4055 and 4057. There is a further restriction
introduced only in the text of Regulation No. 4055
by the word "that" in lieu of "a". Is it a last
minute oversight or was it a legislative intent to
differentiate the terms of the two Regulations by
rendering the former more restrictive as compared to
the latter with regard to beneficiaries? This is an
unresolved problem.

(e)   Third Country Shipowners

According to Article 3 (a) "third country shipowners" are defined as cargo liner shipping companies other than those defined under "Community Shipowners". It can be safely inferred that in case of vessels flying the flag of a Member State belonging to shipping companies established outside the Community and controlled by nationals of Member States, which are chartered by third country shipowners involved in alleged pricing practices, these vessels cannot become subject to Community redressive duties: such vessels are still considered to belong to Community Shipowners despite the chartering to third country shipowners. The third country shipowners are the only liable to Community redressive duties.

(f)   Examination of injury

Pursuant to Article 4, a number of factors have to be met in establishing the injury of Community shipowners. Those are: the freight rates offered by Community shipowners' competitors on the route in question, in particular in order to determine whether they have been significantly lower than the normal freight rate offered by Community shipowners, taking into account the level of service offered by all the companies concerned; the effect of the above factor on Community shipowners as indicated by trends in a number of economic indicators such as sailings, utilisation of capacity, cargo bookings, market share, freight rates, profits, return of capital, investment, employment.

Where a threat of injury is alleged, the Commission may examine whether it is clearly foreseeable that a particular situation is likely to develop into actual injury by taking into account, inter alia, the increase in tonnage deployed on the shipping route in question or the capacity already available or to become available in the foreseeable future in the country of the foreign shipowners.

It is noteworthy, however, that injury caused to Community shipowners by other factors must not be attributed to the practices in question (Article 4 para 3).

(g) Complaint

The mechanism of Commission intervention, which for the most part reflects[17] the provisions of Regulation 2176/84 on dumping in shore based industries, is activated following a written complaint lodged by any natural or legal person or an association not having legal personality acting on behalf of the Community shipping industry who consider themselves injured or threatened by unfair pricing practices. It is noteworthy that despite the concurring views of the European Parliament, the Economic and Social Committee and the ITF and the efforts of the Transport Commissioner endorsing these views, the Council did not finally extend the benefit of the right to lodge a compaint to seamen's unions. The complaint may be submitted to the Commission directly or to a Member State. If, on the other hand, a Member State - in absence of any complaint - is in possession of sufficient evidence of unfair pricing practices and of injury resulting therefrom, it shall immediately communicate such evidence to the Commission. It is evident from the above that the complaint introduces a prima facie case and it has to be a Community complaint; individual elements concerning a company of one Member State are not enough to substantiate a Community complaint which has to involve several Member States. The complaint is lodged in three versions: a) a confidential version, b) a semi-confidential version and c) a non-confidential version (available to anyone). An unfair pricing case does not have a plantiff or a defendant as in normal litigation. The procedure is administrative and not judicial.[18]

(h) Consultations

The consultations provided for in the Regulation shall take place within an Advisory Committee consisting of representatives of each Member State under the chairmanship of the Commission. Consultations may also be in writing only following notification to Member States by the Commission and specification of a period within which they are entitled to express their views or request oral consultation. The consultations will cover the existence of unfair pricing practices, the existence of injury, their causal link and the appropriate measures (Article 6).

(i) Investigation

The Commission has the sole power to investigate but will not initiate cases on its own. If there is sufficient evidence to justify initiation of proceedings, the Commission proceeds immediately to an announcement in the Official Journal of the European Communities indicating a summary of all relevant information and the period for submission of views by interested parties. The Commission is also under the obligation to advise accordingly shipowners, shippers and freight forwarders known to be concerned as well as the complainants. The investigation at Community level in cooperation with the Member States shall cover a period of not less than six months immediately prior to the initiation of proceedings. The Commission is empowered to carry out investigations in third countries and seek all information it deems necessary, checking with shipowners, agents, shippers, freight forwarders and conferences. It is noteworthy that information received under the Regulation by the Council, the Commission, the Member States or their officials is covered by confidentiality if it has been so requested by its supplier (Article 8).

(j) Termination of proceedings - undertakings

Proceedings may be terminated if it becomes apparent after consultation that protective measures are unnecessary. In all other cases, the Commission will submit to the Council a report on the results of the consultation, together with a proposal that the proceedings be terminated. If the Council, acting by a qualified majority within one month, has not decided otherwise, proceedings will stand terminated. The termination will be announced in the Official Journal of the European Communities.

The investigation may also be terminated without imposition of redressive duties, if undertakings offered are judged acceptable by the Commission. The undertakings are those under which rates are revised to an extent such that the Commission is satisfied that the unfair pricing practice or its injurious effects are eliminated (Article 10).

Since undertakings usually provide for price increases that restore the normal terms of competition, they inevitably increase the profit margins that are the object of the measure. This may even further undermine the competitive position of Community undertakings in the medium term.[19]

(k) Redressive Duties

On the other hand, where investigation shows that there is an unfair pricing practice, that injury is caused by it and that the interests of the Community render Community intervention necessary, the Commission shall propose to the Council the introduction of a redressive duty.[20] The Council, acting by a qualified majority, shall take a decision within two months. In deciding on the redressive duties, however, there is a caveat in Article 12 similar to the one provided by Article 3 of regulation 4058/86 whereby the Council shall also take due account of external trade policy considerations as well as the port interests and shipping policy considerations of the Member States concerned.

All relevant information concerning the imposition of redressive duties upon the foreign shipowners shall be covered by regulation, ie, the amount and type of duties, the commodities transported, the name and country of origin of the foreign shipowner and the reasoning. The amount of the duties shall not exceed the differences between the freight rate charged and the normal freight rate referred in Article 3 (c) of the Regulation. Duties shall be collected by the Member States concerned (Article 13). Regulations imposing redressive duties and decisions to accept undertakings shall be subject to review, wholly or partly at the request of a Member State, on the initiative of the Commission or at the request of an interested party. In such cases investigation shall be reopened and the measures may be amended, repealed or annulled.

Redressive duties and undertakings shall lapse after five years from the date on which they entered into force or were last amended or confirmed. A notice to this effect is published in the Official Journal of the European Communities (Article 15).

If the shipowner concerned can prove that the duty collected exceeds the difference between the freight rate charged and the normal freight rate referred to in Article 3 (c), the excess amount will be reimbursed. An application will be submitted to the Commission to this effect via the Member State concerned (Article 16).

(1) Entry into Force

The Regulation entered into force on 1 July 1987.

REGULATION NO. 4058/86 CONCERNING COORDINATED ACTION TO SAFEGUARD FREE ACCESS TO CARGOES IN OCEAN TRADES

The antiprotectionist character of this Regulation may be highlighted by reference to two of its preambular paragraphs where it is stated that "certain countries, by virtue of measures they have adopted or practices they have imposed, have distorted the application of the principle of fair and free competition in shipping trade with one or more Community Member States" and further that "in respect of bulk trades there is an increasing tendency on the part of third countries to restrict access to bulk cargoes, which poses a serious threat to the freely competitive environment broadly prevailing in the bulk trades, whereas the Member States affirm their commitment to a freely competitive environment as being an essential feature of the dry and liquid bulk trades and are convinced that the introduction of cargo-sharing in these trades will have a serious effect on the trading interests of all countries by substantially increasing transportation costs". The legal basis of the Regulation is Article 84 para 2 EEC.

(a) Scope of Application

The Regulation applies to the following transportations:

- liner cargoes in UNCTAD Liner Code trades,
- liner cargoes in non-Code trades,
- bulk cargoes and any other cargo on tramp services,
- passengers,
- off-shore installations (Article 1).

(b)   Beneficiaries (Application Ratione Personae)

The Regulation applies when action by a third country or by its agents restricts or threatens to restrict free access by shipping companies of Member States or by ships registered in a Member State in accordance with its legislation (Article 1). It may be observed that the Regulation does not define what is meant by action which restricts free access. Obviously, direct action (such as the setting up of central freight bureaux) is covered but what about more indirect action (financial privileges or state aids)?

Furthermore, the Regulation may be applied when similar access to cargoes is restricted to shipping companies of another OECD country where, on the basis of reciprocity, it has been agreed between that country and the Community to resort to coordinated resistance (Article 8). This is a clearcut commitment of the Community vis-a-vis its OECD partners in the context of the agreement of the CSG/US dialogue.[21] It is unclear, however, what kind of arrangements will be required for coordinating EEC action with that of OECD countries. For instance, will a formal agreement be required or will a joint declaration or recommendation suffice?

(c)   Coordinated Action

The crunch of the regulation consists in the mechanism of coordinated action provided in Articles 3-5. Coordinated action is triggered by a request of a Member State addressed to the Commission, which in turn will submit a recommendation to the Council within four weeks. Thereafter, the Council may decide on the coordinated action, acting in accordance with the voting procedure laid down in Article 84 paragraph 2 of the EEC Treaty.

It is odd to find such a reference to the unanimity voting rule under Article 84 paragraph 2 EEC on the eve of entry into force of the European Single Act (1/7/86) which in Article 16 para 5 changes the unanimity voting rule to qualified majority rule. Such a reference to the unanimity voting rule may not be attributed to an oversight of the drafters of the Regulation. It indicates clearly the intention that decisions by de facto unanimity will again be sought in Council with regard to the triggering of the coordinated resistance. This intention is corroborated by the provision in Article 3 paragraph 4 expressis verbis that "in deciding on coordinated action, the Council shall also take due account of the external trade policy considerations as well as the ports interests and the shipping policy considerations of the Member States concerned". Insertion of the latter paragraph may be attributed primarily to the Greek delegation, which initially had strong reservations about the countermeasures mechanism of the Regulation. The Greek apprehension was mainly not to upset its traditionally good commercial and shipping relations with COMECON countries by the introduction of a legislative instrument on countermeasures, considered basically a protectionist device that could very well expose certain Community countries to the risk of retaliatory measures by the COMECON countries concerned.

However, there is a counterbalance to decisions for coordinated action taken by unanimity (Article 3 paragraph 3). This is the consequence of the combined effect of Article 6 paragraphs 1-2, whereby if the Council has not decided on coordinated action within two months, Member States are empowered to take national countermeasures unilaterally or as a group or even provisional countermeasures at the national level even within the two-month period. For Member States interested in the speedy application of countermeasures, the above Article provides a leeway to overcome delay in a Council decision.

(d)   Phases - Nature of Coordinated Action

According to Article 4, coordinated action may consist of two phases: a) diplomatic representations to the third countries concerned; and b) counter-measures directed at the shipping company or companies of the third countries concerned or of other countries which benefit from the action taken by the countries concerned, whether operating as a home trader[22] or as a cross-trader in Community trades.

As to the nature of the countermeasures, which may be taken separately or in combination, they may consist of a) the imposition of a quota; b) the imposition of taxes or duties; c) the imposition of an obligation to obtain a permit to load, carry or discharge cargoes.

It is noteworthy that diplomatic representations shall precede countermeasures (Article 4 paragraph 2). This provision again may be attributed to appeasement of Greek apprehensions with the result that countermeasures will be the last recourse only when diplomatic persuasion fails.

Furthermore, the decision of the Council on countermeasures should enlist a number of specifications, namely, the duration of countermeasures, the reason for their imposition, the range of ports or trades to which they are to apply, the flag or shipping company of the third country concerned, the maximum number of sailings to and from Community ports, the maximum volume or value of cargo to be loaded or discharged in ports of Member States, and finally the amount or percentage and basis of the taxes and duties to be levied and the mechanism for their collection (Article 5). With regard to the above mentioned specifications one may comment that they are completely liner oriented in that they take for granted that there will be a frequency of sailings to and from Community ports, which is a characteristic only of liner trades. Quid in the case of tramp trades, where vessels of the third countries concerned call at Community ports only occasionally? Furthermore, quid in the case of Latin American countries with large volumes of commercial relations with the Community but insignificant fleets? In such cases, the maritime countermeasures will have no biting element at all. In order to cover such cases, it would have been more expedient to make provision for commercial countermeasures against the offending country's exports to the Community.

Finally, during the period in which the countermeasures are to apply, the consultation procedure established by Decision 77/587/EEC will be in force in order to discuss the effects of the countermeasures.

(e) Community Countermeasures - National
     Countermeasures

It is noteworthy that most Community countries
have national countermeasures.[23] The exceptions are
Greece, Ireland, Portugal and Luxembourg. In light
of the above and in cases of inaction by the
Council, Member States may apply national
countermeasures unilaterally or as a group, if the
situation so requires (Article 6), provided that the
Commission and the other Member States are notified
immediately.

(f) Entry into Force

The Regulation entered into force on 1/7/87.[24]

THE PACKAGE OF MEASURES ADOPTED VIS-A-VIS THE
COMMISSION'S PROPOSALS

If one takes apart the basic stumbling blocks of
the negotiations, namely, the issue of cabotage and
the issue of beneficiaries, it is remarkable that
for the remaining texts of the four Regulations the
final versions adopted by the Council in December
1986 are not so different in substance from the
original versions contained in the Commission
Memorandum of March 1985. Between these two
versions, however, the Commission proposal was
substantially modified by various proposals put
forward by the Member States in Council. Hence, the
version adopted constitutes in a sense a "retour aux
sources". Despite the differences of opinion among
the various Member States, there was basic agreement
on such issues as moderated liberalism, closed
conferences between most of the Member States. Such
agreement left out Greece supporting positions which
were in most instances at the other end of the
pendulum and constituted a sui generis case, eg, on
the issue of beneficiaries, the support of the open
conference system and the support of unconditional
liberalism. In light of the above situation and
taking into account the fact that Greece represented
by far the biggest fleet in the EEC, it could be
argued that the negotiations were basically
conducted between the West European countries and
Greece, with the United Kingdom acting as a go-
between expressing sympathies to both sides
according to the issue at stake. Without wishing to

oversimplify the issues, it could be argued in the same vein that the final versions of the four regulations seen from that angle could be characterised as follows: Regulations 4055 and 4058 constitute a success for the Greek views and Regulations 4056 and 4057 constitute a success for the other Member States.

THE SINGLE EUROPEAN ACT AND THE MARITIME SECTOR

The process towards achievement of the internal market in 1992, which was set in motion on 1/7/87 by the European Single Act will inevitably trigger new developments in the maritime field. In fact it has been observed[25] that the lack of progress towards integrating the transport sector was partly due to the compartmentalization of decision-making in the Council, with transport ministers scoring points off each other while colleagues in different Councils, interested in finishing the internal market make high-sounding pronouncements about the desirability of such integration. This situation is expected to change as a result of the change in voting procedures which came about pursuant to the provisions of the European Single Act as of 1/7/87. In fact, under the terms of Article 16 para 5, the voting procedure requiring unanimity in Council under Article 84 paragraph 2 of the EEC Treaty is amended to a qualified majority, whereby 54 votes are required out of a total of 76 for a Council decision to be taken.[26] Article 84 para 2 as it stands now reads as follows:
"The Council may, acting by a qualified majority, decide whether, to what extent and by what procedure appropriate provisions may be laid down for sea and air transport...".[27]

There is still provision,[28] however, that decision will not harm the vital interests of a Member State in a given sector and, in this case, unanimity is still retained. Despite this possibility, it is to be expected that achievement of the internal market, facilitated by the new voting rules, will inevitably score points in the maritime transport sector. Moreover, it is to be expected that the upgrading of maritime transport policy would render far-reaching liberalisation of the maritime transport sector an almost inescapable choice.

NOTES

1 With regard to the future treatment of consortia,
  it has been proposed by some shipowner quarters
  to make the following distinction: the activities
  of consortia operating within conferences lie
  within the intent of Regulation 4056. The few
  consortia operated as single commercial
  activities should be treated in the same manner
  as individual shipping companies and should
  therefore require no special treatment under the
  competition rules. In the rare cases where a
  consortium operates outside a conference and is
  under single company operation it will be obliged
  to have a rate fixing role and should be subject
  to a similar group exemption as that provided
  under Regulation 4056. Alan Bott in "The EEC and
  Shipping", Institute of Maritime Law, Conference
  11/2/88, London.

2 "A" item = without debate.

3 It appears that translations of the Regulations
  in some of the official languages present
  problems. It is advisable, therefore, to use the
  English text as the guiding text.

4 Spanish Regulation No. 1382 of 18/1/1985 provides
  for liberalisation of maritime transport from the
  reservation for Spanish flag vessels of the
  transportation of certain commodities save for an
  extremely long list of commodities including,
  inter alia,: tobacco, coal, lignite, crude oil
  and other types of oil, petroleum gas, cotton,
  meat, coffee, wheat, rye, barley, corn, rice,
  cereal, flour, olive oil, soya oil, sunflower
  oil, sugar.

5 The Regulation refers to bilateral agreements
  concluded at governmental level. It leaves
  untouched the area of private agreements
  concluded between companies; the latter
  agreements may still contain cargo sharing
  clauses and be compatible with the Regulation.
  We consider this a serious gap in the Regulation.

6 For a detailed criticism of the shortcomings of the Regulation cf George Close "Free Access to Cargoes and Freedom to Operate" in "EEC Shipping Law", Conference 4-5/2/88, Rotterdam, European Study Conferences Ltd.

7 For the background of the adoption of the competition regulation cf case 167/73 of the European Court of Justice and the so-called Asjes-judgment case n° 209/84, 30/4/1986, Rec. 1986, p.1425-1473; A.J.Braakman "Competition and Merchant Shipping" in "EEC Shipping Law", Conference 4-5/2/88, Rotterdam, European Study Conferences Ltd. Braakman argues that in the Asjes-judgment the European Court confirmed the ruling in the French seamen's case about direct applicability of Articles 85-86 of the Treaty and indicated that as soon as the incompatibility of an agreement with Article 85 para 1 has been found either by a national authority under Article 88 or by the Commission under Article 89 para 2, the national courts must draw all the consequences from it. In particular, they must pronounce the nullity under Article 85 para 2 of the agreement. The main problem with the Asjes regime lies in the possibility of granting an exemption from the cartel prohibition.

8 Braakman, ibid, argues that allegedly there are no anti-competitive restrictions in the tramp vessel services. There are eg. long term contracts for the transportation of certain raw materials. The Dutch social council has stated that in cases where a conference has determined the rates and other conditions for the transportation of bulk cargo, the Commission should bring such transports within the scope of Regulation 4056/86. It is further argued that the definition of tramp vessel services implies that offshore transport, sea towing services and supply-and salvage activities also fall outside the scope of Regulation 4056/86.

9 It is uncertain whether providers of ancillary services (insurers, classification societies, stevedores, shipping agents) are covered by the Regulation or whether they are subject to the ordinary rules of competition. Basically, the Regulation is of direct relevance only to

shipowners and operators. Nicholas Green argues
that non-ship operators may potentially benefit
from certain of the provisions of the Regulation
cf "Regulation 4056/86: Competition Law and
Maritime Transport, in "The EEC and Shipping",
Institute of Maritime Law, Conference 11/2/88,
London.

10 Service contracts are recognized under the 1984
US Shipping Act. The silence of Regulation
4056/86 as to their status under Community Law
opens the door to various interpretations
concerning their legality. We are inclined to
infer from this silence that service contracts
are permissible under Community law.

11 Cf. Nicholas Green "Regulation 4056/86:
Competition Law and Maritime Transport" in "The
EEC and Shipping", Institute of Maritime Law,
Conference 11/2/88, London.

12 It will be interesting to see how this provision
about the 10% turnover will be applied in
practice in case of a company engaged both in
maritime transport activities and other
activities. Such a provision may trigger the
progress of creation of one ship companies (in
cases where they did not exist up to now) in
order to minimize the risk from application of
the 10% turnover provision.

13 Cf. Chapter 4 - Initiatives 1977-1985.

14 Cf. the contrary view, ie, that the case has not
been made by the Commission, is maintained in the
findings of Simon Bergestrand - Rigas Doganis
"The Impact of Soviet Shipping", Allen of Unwin,
1987; cf, also the views to the contrary of the
European Shippers Councils in "Progress towards a
Common Transport Policy - Maritime Transport" -
views of the European Shippers Councils, October
1985.

15 The UNCTAD Secreteriat in a preparatory paper on
Possible Issues and Proposals for Amendments
concerning the Review Conference of the U N Code
of Conduct for liner conferences (June 1987)
argues (paragraph 101, p.33) that under
Regulation 4057/86 unfairness is narrowly defined

as a non-commercial advantage granted by a state and complains that no reference is made to unfair pricing practices which may be based on commercial advantages such as surplus tonnage, soft finance, or cross subsidisation of routes. By and large, Regulation 4057/86 is criticized as being a one-sided attempt to define the concept of fair competition on a commercial basis.

16 Jacques Steenbergen observes that with regard to the basis of comparison which can either be the rate as practiced on the market or a constructed value -if the Community institutions interpret the rule in Regulation 4057/86 as they interpret the equivalent provisions in other commercial policy instruments, the Community will make extensive use of constructed values, especially when there are reasons to believe that few competitors charge normal freight rates: the use of constructed values leads usually to a comparatively higher countervailable margin cf "Unfair Pricing Practices in Maritime Transport" in "EEC Shipping Law, Conference 4-5/2/88, Rotterdam, European Study Conferences Ltd.

17 The Regulation in its operative and procedural part resembles to Regulation 2176/84. The concepts of "normal freight rates" and "lower than normal freight rates" are inspired by the notion of "normal value" first expounded vis-a-vis the EEC in Article VI of GATT and later used in Regulation 2176/84. There are, however, differences between the two Regulations. For a comparison of the differences between the two Regulations cf. Fergus Randolph "Dumping: Unfair Pricing Practices of Non-EEC Lines" in "The EEC and Shipping", Institute of Maritime Law, Conference 11/2/88, London; Jacques Steenbergen "Unfair Pricing Practices in Maritime Transport", in "EEC Shipping Law", Conference 4-5/2/88, Rotterdam, European Study Conferences Ltd.

18 M.Hutchings "Unfair Pricing Practices-Procedure" in "The EEC and Shipping", Institute of Maritime Law, Conference 11/2/88, London.

19 Cf. Jacques Steenbergen, op.cit.

20 It is noteworthy that the original version of the Regulation, as proposed by the Commission, provided under Articles 11-12 for a distinction between provisional duties and definitive duties. Provisional duties were imposed by the Commission within five days on receipt of the request and with a maximum period of validity of four months.

21 This Article was drafted on the assumption that there would be a legally binding CSG/US agreement. However, the 1986 Copenhagen Declaration of the dialogue has no legal force. Despite the absence of such a binding agreement, there is still need of some form of legally binding commitment on behalf of the United States, or, else, Article 8 will be conferring rights on OECD countries without obligations to the Community. Hence, an exchange of letters on behalf of the United States does not confer the character of "reciprocity".

22 According to Article 2 of the Regulation and for its purposes the term "home trader" means a shipping company of a third country which operates a service between its own country and one or more Member States and "cross trader" means a shipping company of a third country which operates a service between another third country and one or more Member States.

23 Cf: Belgium: Law protecting the Belgian Merchant Marine (25/1/84). The Netherlands: Act of 27/10/1982 containing rules concerning the sea transport market (Sea Transport Act) (art.12), and Act of 4/5/1977 Regulating Retaliatory Action in the Field of Maritime Shipping (Maritime Shipping Retaliation Act). France: Law No.83.1119 of 23/12/1983 concerning the measures that may be taken in case of prejudice against the maritime and commercial interests of France. Denmark: Law of 2/12/1977. Germany: Foreign Trade Law 28/4/1961 (sections 6 and 18) as amended on 26/5/1973 and Customs Act 14/6/1961 (Section 21). Italy: Law No.388 4/3/1963 as amended by Law 8/4/1976. Spain: Law No. 6/70-III. United Kingdom: U.K. Merchant Shipping Act 1974, Part III on protection of shipping and trading interests (Section 14). It is noteworthy that retaliatory legislation (either specifically

concerning maritime countermeasures or general commercial countermeasures) exists in other OECD countries such as the United States of America, Japan, Finland, Sweden and Norway. Moreover, the principle of countermeasures is also enshrined in the recently adopted (13/2/87) OECD Decision and Recommendation of the Council concerning Common principles of Shipping Policy for Member Countries (Principles 4-6). Broadly speaking, national retaliatory measures take the following forms: restrictions of loadings/unloadings, customs taxes or levies, fines and/or imprisonment.

24 For a detailed criticism of the shortcomings of the Regulation cf George Close "Free Access to Cargoes and Freedom to Operate" in "EEC Shipping Law", Conference 4-5/2/88, Rotterdam, European Study Conferences Ltd.

25 "The Unfinished European Integration", Netherlands Scientific Council for Government Policy, No.28, 1986, The Hague, pp. 94-95.

26 Cf. Article 148 para 2 of the EEC Treaty as amended by Article 11 of the Act of Accession of Spain and Portugal.

27 Cf. Chapter 4, for the previous version of Article 84 before its amendment by the European Single Act, Article 16 para 5.

28 A Member State can still require a unanimous decision but only under the conditions of Article 75 para 3 of the Treaty which the Single Act declared applicable, according to Article 16 para 6. More particularly, Article 75 para 3 states that: "By way of derogation from the procedure provided for in para 1, where the application of provisions concerning the principles of the regulatory system for transport would be liable to have a serious effect on the standard of living and on employment in certain areas and on the operation of transport facilities, they shall be laid down by the Council acting unanimously. In so doing, the Council shall take into account the need for adaptation to the economic development which will result from establishing the common market".

CHAPTER 9

THE IMPLICATIONS OF THE 1986 PACKAGE OF MEASURES FOR THE INDIVIDUAL EC MEMBER STATES

Although Regulations 4055/86, 4056/86, 4057/86 and 4058/86 constitute a package of measures their implications for each of the EC Member States have first to be assessed separately in relation to the main characteristics of current national maritime policies. It would then be easier to produce an overall assessment.

IMPLICATIONS OF REGULATION 4055/86

This Regulation is bound to cause significant adjustments in the maritime policy of those Member States which resort to unilateral or bilateral cargo reservation practices in their international trades. As reported in Chapter 3 these countries are Belgium, France, Germany, Italy, Portugal and Spain.

It has to be remembered of course that under Articles 2, 3 and 4 of this Regulation there exist interim periods for the abolition of all national restrictions existing prior to July 1st 1986. Thus the necessary adjustments in the maritime policy of these countries are not going to materialise in the near future. Furthermore, the practical experience from the application of Regulation 4055/86 so far has revealed a great reluctance on the part of individual Member States to comply with its provisions.

A notable case is that of the cargo sharing agreement between Italy and Algeria which was initialled on January 30, 1987 and signed on February 28, 1987, i.e. after the provisions of Regulation 4055/86 had come into force. The Italian government informed the Commission on the existence of that agreement in March 1987 and the latter reacted by treating the submission of this information as constituting action by a Member State under Article 6 of Regulation 4055/86 when its shipping companies face difficulties in participating in sea transport to or from a third country. Hence, the Commission proceeded and submitted to the Council a draft decision specifying that Italy could not ratify the above agreement unless:

(a) it ratified as soon as possible the UN Liner Code in accordance with EEC Regulation 954/79,

(b) the arrangements for cargo sharing were put into conformity with EC law in certain specified ways,

(c) these arrangements ceased to have effect as soon as the Liner Code became applicable to the conference traffic between Italy and Algeria, and at the latest 3 years after the date of the proposed Council decision, and

(d) Italy consulted the Commission before ratifying the modified agreement.

Italy reacted to the Commission proposals by arguing that its agreement with Algeria had been negotiated before Regulation 4055/86 come into force, and consequently was not covered by the provisions of Article 6. The Italian government also claimed that the agreement per se did not contain a cargo sharing system, because it did not specify fixed shares but instead left the task of sharing out to the shipowners of the two countries!

These arguments although unsustainable under EC law found a sympathetic reception among those EC governments that have bilateral cargo-sharing agreements with third countries or are exploring the possiblities of new ones. This resulted in acrimonious discussions in the Council and it was the pressure exerted by the Commission as guardian of the application of Community law, and of the Greek government (which represented considerable cross-trading interests) that led to the adoption of a compromise Council Decision on September 17, 1987.

That decision authorised the Italian government to ratify its agreement with Algeria subject to the following conditions:

(a) Italy would accede as soon as possible to the UN Code in accordance with the provisions of Regulation 954/79,

(b) will reiterate to Algeria that the provisions of the Agreement will be implemented in accordance with Community law, and

(c) will report to the Member States and the Commission within not later than one year of notification of the Council Decision on the implementation of the Agreement.

The Commission found this decision weak and in violation of Articles 5 and 6 of Regulation 4055/86. Consequently it has initiated proceedings before the Court of Justice of the European Communities for its annulment. At the time of writing no ruling had been delivered by the Court on this matter. When the above Decision was taken by the Council Italy announced that it had initiated the necessary proceedings for ratification of the Liner Code but no such event had taken place at the time of writing.

The foot dragging by the Member States concerned in respect to the application of the provisions of Regulation 4055/86 manifests itself also in their reactions to requests of relevant information by the Commission. Under Article 4(3) of Regulation 4055/86 Member States have an obligation to report to the Commission initially every six months and subsequently every year on progress of the adjustments made to cargo-sharing agreements existing prior to the coming into force of this regulation. The Commission had not reported on whether Member States had complied with this obligation in the first year of the application of that Regulation. Presumably, Member States involved in cargo-sharing agreements had not done so. According to a document submitted by the Commission services to the Council Transport Group on 12 July 1988 on this matter, two Member States had not complied with the above obligation although more than a year had elapsed since the Regulation had to come into force. These countries were Spain which had given no reply at all to requests of information from the Commission and Belgium which had given an incomplete reply. Moreover, with respect to existing agreements the replies given by Belgium, France, Italy and Portugal do not clarify whether these apply to bulk as well as to liner trades.

In its reply Germany indicated the existence of
agreements with Argentina, Brazil and Ivory Coast,
but produced a unilateral interpretation that these
do not consitute cargo-sharing, since cargo is
reserved in favour of the third country!

Portugal went even further in interpreting its
agreements with a large number of third countries as
non-cargo-sharing by alleging that these are based
on the "principle of balance" meaning that
shipowners of each party have equal rights on the
carrying of cargoes, and that this principle does
not constitute cargo-sharing! The Commission
document of July 1988 also refers to new agreements
concluded after the 1st of January 1987. Apart from
the Italy-Algeria agreement referred to above, the
document reports on agreements signed or initialled
by Belgium and South Korea, Brazil, Zaire and Togo,
and between France and Mauritania, and on the
conclusion of negotiations between Germany and the
Soviet Union. With respect to the Belgium-South
Korea agreement the Commission states that
consultations are taking place with the former with
the purpose of modifying the agreement in accordance
with Regulation 954/79 since the Liner Code has come
into force between these two countries.

On the other hand, the Commission has indicated
to the Belgian government that the other three
agreements are not in conformity with Regulation
4055/86. The view of the Belgian government is that
these agreements constitute no cargo-sharing. A
similar view has been expressed by the German
government with respect to the shipping agreement it
has negotiated with the Soviet Union. Finally,
France had not replied by mid 1988 to the enquiries
of the Commission concerning its agreement with
Mauritania.

The impression derived from the responses to the
Commission's enquiries of the above Member States
involved in bilateral cargo reservation agreements
is that they are trying to by-pass the enforcement
of Regulation 4055/86 by questioning what
constitutes cargo-sharing. It remains to be seen
what the Commission will do to enforce Community law
in this area. Judging from its response to the
Italy-Algeria agreement the most likely course of

action would be that leading to the European Court of Justice.

The reluctance of the Member States concerned to adjust their bilateral shipping relations with third countries to the new Community "maritime order" is also reflected by the fact that none of them has informed the Council and the Commission according to Article 4(4) on the difficulties arising in the process of adjusting their bilateral agreements.

A good example of such difficulties is the widely reported use of central freight bureaux by a number of West African countries (eg. Senegal, Ivory Coast, Togo, Benin, Cameroun) through which they practice pre-shipment control of cargoes. In addition the countries of Central and West Africa signed in April 1987 an agreement, known as the Hamburg Protocol, with the governments of Belgium, Germany, and the Netherlands for cargo allocation in their bilateral liner trades. This Protocol was subsequently translated into a specific cargo-sharing agreement, the Kinshasa Agreement, between the shippers of those countries (who represent government organisations) and the West African conference, which includes liner companies of the above EC countries. It is notable that these countries did not make use of the relevant EC Regulations to deal with whatever difficulties the practices of Central and West African countries create, but instead reverted to arranging a solution outside the Community framework.

This approach by Belgium, Germany and the Netherlands triggered off the reaction of the Danish government which tabled a formal complaint to the Council for violations of Regulations 4055/86 and 4058/86. The Danish government was particularly concerned since the Kinshasa agreement was detrimental to the interests of Danish liner companies which operate as outsiders in the Central and West African trades. Furthermore, the Danish Shipowners' Association and the European Shippers Councils lodged a complaint with the Commission claiming that the Kinshasa Agreement was in violation of the provisions of Regulation 4056/86. The implications of the Kinshasa Agreement as far as the other Regulations are concerned are examined below.

Despite the evasive tactics of the individual Member States affected it is unavoidable for them that they would have to comply with Regulation 4055/86 as has been repeatedly demonstrated in the removal of trade berriers in other sectors of economic activity in the Community. In the meantime these countries have an opportunity to utilise the time at their disposal, (either provided for by the Regulation itself or resulting from their foot-dragging) to improve the competitiveness of their shipping industries so as to be able to survive the abolition of cargo-reservation arrangements existing currently in their favour.

One possible line of action would involve the removal of impediments to improved competitiveness resulting from national restrictions on the employment of factors of production such as the exclusive employment of national seafarers or the ordering of vessels at national shipyards. As seen in Chapter 3, France, Ireland, Portugal and Spain do not allow the employment of non-nationals on board ships in their national registries. Shipowners in Italy, Portugal and Spain have no recourse to the more competitive Far Eastern shipyards for ordering new vessels.

In parallel with the removal of these restrictions, the governments of these countries could resort to the use of more subsidies, either through the provision of direct aid or through the exemption from the payment of taxes and social security contributions.[1] Already some Member States have taken steps in the above directions through the creation of new parallel registers, in response to the competition faced internationally by their shipping industry.

Other Member States have taken similar measures within the framework of their existing registry. Eg. the government of the Netherlands obtained very recently approval from the Commission for a package of measures that constitute a favourable treatment of its shipping sector in comparison to other sectors of its economy.[2] The measures included an exemption of 35% of seafarers' salaries from income tax with the objective of lowering the operating costs of Dutch shipowning companies. In addition, the employment of non-domiciles from developing countries will become more flexible. The approval granted by the Commission in this case can be taken to indicate a lenient view with respect to the special treatment of the shipping sector in the Member States in relation to the provisions in the Treaty of Rome concerning state aids (Articles 92 and 93).

The removal of the barriers to trade in maritime services as a consequence of the enforcement of Regulation 4055/86 would be expected simply to accentuate the established trend for the special treatment of the maritime sector in the individual Member States. The pressures for such action would be particularly strong in those Member States which practice unilateral or bilateral cargo reservation practices in their international trade.

Thus the enforcement of Regulation 4055/86 is likely to contribute to the reshaping of the industrial policies of individual Member States with respect to their shipping industries through the replacement of barriers to trade in maritime services by subsidies. This replacement would theoretically be expected to produce a lower degree of distortion in the allocation of resources since the prices paid by the consumers of maritime services in the respective countries would not be artificially higher than those determined internationally by market forces. It is not surprising therefore, that shippers' groups in all Member States are strong advocates of the firm enforcement of the provisions of Regulation 4055/86.[3]

The likely removal of the obligations imposed upon the maritime sectors in the aforementioned Member States to rely exclusively upon their national labour market and shipbuilding industry would also lead ceteris paribus to a more competitive environment for the latter. Needless to say that the enforcement of the provisions of Regulation 4055/86 would offer greater opportunities for competitive access to trades to those shipowners in EC Member States that are already fully exposed to the forces of international competition.

An important side effect of the application of Regulation 4055/86 would be the removal of one competitive disadvantage for the ports of those countries that resort to cargo reservation practices in their international trades. The extent to which the higher freight rates resulting from those practices divert at present trade to ports of other nearby countries and the subsequent use of land transport is unknown. Nevertheless, it can safely be inferred that the abolition of cargo reservation practices will create a more competitive environment for the ports of the Member States.

IMPLICATIONS OF REGULATION 4056/86

The application of Regulation 4056/86 is expected to affect maritime policy in Member States in two ways:

(a) directly, by filling in the vacuum in national competition policy that has been created by the reluctance of individual states to get involved in the regulation of liner conferences[4], and

(b) indirectly, through its interaction with the other three Regulations which in themselves affect the external maritime relations of the Member States.

Regulation 4056/86 has[5] now clarified the standing of liner conferences. In essence, it has accepted the system of closed conferences and in parallel it strikes a balance between the interests of liner conference carriers, independent operators and transport users. The conditions and obligations under which exemption is granted from the application of Articles 85 and 86 of the Treaty of Rome undoubtedly has strengthened the bargaining power of transport users. That power has also been strengthened by the exemption under Article 6 of the agreements between the transport users themselves which may be necessary for the purpose of dealing with conferences.

Already the European Shippers' Councils and the British Shippers' Council have taken action under the provisions of Regulation 4056/86 against the agreements between the North Europe-US Atlantic Conferences and some important outsiders known as the Eurocorde agreements, which in their view restrict competition by creating a near-monopoly situation.[6]

Following that complaint the Commission opened formal proceedings under Article 10 of the Regulation so as to terminate any infringement that might exist of the provisions of Articles 85(1) and 86 of the Treaty.

Subsequently the conference carriers and one of the outsiders involved in the Eurocorde agreements applied for individual exemption under Regulation 4056/86. The case is still pending with the Commission.

Interestingly enough the above agreements have been given clearance by the Federal Maritime Commission under the provisions of the U.S. Shipping Act 1984.

Similarly, the conditions and obligations attached to the exemption granted constitute a concrete measure for safeguarding the position of outsiders in the liner trades, especially the provisions in Article 7 referring to acts of third countries that close the trade to outsiders or restrict their operation. Thus, the policies of the individual Member States in connection with the position of outsiders expressed in international conventions such as the UN Code of Conduct have taken through Regulation 4056/86 a more specific and substantive form.

This provision forms a crucial link between this Regulation and Regulations 4055/86 and 4058/86: Exemption is granted to liner conferences subject to there being effective competition from outsiders. If this is prevented from materializing due to bilateral agreements between individual Community countries and third countries that do not comply with Regulation 954/79 and 4055/86, or due to unilateral restrictive action by third countries that should have been dealt with through the coordinated steps envisaged by Regulation 4058/86, the exemption is withdrawn.

It is interesting therefore to note that the Danish Shipowners' Association approach to the problems its members face in the Europe -Central and West Africa trades involves a recourse to Regulation 4056/86.[7]

Since a complaint has been lodged the Commission (DG IV) is obliged to initiate the proceedings under Article 10 to bring to an end any violation of Articles 85(1) and 86 of the Treaty.

Although the contentious issue of the Kinshasa agreement has yet to be resolved according to Community law, the pressures generated by the need to comply with this Regulation would eventually compel those Member States that are involved with bilateral cargo-sharing agreements with African countries to comply with Regulation 4055/86.

An important outstanding question still to be resolved concerns the status of consortia in relation to the EC competition rules.

The use of consortia in the liner trades has been gaining momentum over the recent years as a result of containerisation and the increasingly capital intensive form of production of maritime services in those trades. The issue at stake centers on whether consortia are compatible with the rules on competition and can be granted an a priori block exemption, under the terms of Regulation 4056/86. This issue is of major importance to the liner trades since consortia are substituting the traditional conference system as an organisational framework for co-operation and rationalisation between liner shipping companies. However, no common definition on what constitutes a consortium has been put forward by the shipping industry itself or the member governments. At the time of the adoption of the 1986 Regulations the Commission undertook at the request of the Council to consider whether it was necessary to submit proposals for the treatment of consortia in relation to the EC competition rules. The Commission has yet to produce such proposals. This delay must be attributed to the complexity of the issue.[8]

Furthermore, as seen from the Annual Report 1987-88 of the European Shipowners' Organisation (CAACE) the position of shipowners on the above issue is not unified.[9] The majority of the members of CAACE, which represent countries with a strong presence in consortia in the liner trades argue against subjecting them to additional regulation in the EEC. On the other hand, the Union of Greek Shipowners representing cross-trading interests and independent operators argues that there can be no general a priori exemption since there exist different types of consortia. It supports therefore a case by case approach whereby exemption could be granted on an individual basis.

According to a Council Transport Working Group document of January 11, 1988 the Commission has been pressed by the governments of Denmark, Germany and the United Kingdom to produce a proposal for the exemption of consortia in view of the Review Conference of the Liner Code in 1988. However, given the complexity of the issue and the conflicting interests of Member States it is likely that the problem of consortia will only be resolved in the context of phase two of the EC maritime policy as part of a package of measures.

IMPLICATIONS OF REGULATION 4057/86

This Regulation also adds a new dimension to the shipping policy of individual Member States, that of anti-dumping measures which did not exist before. Dumping has been replaced in this case by the term "unfair practices" but the approach here is by and large the same as the one used in anti-dumping legislation concerning trade in goods.[10] In assessing the impact of this Regulation on national maritime policy it should be recalled that the dividing line between anti-dumping measures and protectionism is very fine indeed. To a large extent the effects on national maritime policy would depend on how the Commission and the Council intend to deal with the actual complaints brought forward by Community liner companies against carriers from third countries.

On an a priori basis the application of this Regulation generates a shift in the national maritime policies in favour of the national carriers and at the expense of transport users. As mentioned in Chapter 8, this Regulation cannot be invoked and misused by shipping lines so as to avoid the application of Regulation 4056/86. This link with the competition rules constitutes an important safeguard for the consumers of maritime services and could act as a break to any attempts to apply this Regulation in such a way that it degenerates into an instrument of protectionism.

The first test case brought under the terms of Regulation 4057/86 involves the South Korean shipping line Hyundai Merchant Marine. A complaint against that company for allegedly unfair practices was lodged soon after the Regulation became operative in July 1987 by eight liner operators, members of the Australia-Europe conference, supported by an outsider.[11] The complaint was that Hyundai charges "uneconomic" and "unfair" freight rates on the southbound trip from North Europe to Australia and that this is the result of the Korean government's policies of subsidies and protectionism. Following the complaint, the Commission initiated the proceedings of investigation envisaged by this Regulation and in October 1988 came to the conclusion that Hyundai had damaged European shipping lines by unfairly undercutting freight rates. Consequently, it recommended to the Council the imposition of a redressive duty of 26%. The Council had not decided at the time of writing on this recommendation.

European shippers ever since the above complaint was lodged have contested it strongly and backed Hyundai's arguments to the effect that the claims by the European shipping lines were invalid.[12] They argued instead that the imposition of a duty would cause a withdrawal by Hyundai from the North-Europe-Australia trade, an event that would affect adversely exports to Australia of high volume-low value cargoes, such as chemicals. The shippers also argued that the acceptance of the complaint of the European shipping lines would lead to a new set of relationships between the conference and the various independents operating in the Europe-Australia trade, to the detriment of competition. It is clear from the recommendation pending in the Council that the Commission has tilted the balance in favour of the interests of the European shipping lines and to the detriment of the transport users.

IMPLICATIONS OF REGULATION 4058/86

For the majority of Member States -which already had national countermeasures legislation[13] before this Regulation was enacted- its direct result would be to strengthen the impact that the existence of such legislation might have in preventing protectionist acts by third countries. The preventive impact would be expected to increase if the third country considers it likely that its actions are going to produce concerted countermeasures by a group of countries than the single country affected on its own.

For Greece, Ireland and Portugal (Luxembourg has no merchant fleet yet) the Regulation adds a new dimension to their international maritime policy. They now have a mechanism for initiating countermeasures if their merchant fleets are adversely affected by protectionist measures of third countries.

This Regulation also strengthens the position of all the EC Member States in the context of the CSG-US dialogue, since the American side had persistently asked in the past for the enactment of such legislation by the CSG member countries as proof of their intention to act in a concerted way to face protectionism. However, the usefulness of this Regulation for an individual Member State rests upon the degree of solidarity the other EC Member States are willing to provide. This degree would vary depending on their trading interests with the offending third country.

Moreover, in some instances this Regulation could turn out to run counter to the interests of Member States, such as Greece, the United Kingdom, and Denmark, with strong cross-trading interests. These interests might be affected adversely if a trade war in maritime services erupts between another EC Member State and a third country and Regulation 4058/86 is activated as a consequence. This danger might explain why Greece had not enacted any national countermeasures legislation so far.

The first test case where this Regulation has been applied is that of the aforementioned Central and West African cargo reservation practices.

Following the complaint from Denmark concerning the Kinshasa Agreement, the Commission proposed to the Council the activation of Regulation 4058/86. In the Council Transport Group only three countries (Denmark, Greece and the United Kingdom) supported the firm implementation of this Regulation whilst the others were reluctant to take any action for fear that this might jeopardise their trading interests. The reluctance of the governments of Belgium, Germany and the Netherlands in particular was also connected with the fact that they had already negotiated separately with the African side for the purpose of safeguarding the interests of their national shipping lines and had concluded the Hamburg Protocol.

A compromise was found in October 1987 and it was decided[14] that the first stage of coordinated resistance envisaged in the Regulation should be activated, namely the resort to diplomatic representations. These representations were, however, to take the form of consultations with the African countries in the context of the Lome III Convention. The link with that Convention was proposed by the Commission because it contains provision (Articles 86 to 91) dealing with the shipping relations between the EC and the ACP countries. This move purported also to placate the fears of those Member States concerned about their trading interests with the African States, since the Decision provides that the consultations should replace and supercede all other dipomatic initiatives of the Member States.

Following that Decision, the problem of the Central and West African trades was placed on the Agenda for the 29th meeting of the ACP/EEC Committee of Ambassadors on December 18, 1987. Subsequently, a number of meetings took place between experts of the EC countries and those ACP countries which are members of the Ministerial Conference of West and Central African States on Maritime Transport. The discussions have not produced any concrete results so far. There has been an agreement on principle which provides for the abolition of the freight booking offices and their replacement by a monitoring system of the whole liner trade. The African side appears, however, to be back tracking and insists on a share of 40% of the whole trade (both liner and bulk).

OVERALL ASSESSMENT

The four Regulations considered together are likely to press the formulation of maritime policy in the individual EC Member States in two opposite ways.

On the one hand, they are exerting pressure for the liberalisation of their international shipping trades where these are still closed, as well as for the creation or preservation of a competitive environment for shipping firms to operate. This liberalisation of the shipping markets will consequently necessitate the abandonment of national restrictions upon EC shipowners concerning their choices in the employment of factors of production - where these still apply- so that they can survive from their full exposure to international competition.

On the other hand, the package preserves restrictive practices such as the closed conference system and contains anti-dumping provisions that can easily be abused as a means of protectionism.

The balance to be achieved between these two opposite pressures will depend, of course, on the way the four Regulations are going to be applied in practice. The experience so far has shown that the majority of states is not keen on the firm implementation of those aspects of the Regulations that involve the further liberalisation of their international maritime relations and the resistance of protectionism by third countries.

NOTES

1 Goss, R.O., "Social Costs, Transfer Payments and International Competition in Shipping", Maritime Policy and Management, Vol. 12, No 2, 1985.

2 Lloyd's List, November 28, 1988.

3 Curzon Price, V. "Industrial Policies in the European Community", Trade Policy Research Centre, The Macmillan Press, London 1981. Wallace, H., W. Wallace and C. Webb, "Policy Making in the European Community", John Wiley and Sons, 1983.

4 House of Lords, Select Committee on the European Communities, Chairman Viscount Rochdale, "Competition Policy: Shipping", HMSO. London, 1983.

5 Kreis, H.W.R., "Maritime Transport and EEC. Competition Rules", Antwerp International Congress on EEC Maritime Regulation, November 25-26, 1988, Journal of Law and Economics, Vol. XXIII, No 5, 1988.

6 Lloyd's List, August 8th, 1987. American Shipper, October 1987, U.S. Journal of Commerce of January 20th, 1988.

7 Lloyd's List, July 24th, 1987.

8 Kreis, H.W.R., "Maritime Transport and EEC Competition Rules", op.cit.

9 CAACE, "Annual Report" 1987/1988.

10 Sturmey, S.G., "Competition in Shipping: Distortion EEC-Style?", Greek Shipping Intelligence, July 15th, 1988.

11 The conference members were Associated Container Transportation (Australia) Ltd, P&O Containers, Compagnie Generale Maritime, Hapag-Lloyd, Nedlloyd, Lloyd Triestino, East Asiatic Co and Compania Naviera Marasia. The outsider was the Belgian company A.B.C. Containerline.

12 Lloyd's List, July 14th, 1988, November 18th, 1988.

13 See Chapter 8.

14 Council Decision of October 20, 1987 concerning coordinated action to safeguard free access to cargoes in ocean trades with West African and Central African States.

CHAPTER 10

THE IMPLICATIONS OF THE 1986 PACKAGE OF MEASURES AT COMMUNITY LEVEL

The identification of the implications of the 1986 package of Regulations involves essentially an assessment of its contribution to the process of European integration. In particular, it has to be examined how far and in which direction does the package go in formulating a common EC maritime transport policy.

INTEGRATION OF MARITIME MARKETS

As seen in Chapter 8 the package has initiated a process leading to the elimination of barriers to international trade in maritime services between EC Member States, as well as between Member States and third countries as far as Community shipping companies or vessels registered in Member States are concerned.

Thus, the package has laid the foundations for the creation of a common market in maritime services. Needless to say, that the creation of such a market in the real sense has a long way to go given the complexity of problems in harmonizing transport policy in general, and maritime in particular and the sensitivities of Member States in preserving national jurisdiction in transport policy formulation[1]. It is indicative that the issue of cabotage has yet to be resolved, and that many governments are drugging their feet as far as the implementation of Regulation 4055/86 is concerned.

It should also be stressed that, unlike the Community initiatives in other modes of transport, the abolition of barriers to trade in maritime services has not been linked to any harmonisation of technical or social conditions in the production of those services.

This must be attributed to four factors:

(a) The fact that technical or social standards in the maritime sector are governed by international conventions elaborated in the framework of IMO and ILO and incorporated into the national laws of Member States.

(b) The urgency of action to face the external pressures on Community shipping resulting from protectionism and flag discrimination practices of third countries, and

(c) The reluctance of a number of Member States (notably Denmank, Greece, and the United Kingdom) to accept harmonisation of technical and social conditions as a precondition to the liberalisation of shipping markets.

(d) The absence of detailed provisions for maritime transport in the relevant title of the Treaty.

The interaction of these factors shaped the priorities of the Commission initiatives[2] and the direction of negotiations at Council level that produced the 1986 compromise. In a sense, the Community did not adopt a maximalist approach in shaping EC maritime policy, but tried to bring the formulation of maritime policy into a Community framework by concentrating in areas where Member States could easily identify the existence of common interest. This gradualist approach is no different to the experience from the development of common EC policies in other sectors of economic activity.[3]

HARMONISATION OF EXTERNAL MARITIME RELATIONS

The area of maritime policy where Member States were more readily willing to accept an important Community involvement was that of external maritime relations. This is the area where

(a) Community measures had already been adopted in the past,

(b) Member States had accepted the applicability of the Treaty and

(c) there were problems requiring immediate attention, such as the acts of protectionism by third countries, which could be dealt with more effectively through joint Community action. Thus, the package introduces the element of solidarity in the international maritime relations of Member States.

In essence, the package reaffirms the commitment of the Member States and the Community as a whole to the promotion of free and fair competition in international maritime transport. This commitment which had been expressed in the past in various fora such as the OECD and UNCTAD is given substance through the provisions of Regulation 4058/86 for coordinated action to safeguard free access to cargoes in ocean trades. This leads to an enhancement of the role of the Community and especially of the Commission in international maritime negotiations.

A vivid example of such an enhancement can be seen in the on-going negotiations concerning the activities of Central and West African countries referred to in the previous Chapter. As reported in that Chapter, the Commission has been negotiating with the African countries concerned on behalf of the Community as a whole, whilst previously these countries had been involved in negotiations with individual EC Member States.

This enhancement is also detected in the exploratory talks on maritime affairs between the Commission and the maritime authorities of the Soviet Union that took place in Leningrad in September 1988 following an initiative of the latter.

It is worth mentioning also in this respect that the Commission participated officially for the first time in the recent negotiations in the context of the UN Liner Code Review Conference in Geneva (27th October - 18th November 1988). Following an agreement of the twelve EC Member States as well as of the remaining Group B countries, the Commission representative was allowed to make an official declaration on EC policy at the Review Conference.

Member States, however, did not surrender completely to the Community their competence for the adoption of national countermeasures. Article 6 of that Regulation, introduces "escape clauses" whereby Member States may act unilaterally if the Council has not adopted a proposal from the Commission within a period of two months or in cases of urgency.

There are other areas where the package leads to the harmonisation of external maritime relations: (i) cargo sharing agreements whith third countries, (ii) unfair pricing practices by third country shipowners in international cargo liner shipping, and (iii) acts of third countries which prevent the operation of outsiders in a liner trade.

The adjustment of existing cargo sharing agreements with third countries and the prohibition of future ones according to the provisions of Regulation 4055/86 must be seen as a basic prerequisite for the creation of a common market for maritime services since the carriage of goods between Community Member States and third countries represents the largest proportion of their trade in those services. This can be seen from the data presented on Table 10.1 which refer to the volume of seaborne imports by certain EC Member States in 1985. The Member States covered are those for which data were available. It is interesting to note that only in the United Kingdom -which is an island state- does the percentage of seaborne imports from other EC Member States reach 40%. In the remaining Member States it is much less than that.

TABLE 10.1
TONNAGE IMPORTED BY SEA BY EC MEMBER STATES IN 1985
IN THOUSAND METRIC TONNES

IMPORTING COUNTRY	INTRA EC	TOTAL	PERCENTAGE INTRA EC/TOTAL
BELGIUM/LUX.	15.355	73.047	21.02
FRANCE	29.462	152.508	19.32
FRG	23.378	84.984	27.50
NETHERLANDS	41.858	244.061	17.15
UN. KINGDOM	54.067	136.806	39.52
SPAIN	8.123	79.700	10.19

Source: OECD

Therefore, no real progress would have been made towards achieving the goal of a Common market in maritime services, if the abolition of barriers had been restricted to intra-Community shipping services only. Furthermore, if traffic with third countries had not been included in the provisions of the Regulation, the abolition of intra Community restrictions might have led to distortions in the competition between the ports of Member States. The framework instituted through Regulation 4057/86 for a Community wide response to unfair pricing can be seen as the only direct EC involvement in industrial policy formulation for the maritime sector.

The gradual abolition of barriers to trade in maritime services has not been linked to the adoption of measures at Community level that would promote structural changes so that the Community producers of maritime services would be able to survive increased competition. There are two reasons for this: First the Commission has been of the opinion, reflected in its 1985 Memorandum that national industrial policies for the maritime sector of the Member States, mainly the government subsidies listed in our Table 3.1 do not result in serious distortions in intra-Community trade[4]. The second reason is that a large proportion of the tonnage under Community flags, mainly from Denmark, Greece and the United Kingdom, is employed in cross-trading, mainly as tramps, and consequently has been fully exposed to the forces of free competition.

The cross-trading section of Community shipping must therefore have undergone the necessary structural adjustments to be able to survive its prolonged exposure to free competition. This second reason must also explain the reason why Regulation 4057/86 covers only liner shipping.

This Community involvement in industrial policy for the liner trades sector is basically of a negative nature in the sense that it attempts to alleviate the effects of international competition through the imposition of redressive duties. Thus, this kind of policy might slow down the process of structural adjustment that would be necessary for the Community liner trades sector to survive international competition[5].

COMPETITION RULES

The introduction of an international dimension into the competition rules for liner shipping represents a continuation of past Community initiatives vis-a-vis the UN Liner Code as expressed through Regulation 954/79.

In any case, the exclusion of liner trades to and from third countries from the scope of Regulation 4056/86 would have made the application of competition rules meaningless since, as indicated in Table 10.1, the largest percentage of the EC seaborne trade is external. Furthermore, such an exclusion would have ignored the interests of the consumers of maritime services in the Community, i.e. the importers or exporters of goods.

This extra-territorial dimension in the provisions of Regulation 4056/86 also enhances the role of the Commission in international maritime relations. Thus the Commission has been granted a role in international liner shipping similar to that played for many years by the Federal Maritime Commission in the United States[6]. The Commission has now the responsibility of regulating the activity of conferences not only within the Community but also between the Community and third countries. Hence, for the first time now the behaviour of third country carriers is subjected to Community control through the Commission.

The application of the competition rules to the liner trades is the only area in maritime policy where the Member States have surrendered full power to the Commission. This is not a new phenomenon in the process of Community integration, since in competition matters the Commission is given full authority under the Treaty. Another reason is that in those matters the governments of the Member States are more than willing to "pass the bucket" to a supranational authority and avoid the highly controversial issues inherent in any regulation of the behaviour of firms. Here is a case that the regulator has to balance the conflicting interests of carriers and the users of their services, as well as of the employees of those groups. Any balancing act produces political costs, which national governments are glad to avoid through the projection of final responsibility to a supranational authority, such as the Commission. The end result, however, is that the Commission has now acquired important powers of investigation and of the imposition of fines which are independent of the desires of individual Member States reflected in the deliberations of the Council. These powers make Regulation 4056/86 the most concrete of the maritime policy measures adopted in 1986.

In relation to the new powers acquired by the Commission on competition matters in maritime transport it is worth remembering its response to the first test cases before it, notally the Eurocode agreements referred to in the previous chapter.

In contrast to the U.S. Federal Maritime Commission which had already given its approval, the Commission was unwilling to grant a block exemption[7], but instead opened formal proceedings according to the provisions of Article 10 of Regulation 4056/86.

This reaction led the conferences involved and one of the outsiders to apply for individual exemptions. The case is still pending.

Hence, the first impression emerging is that of a more strict competition policy developing at European level than the one pursued on the other side of the Atlantic, following the 1984 U.S. Shipping Act. That stricter approach must be related to the fact that Community law in contrast to American law has accepted the system of closed conferences, but on the other hand has put a duty on the Commission to see that actual or potential non-conference competition is preserved.

SOURCE OF CONFLICTS WITHIN THE COMMISSION

The linkage between the four Regulations of the package is likely to produce conflicts between the various Directorates-General within the Commission.

The extra-territorial dimension of the conditions for the exemption of liner conferences from the application of the competition rules necessitates an interaction between the

Directorates-General responsible for competition policy, transport policy, external relations and relations with developing countries, respectively, DG IV, DG VII, DG I, and DG VIII. It is far from certain that, when the Commission is called upon to act on a complaint by an outsider that a trade is closed to him as a result of action by a third country, all these Directorates-General will proceed in the same direction in formulating a Commission response.

DG IV would be keen to activate the provisions of Regulation 4056/86 so that outsiders would be able to have competitive access in the trade concerned. DG I or DG VIII would be more concerned with avoiding any disturbance in the economic and political relations between the Community and the third country concerned.

Finally, DG VII would try to arrive at an amicable agreement with the offending third country which would compromise its demands for a significant share in the trade with the general guidelines of Community law, so that maritime trade is not disturbed. These different priorities would be expected to strain the relationships between the above Directorates-General.

Indeed, the information emanating from the various Commission services on policy formulation concerning the Danish complaint on the Central and West African problem discussed in the previous Chapter points in that direction.

Another recent example is the complaint brought against Hyundai Merchant Marine. It was reported in the press that DG IV was not keen to endorse the position adopted by DG VII which accepted the validity of that complaint and proposed the imposition of a redressive duty according to the provisions of Regulation 4057/86. The reluctance of DG IV is related to its duty to see that actual or potential competition from outsiders exists in the liner conference trades as required by Regulation 4056/86.

CONCLUSIONS

The main implications of the 1986 Package at Community level appear to be the strengthening of its international role in maritime affairs combined with a commitment to a liberal international maritime regime and the direct involvement of the Commission in the regulation of the behaviour of carriers in the liner trades. Moreover, the package would lead to the creation of a common market in those international maritime services which relate to the external trade of the Member States. The creation of that market has not been linked in any real sense with any measures aiming at the approximation of technical or social conditions in the production of maritime services.

Although the Council expressed in December 1986 its desire to proceed with stage two of the EC maritime policy that would relate to the supply side of maritime services within the Community, in essence the liberalisation of the maritime markets is proceeding independently. Thus, it looks likely that any approximation of the above conditions would be brought about by market forces rather than prior Community action.

NOTES

1 Cosgrove Twitchett C. "Harmonisation in the EEC", St. Martin's Press Inc., New York 1981, Chapter 5.

2 See Chapter 5.

3 Wallace H., W. Wallace and C. Webb, Editors "Policy Making in the European Community", Second Edition, John Wiley and Sons, 1983. cf also, Chapter 4 "Assessment of Community Initiatives".

4 See Commission of the European Communities "Progress towards a Common Transport Policy: Maritime Transport" COM(85)90 final, paragraph 39.

5 Curzon Price V. "International Policies in the European Community", Trade Policy Research Centre, London 1981.

6 Frankel, E.G. "Regulation and Policies of American Shipping" Auburn House Publishing Company, Boston Mass., 1982. Goss, R.O. "Studies in Maritime Economics", Cambridge University Press, London 1970, Chapter 2. Shashikumar, N. "U.S. Shipping Act of 1984: A Scrutiny of Controversial Provisions", Maine Maritime Press, Castine, Maine, 1987.

7 Kreis H.W.R., "Maritime Transport and EEC Competition Rules", Antwerp International Congress on EEC Maritime Regulations, November 25-26, 1988, Journal of Law and Economics, Vol. XXIII, No 5, 1988.

CHAPTER 11

THE IMPLICATIONS OF THE 1986 PACKAGE OF REGULATIONS AT INTERNATIONAL LEVEL

The adoption of the 1986 package has taken place at a time when governments in many countries appear to be upgrading the relative importance of their national maritime sector in economic policy formulation. This may be due to the effects of the prolonged international shipping crisis which has highlighted the significance of shipping as an earner of foreign exchange and generator of employment. Shipping is now looked upon much more as a sector on its own merits rather than as a trunk industry subservient to other sectors. This coincidence increases in itself the likelihood of conflict situations arising in international maritime relations between the Community as a whole and third countries.

Furthermore, in assessing the implications of the 1986 package at international level it should be borne in mind that the Commission now possesses clear-cut powers for autonomous action in competition mattters. Thus, if conflict situations with third countries arise in those matters these would not be subject to the direct political control of Member States and the Council. In relation to this elevated role of the Commission in international maritime affairs it is worth noting that, following a long period of continuous erosion of the conditions of free competition in the international shipping markets, there is now tangible evidence of a reaction from the Western developed countries to protectionism[1] and flag discrimination practices, through coordinated initiatives aiming at the creation of more liberal conditions. A notable example is the OECD Council Recommendation on common principles of shipping policy which was adopted in February 1987. It commits OECD Member States according to Principle 1 to promote the free movement of shipping in international trades in free and fair competition.[2]

Moreover, under Principle 2 Member Countries should "actively oppose the imposition of regimes which restrict the access to cargo moving internationally by shipping companies adhering to the principle of free competition on a commercial basis". However, this commitment is somewhat undermined by the statement that "in the case of state-trading countries and their carriers, it is necessary to take account of non-commercial and non-reciprocal practices with the aim of arriving at a situation of reciprocity and equality of opportunity". The adoption of this fallback position, which opens the door for the conclusion of new cargo-sharing agreements with state trading countries, may be attributed to the real difficulties experienced by western shipping companies in being able to participate in the carriage of goods to and from these countries. An additional reason may be the reluctance of various western countries, with limited cross-trading interests, to open up their bilateral trades with the state trading countries to third country carriers.

Equally important in this respect is the position adopted by the developed market economy countries, known as the group B vis a vis the UN Code of Conduct Review Conference in October-November 1988 which opposes the initiatives of various developing countries (Group 77) and of the UNCTAD Secretariat to extend its cargo sharing principles to the dry and liquid bulk trades, and to restrict the operation of outsiders in the liner trades. It is indicative of the intentions of the UNCTAD Secretariat that Chapter IV of its working document for the 1988 Review Conference[3] notes the rapid growth in the market share of non-conference lines in many trades (by as much as 55% in some cases) and claims that it has frustrated one of the main objectives of the Code, namely the participation to a substantial degree of the national shipping lines of developing countries in their national trades. It also argues that the role of outsiders has had a destabilizing effect in the liner trades and calls for a regulation of their activities in such a way that it would effectively bar them from those trades.

The development of the Community maritime policy has also coincided with the Uruguay round of negotiations for trade liberalisation under GATT which has raised the possibility of its extension to cover trade in services including shipping.

Another general observation that has to be made before examining in detail the international implications of the individual Regulations concerns the on-going CSG-US dialogue. That dialogue which, inter-alia, involves the Commission itself has so far produced two joint statements, in Copenhagen in 1986 and in Washington DC, in November 1987, whereby all sides state their common interest in the prevention of the spread of protectionism in maritime transport. That dialogue, however, has produced so far only a few concrete results, the successful resistance to cargo reservation practices by Indonesia and joint representations to Peru and Sri Lanka.[4] It should also be remembered that one of the original purposes for the setting up of CSG was the concern of European and Japanese governments about the extraterritorial regulatory activities on shipping by the Federal Maritime Commission under US law.

IMPLICATIONS OF REGULATION 4055/86

The application of the principle to provide services to maritime traffic between EC Member States as well as between Member States and third countries reaffirms the existing commitments of the Community against protectionism and cargo reservation practices. Hence, the adoption of this Regulation is likely to increase the pressure on other members of the CSG-US dialogue and the OECD, especially the United States, to refrain from resorting to new bilateral cargo-sharing agreements with third countries.[5] Resorting to these agreements has been for the United States a second-best solution when unilateral action by third countries inhibits the operation of American carriers, and the cost of an open trade war is considered too high. How strong this pressure will be on the non-EC partners to the CSG-US dialogue and the OECD will depend on how Regulation 4055/86 is implemented.

The reluctance of many EC Member States to adhere to the provisions of this Regulation concerning the transparency of information on their bilateral cargo-sharing agreements with third countries and its outright violation by the Italy-

Algeria agreement as described in Chapter 9 raise doubts as to the credibility of Community action to liberalise international maritime trade.

These developments have occured against the background of the review taking place currently within the OECD concerning the maritime transport provisions of its Invisibles Code and of Member countries relevant policies so that the objective of liberalising maritime transport be achieved.[6] Perhaps there might be a feedback into the EC from the OECD deliberations leading to a stricter adherence to Regulation 4055/86 by the Community Member States.

The credibility of the Community Member States' commitment to refrain from the Conclusion of bilateral cargo-sharing agreements is also undermined by the possibility that individual Member States have in concluding future cargo sharing agreements with third countries in the liner trades under the provisions of Regulation 4055/86 itself. In particular, Article 5 has introduced the notion of "exceptional circumstances" where the liner shipping companies of Member States would not otherwise have an opportunity to participate in a trade to and from the third country concerned. Of course, the possibility exists for the Council adopting counter-measures under Regulation 4058/86 if a third country seeks to impose a cargo sharing arrangement on a Member State. However, as the experience from the Italy-Algeria case indicates, it is very doubtful whether the Member State affected would seek the adoption of countermeasures by the Council given its broader trade and political considerations, or that the qualified majority of the Council Members would be willing to do so for that matter.

On the contrary, it might be the Member State itself seeking the conclusion of the bilateral cargo-sharing agreement, as appears to be the case with a number of bilateral agreements reported recently to the Commission.[7] Consequently, this notion of "exceptional circumstances", because of its vagueness, is likely to be used as an escape clause for the proliferation of cargo sharing agreements in the liner trades. In fact, a Member State resorting to a bilateral cargo-sharing agreement under this Regulation could easily justify its action to other OECD Members under Principle 2 of the 1987 Recommendation, if that agreement was concluded with a state-trading country, which is usually the case. Moreover, recourse to such agreements will gain further ground if the recent reports that the United States is in the process of concluding a cargo sharing agreement with China are proved correct. The only real constraint in this case is the obligation that these agreements must be in accordance with Community law and that there should be no discrimination against liner shipping companies from other EC Member States.

The special treatment afforded by this Regulation to existing cargo sharing agreements in liner trades is likely to cause some friction with the United States. These agreements will have to be adjusted according to the obligations of Member States under Regulation 954/79.

The United States on the other hand is firmly opposed to the UN Code and the enactment of Regulation 954/79 has been a cause of friction with EC Member States since in the American view it constitutes a regressive step vis a vis the efforts by market economy countries to liberalize international maritime trade.

IMPLICATIONS OF REGULATION 4056/86

The main impact of this Regulation on the international front is likely to come from its extra-territorial application in terms of the requirement that actual or potential non-conference competition is not precluded in any given liner trade. The preclusion of such competition by the closure of trade by a third country would lead to the withdrawal of group exemption for the Conference lines operating in that trade. In that case the conference lines might face fines if they cannot obtain an individual exemption. In turn, it is likely that a conflict situation will develop between the Community and the third country concerned. Indeed, as discussed in Chapter 8 this likelihood is foreseen in Article 9 of this Regulation which provides for consultations between the Commission and the competent authorities of the third country concerned with the aim of reconciling the opposed interests.

It is too early yet to judge on how such conflict situations will be dealt with in practice. The Danish complaints against cargo allocation and restrictions of free access to outsiders in the trades between Europe and Central and West Africa also involve Regulation 4056/86. This problem is at the moment being dealt with in the context of Regulation 4058/86 and the Lome III Convention, but given the footdragging by the African side reported in the previous chapters it is likely that a direct involvement of Directorate-General IV will become unavoidable.

Apart from the potential problems with various third-world countries which practice protectionism that might arise as a result of the implementation of Regulation 4056/86, conflict situations might also be created between the EC and non-EC Members of the OECD. A notable case is the Eurocorde pricing agreements[8] which are subject to an investigation by the Commission following the filing of a complaint by the British Shippers Council. These agreements have already been approved by the Federal Maritime Commission in the United States under the terms of the 1984 Shipping Act. This difference between the two sides of the Atlantic in approaching the same issue is the result of the fundamental differences in the philosophies of the two regulatory regimes of activity in the liner trades.

The EC side, as already discussed has accepted the system of closed conferences and loyalty agreements whilst the American side allows the operation of open ones only and prohibits loyalty agreements. Consequently, the Commission in order to ensure the preservation of a competitive regime in a given trade is very sensitive vis a vis pricing agreements that might lead to the extinction of actual or potential competition. On the other hand, the Federal Maritime Commission is obliged to scrutinize pricing agreements if these are linked to measures that coordinate the activity of carriers, such as the allocation of calls and capacity among members, since these measures might lead to restrictions in competition.

The implementation of Regulation 4056/86 in cases such as the Eurocorde agreements is likely to strain maritime relations between the Community and other non-EC European states. Eg. the Nordic countries restrict the application of their competition laws to activity within their national territorial boundaries. On the other hand, certain shipping lines which are parties to the Eurocorde agreements are established in those countries, and the imposition of fines by the Commission might lead to a diplomatic row.

Another potential source of conflict with the non-EC members of the OECD is the different treatment afforded to consortia. The issue has still to be resolved in the EC and the indications are that the Commission is likely to adopt a case by case approach leading to the granting of individual exemptions rather than a block exemption.[9] The 1984 US Shipping Act, on the other hand, treats consortia as single entities, and if they operate within a conference they are bound to the regulatory regime for conference activity.

Despite the problems of extraterritorial jurisdiction that Regulation 4056/86 might create, its emphasis on the preservation of actual or potential competition in the international liner trades must be seen as a stumbling block to the pressures from many developing countries to restrict the operation of outsiders and extend the scope of the UN Code of Conduct to the whole of liner trades. Thus, the adoption of Regulation 4056/86 must be seen as an important international development in view of the Review Conference for the UN Liner Code.

IMPLICATIONS OF REGULATION 4057/86

The dividing line between anti-dumping measures and protectionism is very fine indeed as shown by the history of anti-dumping legislation and of test-cases in various sectors of economic activity. This statement can most certainly be made about Regulation 4057/86 which can easily be turned into a protectionist instrument in favour of the Community liner companies.

The fact that an operator offers lower rates might not necessarily be due to unfair pricing as a

result of governmental protection. It could also be
due to the employment of factors of production from
different markets which present lower opportunity
costs[10] or to a more efficient organisation in the
production of transport services. In fact in the
case of liner shipping services, which are produced
as part of an integrated multimodal system, lower
rates might be due to a higher degree of efficiency
in the organisation of the whole system or in the
operation of the land based part of the system.
Also, these might be due to a different standard of
service being offered and a different cargo mix
being carried by the operator.

Whether Regulation 4057/86 will turn out to be
an instrument of protectionism or a means of putting
pressure on third countries to abandon restrictive
practices in shipping will depend on how this is
going to be applied. As mentioned in previous
chapters in the first test case, concerning the
Korean company Hyundai Merchant Maritime the
Commission has recommended to the Council the
imposition of a 26% redressive duty on all the
container shipments of that company from Europe to
Australia. The Commission has linked the alleged
freight rate undercutting by Hyundai to a number of
non-commercial advantages derived from the
application of Korean government maritime policy,
and especially (a) its cargo reservation scheme
under Article 16 of the Korean Maritime
Transportation Fostering Act, (b) the discrimination
against the shipping activities in Korea, such as
freight forwarding, maritime transportation,
shipping agency etc by non-Korean companies, under
Articles 34 and 35 of the Korean Maritime
Transportation Business Act and (c) the subsidies
granted under the 1984 Shipping Industry
Rationalisation Plan.

In its defence, Hyundai found strong support
from the British Shippers Council which, inter-alia,
claimed that in terms of standard type of equipment
and reliability the service offered by Hyundai was
vastly inferior[11] and thus the reference by the
complainants to rate-undercutting constituted
irrelevant evidence. The British Shippers Council
pointed out also to the increased share of the
Europe-Australia trade (66.8% from 66.6%) enjoyed by
the conference members despite the rates offered by

Hyundai. From their side, the conference member lines alleged that the service offered by Hyundai was similar to that provided by ABC Container Line, an EC incorporated outsider who was a party to the complaint lodged with the Commission.

It is too early to judge on the Korean government's reaction to the possible adoption by the EC Council of the above Commission's recommendation, and whether a trade war in maritime services would erupt. In such an event it would be surprising if the Korean side did not counter argue that subsidies to shipping also exist in many EC Member States, as described in Chapter 3.

The Hyundai case is developing into an EC-Korea confrontation at a time when the latter is seeking membership of the OECD and has initiated a programme of liberalisation for its shipping industries.[12] Whether this confrontation will cause a reversal or slow-down in that programme is difficult to say.

The only other experience so far on the implications of Regulation 4057/86 is related to the pricing activities of three Soviet shipping lines, Far East Shipping Company, Black Sea Shipping Company and Baltic Shipping Company operating in three routes from Europe to the Far East, the West Indies and East Africa. As reported in the press[13] following investigations conducted by Belgium, France, West Germany, the Netherlands, and the United Kingdom on the activities of these companies, in the context of the monitoring system established by Council Decisions 774/78, 4/79, 1181/80 82/870, 84/656, 86/646[14], the European lines involved in those trades were preparing the lodging of a complaint with the Commission alleging predatory pricing by the Soviet lines. Events, however, did not follow that course, but instead the Soviet lines came to an agreement with the European shipping conferences concerned and any action under Regulation 4057/86 was abandoned. Details of this agreement have not been made public, but this event shows that Regulation 4057/86 may not necessarily lead to a trade war in maritime services. It illustrates though at the same time that its application might be restrictive on international competition in the liner trades to the detriment of consumers' interests.

The   EC legislation on unfair practices in
shipping is not unique among OECD Members.[15] The
United States also possesses a strong arsenal of
measures that the Federal Maritime Commission can
take   under   American legislation against foreign
carriers that are considered to adversely affect the
operations of US carriers in the United States ocean
borne trade. The FMC has acquired powers of
investigation and imposition of penalties against
foreign carriers under Subtitle A, Title X of the
1988 US Trade Bill.

The   penalties   can   take   the   form   of
(a) limitations on sailings to and from US ports or
on   the   amount   or   type   of   cargo carried,
(b) suspension of tariffs filed with the Commission,
(c) suspension of the right of the offending carrier
to operate   under   agreements   filed   with   the   FMC
authorizing preferential treatment at terminals,
space chartering, etc., and (d) a fee, not exceeding
US$ 1 million per voyage.

Thus, we are witnessing a proliferation of
legislation   covering   unfair   practices   in
international maritime transport. Whether this is
going to encourage the promotion of the free
movement of shipping in international trades
according to 1987 OECD Council Recommendation will
depend on whether the above legislation acts as a
deterrent to protectionism by third countries or
turns into an instrument of protectionism by those
that have enacted it.

IMPLICATIONS OF REGULATION 4058/86

The adoption of this Regulation meets one of the
basic demands in the CSG–US dialogue, namely that
the European side should have created the legal
framework   for   coordinated   resistance   to
protectionism. The 1984 US Shipping Act and the
1988 US Trade Bill also contain privisions giving
the Federal Maritime Commission the authority to
resort to countermeasures against carriers from
countries engaged in protectionism.   Hence, its
adoption and implementation would have been expected
to put pressure on the American side or the non-EC
Member States of CSG to refrain from concluding
cargo-sharing agreements with third countries. In

the recent past the Federal Maritime Commission threatened retaliation against Peruvian-flag carriers and has announced a series of investigations against carriers from Korea, Taiwan, and China, because these countries discriminate against US-flag lines.[16]

If the information about the planned China-US cargo sharing agreement proves correct then the adoption of this Regulation may prove to count for very little in the development of OECD solidarity. The search for a bilateral solution to problems experienced by the shipping companies of one country due to acts of another country might yet prove to be the mode rather than the course to coordinated resistance in the context of an agreed multilateral legal framwork.

The application of this Regulation is restricted by three parameters:

a) The acceptance of cargo sharing in the context of the UN Code of Conduct and Regulation 954/79. Thus, action by third countries will not invite countermeasures if it affects cargoes in the Codist trades and is taken according to the provisions of the Code .

b) The provision under Article 1 that the procedure for coordinated action "shall be without prejudice to the obligations of the Community and its Member States under international law", and

c) The elements of solidarity and reciprocity envisaged vis a vis other OECD countries under Article 8.

The distinction between Codist and non-Codist trades in this Regulation sets a boundary beyond which the Community is in principle not prepared to proceed in accommodating the demands of third world countries for cargo allocation. Many of these countries have interpreted in practice the Code to cover the whole of liner trades rather than those served by liner conferences between contracting parties to the Code. This extensive interpretation propounded by the Group of 77 in UNCTAD is not shared by Group B countries (including the EC) militating in favour of the restrictive interpretation of the cargo sharing formula of the Code, whereby its application is limited to liner conference trades between contracting parties. In fact, Group B countries pray in aid to their reading of the Code arguments drawn from its text. Thus, the above distinction can be seen as a signal from the Community to those countries that such an arbitrary interpretation is a "casus belli".

However, as the experience from the way the Community's handling of the Central and West African cargo reservation case so far demonstrates it is unlikely that the EC will adopt in the end a firm stance leading to a trade war in maritime services. Apart from the conflicting interests of the individual Member States involved, an additional reason for a flexible approach in the implementation of Regulation 4058/86 towards developing countries is parameter (b) above. The main obligation of the Community under international law in this case concerns the maritime provisions of the Lome III Convention. The relevant title there (Title V) contains a declaration by both the ACP countries and the EC that the objective of cooperation between the EC and the ACP countries in the field of shipping "shall be to ensure harmonious development of efficient and reliable shipping services on economically satisfactory terms by facilitating the active participation of all parties according to the principle of unrestricted access to the trade on a commercial basis" (Article 86). Nevertheless, the Convention acknowledges the aspirations of the ACP states for greater participation in shipping and in particular bulk cargo shipping but this is linked to the ideas of efficiency in the shipment of cargoes and of the preservation of competitive access (Article 88).

A reference to shipping to be found in the context of the trade and economic cooperation agreements with Brazil (1980) and the Andean Pact countries (1983) does not go beyond an exchange of letters of intent that the problems arising in the maritime relations between the EC and the countries concerned will be examined in a cooperative spirit. Therefore, this reference is of little practical use.

The cooperation agreement with China (1985) constitutes a general framework within which special agreements on specific economic sectors, such as shipping, are to be concluded. The EC Commission is in the process of preparing a draft text for such an agreement in consultation with interested economic groups within the Community.

The flexible application of Regulation 4058/86 vis a vis the ACP countries is likely to decrease its value as a deterrent. The value of any countermeasures legislation consists in its ability to prevent a trade war in the first instance through its existence rather than its actual use. Consequently, the way that this Regulation is being applied in conjunction with the experience on the implementation of Regulation 4055 is likely in the long run to increase friction between the Community and the ACP countries, because the latter note the Community's lack of resolve in fighting protectionism and push for more concessions than the Community can actually yield.

The flexible approach to the ACP group might be misinterpreted by other countries, notably the Eastern Bloc or the developed East Asian Countries to mean an equal lack of resolve by the Community towards them. In this case, however, as the Hyundai case has shown, the Community's political and economic priorities are likely to be very different and a hard approach be adopted.

Hence, the implementation of Regulation 4058/86 and the other three Regulations for that matter, is not going to be uniform in all international fronts. An additional reason for this lack of uniformity is its provision that countermeasures may be adopted by the EC, on the basis of reciprocity, when discriminatory acts by third countries affect companies in other OECD countries as well. A corollary to this provision is that in practice no countermeasures are possible if the offending country belongs to the OECD. This provision necessitates the conclusion of relevant agreements between the Community and other OECD countries. No such agreement has yet materialized and progress in this direction is very much dependant on the cohesion of the CSG group.

This element of solidarity towards the other OECD states, which first appeared in Regulation 954/79 sets the foundations for the creation of a free trade area in maritime services within the OECD. It appears that such a possibility might be the end result of a failure to combat protectionism by non-OECD. countries. Furthermore, the US administration has indicated in the recent past that if its efforts to bring services under the auspices of GATT fail, its attention will be focused on creating a "regional" market among countries that practice liberalism rather than a global one.[17]

The key ingredient for the successful creation of such a free trade area, as clearly stated in this Regulation is that of reciprocity. This is not just relevant to shipping but is becoming a major issue in the process towards the completion of the EC internal market both within the Community and in the policies of its trading partners. The latter express fears that the completion of the economic integration of the Community might lead to increased barriers to goods and services originating from third countries. The creation of "Fortress Europe" could affect shipping directly through an emphasis on the protectionist ingredients of the 1986 package of Regulations and indirectly through the general dislocation of trade in goods that would result in such an event.[18] It is indicative of the fear the concept of reciprocity is generating that the Norwegian shipping industry is now pushing for the establishment of a formal relationship between Norway and the EC in the form of a special agreement in the maritime field until Norway's accession to the Community.[19]

OVERALL ASSESSMENT

From the above analysis it may be concluded that the 1986 package of Regulations is likely to increase tensions in international maritime relations. Whether this impact is going to be compensated by a stand still or roll-back in protectionist activity will depend on how these Regulations are applied.

NOTES

1 OECD "Maritime Transport 1983", Paris 1984, Chapter 5. Ademuni-Odeke "Protectionism and the Future of International Shipping", Martinus Nijhoff Publishers, Dorddrecht, 1984. See also Chapter 3.

2 OECD Council Recommendation on Common Principles of Shipping Policy of 13th February 1987, C(87) 11(Final).

3 UNCTAD, "Issues for the Review Conference", T.D./CODE 2/4.

4 See Lloyd's List, "G.C.B.S. Accuses the U.S. of Blatant Protectionism", 22-3-1984.

5 OECD, "Maritime Transport", 1986, Paris 1987.

6 OECD Joint Working Group Maritime Transport Services, "Interim Report to the CMIT and Maritime Transport Committees", Paris, 8th September 1988.

7 Meeting Document, DG VII/A-1, Brussels, 12th July 1988.

8 See Chapter 10.

9 Kreis, H.W.R., "Maritime Transport and EEC Competition Rules", Journal of Law and Economics, Vol. 23, No 5, 1988.

10 Goss, R.O. "Social Costs, Transfer Payments and International Competition in Shipping", Maritime Policy and Management, Vol. 12, 1985.

11 Lloyd's List, July 14th 1988 and November 18th 1988.

12 Yoon, S., "Trying a New Route to Shipping Company Solvency", Seatrade, March-April 1988.

13 Lloyd's List 14th August 1987.

14 See Chapter 4.

15 See Chapter 3.

16 Seatrade Week, April 24th 1987.

17 See "Trade in the 1980's: Three Views", An
   Interview with Geza Feketekuty, Senior Assistant
   U.S. Trade Representative, Economic Impact,
   Washington DC 1984.

18 Lloyd's List, 1st November 1988.

19 Speech by Mr Nils Astrup. President of the
   Norwegian Shipowners Association at a dinner for
   the EC Ambassadors.

CHAPTER 12

FUTURE DEVELOPMENT IN EC MARITIME POLICY

In developing the four Regulations in December 1986 the Council also stated that these represented only a first stage in the elaboration of Community shipping policy and that future policy should aim "at maintaining and developing an efficient, competitive Community shipping industry to ensure the provision of competitive shipping services for the benefit of Community trade". In that respect the Council invited the Commission to submit proposals on fiscal, social and technical measures needed to promote the Community fleet. The Council also made a statement to the effect that the Commission should study the competitive situation in the passenger and tramp sectors as well as joint ventures, consortia agreements and agreements between transport users, and submit a report on whether block exemptions should be provided. On its part, the Commission urged the Council to take up as a matter of priority its proposal for the improvement of the consultation procedure established by the latter's Decision 587/77.

It is indicative of the lengthly and cumbersome nature of the decision making process within the Community on matters of integration, that whilst almost two years had elapsed since the adoption of the package no tangible progress had been made on any of the above matters, apart from the preliminary position expressed by Directorate-General IV on consortia.[1]

To start with, the orientation of the measures suggested by the Council is inward looking which makes it much more difficult to produce compromises compared to the adoption of external measures as was the case with the 1986 package. The range of conflicting interests among Member States involved in inward looking measures such as fiscal matters is much greater since they touch directly upon their national economic policies and domestic institutional arrangements. Furthermore, any measures that might result in a more favourable treatment of a specific sector within the Community vis-a-vis other sectors in the areas of fiscal or social policy are likely to produce a lively debate within the Commission on the merits and direction of such action. This is bound to cause considerable delays in the formulation of the official Commission proposals to be submitted at Council level.

Although no formal Community measures have been adopted, there has been considerable debate both public and private within the Commission to the effect that if this is assessed in conjunction with the orientation given by the Council and Commission statements of December 1986, one can speculate on future course of action.

THE FATE OF ANNEXES II-3 AND II-4

Neither the Commission nor the Council has shown any real interest in pushing ahead with the adoption of the measures contained in the above Annexes to the 1985 Commission Memorandum[2] which were left aside by the Council in 1986.

The proposal of strengthening the consultation procedure among Member States on their maritime relations with third countries (Annex II-3) seems to have been forgotten since every Member State appears to be keen to preserve a high degree of freedom in its bilateral shipping relations with third countries. This unwillingness to accept prior consultation before the conclusion of bilateral shipping agreements is reflected in the behaviour of several Member States in respect to the implementation of Regulation 4055/86 which is described in Chapter 9. Thus, it is most unlikely that the proposals in Annex II-3 will be transformed into a Regulation in the foreseeable future.

A similar treatment has been afforded to the proposals in Annex II-4 concerning the definition of a "national shipping line". The general consensus appears to focus on leaving the competency for such a definition with the individual Member States.

THE ISSUE OF CABOTAGE

The issue of the abolition of national cabotage restrictions that exist in half of the Member States is such a contentious issue that it became necessary to separate[3] it from the other proposals contained in the original Annex II-2 so that progress could be made in enacting stage one of the Community's maritime policy in 1986. The issue remains still highly contentious and there are no signs of any breakthrough in the stalemate to which the discussions within the Council have reached.

The U.K. government has been pushing hard for the adoption of the original proposal in Annex II-2 on the abolition of cabotage restrictions but its initiatives are meeting with strong opposition from the "Southern front" of Member States, namely France, Greece, Italy, Spain and Portugal. The U.K. government, supported by other Northern European countries which have no cabotage restrictions, claims that these are in conflict with the objectives of a single European internal market and the general commitments towards liberalising maritime transport. The "Southern front" countries differ in the arguments they put forward in adopting the same negative stance. Greece emphasizes the strategic arguments involved in cabotage restrictions concerning services to its islands in the Aegean sea. Other countries consider the adoption of positive measures leading to the improvement of the competitiveness of their fleets as a sine-qua-non for any concessions on cabotage.

In the meantime the U.K. government was given under an amendment to the Merchant Shipping Act in April 1988 new powers for retaliatory action against inter-alia other EC Member States which preserve cabotage restrictions in favour of their national shipowners, and refuse UK shipping companies access to their domestic traffic.[4] That action would essentially take the form of outlawing the activities of companies from the other states in the carriage of goods and/or passengers between ports in the United Kingdom, between British ports and offshore installations on the UK Continental shelf, or between those installations themselves. The outlawing could also cover cruises beginning and ending in UK ports.

So far, the U.K. government has not activated these powers, but given the stalemate in the Council deliberations such an event cannot be ruled out. This development is of particular interest from the angle of the integration process within the Community since the concept of reciprocity is introduced explicitly into the national policy of a Member State vis-a-vis other Member States with the ultimate aim of forcing the latter to proceed towards the liberalisation of a specific market. A regressive step is taken so as to encourage progress!

The only reactions to this British initiative have come so far from Greece and the Netherlands. The Greek government reiterated in the European Parliament in June 1988 its opposition to the relaxation of its cabotage law stressing its importance for national defence. This stance found strong support from both Greek shipowners and trade unions.[5] On the other hand, Dutch shipowners have indicated that they will challenge the legality of any move by the British government to restrict entry to its national cabotage trades.

A BRAINSTORMING EXERCISE: THE ANTWERP SYMPOSIUM

Suggestions for possible Community action on the supply side of its shipping industry were already present in the submissions released in 1985 in relation to the Commission's Memorandum and Proposals by both the shipowners' (CAACE) and trade unions side (ITF).[6] A full airing of these views was given in the context of the Shipping Symposium that was organised in Antwerp on May 5-6, 1987 jointly by the Commission and the Belgian Presidency of the Council. In a Discussion Paper prepared for the purposes of the Symposium, the Commission services raised three fundamental sets of questions:

(A) In view of the steady increase in flagging-out from the national registries of EC Member States can incentives to remain under national flags be effective? And are there disincentives which can be applied to prevent flagging out?

(B) What does the development of "offshore registries" mean for the conditions under which

Member State fleets operate, particularly in terms of the genuine link, employment and the application of national and international regulations? Should the Community monitor the development of these registries? Should the Community consider the establishment of certain conditions for the development of such registries? If so, what criteria should apply?

(C) Has the time come to consider the development of a European flag? If so, should it adopt:

a) a minimum approach which would be the establishment of such a flag as a symbol of the European identity of EC shipowners with the right to carry the flag alongside the national flag, tied to certain criteria such as genuine link, technical standards, social and manning standards, and environmental standards?

b) a more radical approach, replacing the flags of registries of individual Member States by a single coherent system of rules and regulations?

c) or are there other alternatives?

Should the European flag be linked to certain incentives to encourage operators to use it?

In relation to the incentives necessary for the securing of the future of Community shipping the Commission's discussion paper also raised the thorny issue of approximation of operating conditions for shipping. The paper pointed to the acknowledgment by the Council in December 1986 of the need for such an approximation. It highlighted the objectives to be the elimination of distortions in competitive capabilities in view of the creation of the internal market and the strengthening of Community shipping vis-a-vis external competition. Specific areas of approximation of operating conditions were pointed at, such as the common approach to the taxation of and subsidies to shipping activity, approximation of conditions in the social area and the creation of a favourable personal income tax regime for Community seafarers as a way of reducing employment costs.

In relation to the incentives to halt the decline of the Community fleet the discussion paper touched upon the issue of whether assistance to EC shipowners for the building of new ships should be given regardless of where they build them or be linked to ordering in Community shipyards in the context of an overall Community industrial policy.

The Symposium participants included representatives from the Community institutions, the governments of Member States, shipowners associations, trade unions and shippers. Judging from the reports produced by the chairmen of the three sessions into which the Symposium was organised,[7] the closing speech by Commissioner Clinton Davis and press reports, it can hardly be said that its results were dramatic.[8] With the exception of trade unions, all other sides reiterated their belief that the solution to problems facing the European shipping industry does not lie in any resort to protectionism by the European side but rather in the application of measures to strengthen the competitive position of the fleets of Member States vis-a-vis their non-EC competitors.

Shippers' representatives, in particular, stressed the international dimension of maritime activity and pointed to the interest that the Community has in maritime services being provided at the lowest possible cost for a satisfactory level of service.

The representatives of CAACE also rejected the solution of protectionism and pointed out to the need for remedial action in relation to the following disadvantages they face in comparison to their non-EC competitors: (i) higher direct labour costs, (ii) higher social security charges, and (iii) high tax levels.

The trade union side was in agreement with the shipowners representatives for the need for supply side measures (the term coined is "positive measures") and especially the granting of a special fiscal and social security status for the shipping industry. However, they also argued in favour of the reservation of certain cargoes for ships under the flags of Member States.

Whilst all government representatives were of the anti-protectionist school of thought, and agreed on the need for transparency of operating conditions within the Community, there was strong disagreement on whether priority should be given to their approximation.

There was strong disagreement between the shipowners and the trade unions side on the question of the position that the Community should adopt in relation to open registries and the new off-shore registries.[9] The representatives of CAACE considered the use of these registries as a fact of Community shipping life and that it would be futile to try and revert to the old institutional arrangements. If shipowners had not flagged out they would not have been able to survive the shipping crisis, since these registries they pointed out to savings in costs on crewing in the range of US dollars 500 thousand per ship per annum for handy-sized tankers or bulk carriers. On the other hand, seafarers' representatives expressed their strong opposition to the use of open registries "on the grounds of inadequate social standards and denial of trade union rights". Their opposition to the new off-shore registries was not of the same strength. They considered them as "second-class flags" and a second best solution to the problems of the shipping industry. However, they declared their intention to keep an open mind and to pronounce their final judgment according to developments in manning arrangements.

The idea of creating a European flag received a lukewarm reception from all sides. The shipowners side in particular stated that such an institutional arrangement might be welcomed by them if it could lead to lower running costs for their ships. They also felt that in respect to standards the EC should not create a new tier of responsibility between those of the national authorities and the IMO-ILO arrangements.

The Symposium also paid great attention to possible means of achieving a better balance between supply and demand in the international shipping industry. A number of possible measures on the supply side were discussed and the Commission undertook to study in detail the options available. Possible options which were discussed and considered being worth further examination were the following:

(a) The establishment of a ship scrapping fund to reimburse owners with the difference between the scrap value and the second-hand value of the ship.

(b) The setting up of a ship scrap guarantee fund. This would provide creditors with the necessary guarantees that would enable shipowners to remote existing mortgages from ships and sell them for scrap, and

(c) The use of resources from the EC Regional Development Fund to help establish scrapping yards in the Community's territory.

The Symposium did not go far enough, however, in examining in detail the problem of financing of the above measures which is always a major stumbling block in the adoption of sectoral restructuring schemes.

THE COMMISSION'S PROGRESS REPORT

In its progress report to the Council relating to positive measures to assist the Community fleet on January 11, 1988 the Commission admitted that it had not reached the stage where it could submit a concrete set of proposals. The report points out to the proliferation of open registries and the increasing tendency to create offshore or parallel or dual national registries. The Commission views these developments with great concern since they are in the opposite direction to the approximation of operating conditions for Community shipowners. The Commission also expresses its concern that, as Member States seek to support their national fleets through these new registries, distortions to competition and discrimination on the grounds of nationality might arise. In this context the report mentions a letter sent by the Commission to the Permanent Representatives of Member States requesting relevant information on new national registries.

The report also refers to the possibility of creating a Community ship registry with the European flag among the possible options for Community action in support of its shipping industry. It considers that this option could be attractive only if it would be linked to possible measures of support such as the favourable fiscal treatment of Community shipowners.

PRESSURE FROM THE SHIPOWNERS SIDE

The lack of progress at Commission level has given rise to a repeat of calls for measures from various groups of European shipowners. In February 1988 the Central Committee of French Shipowners (CCAF) called in its Annual Report for urgent action by the Commission leading to the harmonisation of fiscal and social charges faced by Community shipowners. French shipowners were also critical of the Commission's attempt to implement Regulation 4055/86 in the case of the Italy-Algeria bilateral cargo sharing agreement and expressed concern about the Danish complaint supported by Greek shipowners on the Central and West Africa case.[10]

In a new comprehensive policy statement submitted to the Commission in May 1988 CAACE also urged the adoption of Community measures in aid of shipping as a matter of urgency. CAACE proposals included (a) the abolition of income tax for seafarers, (b) a favourable fiscal treatment of shipping with the view of strengthening the financial position of the EC shipping industry vis-a-vis its competitors and aiding re-investment of profits, (c) the elimination of existing requirements for employers' social security contributions related to the employment of seafarers serving on EC flag vessels, and (d) other measures that would contribute to the improvement of competitiveness such as the covering by the public purse of crew repatriation and training costs and the adoption of flexible crewing provisions.

On the question of the Community register, CAACE pointed to the fact that the Commission had not yet clarified the concept and suggested that it would have a useful role to play only if it were to create a situation whereby the shipping companies of all Member States have the same competitive climate as exists in off-shore and international registers. The above policy statement was the result of compromises among EC national shipowners associatons within CAACE. Thus, the French shipowners call for harmonisation of fiscal and social charges is not reflected in the CAACE submission apparently having not gained support among a large enough number of its members.

The attempts at compromise within CAACE were not successful enough to cover some fundamental differences between Greek shipowners and the rest of the European shipowners on stage two of the EC maritime policy as well as the implementation of the 1986 package. Thus, the CAACE submission also contained a number of reservations from the Union of Greek shipowners (UGS)[11] which represent approximate a third of the EC fleet. Basically, UGS considers that the firm implementation of all Regulations included in the first stage of the EC shipping policy is a pre-requisite to positive measures, and that it would be unrealistic to try and impose measures at Community level in order to solve problems encountered in some countries only. Consequently, UGS believes that the only legal instrument that should be used at Community level in regard to positive measures for shipping is a Council recommendation. UGS in its reservations also raises the issue on the legal status of the new dual registries in relation to the Treaty of Rome and the December 1986 Regulations and asks for its clarification prior to the adoption of any positive measures.

AN INITIATIVE WITHIN THE EUROPEAN PARLIAMENT

The idea of a European ship register found strong support in a working document to the European Parliament Transport Committee submitted by Euro-MP Manfred Ebel of West Germany.[12] That document proposes that a Community ship registry be established covering all vessels flying the flag of a Member State provided that the national rules of the Member States are harmonised in all areas affecting costs. Harmonisation should be at a level that would allow the Community shipping industry to survive international competition.

In relation to crew costs this document proposes drastic reductions in income tax for European seafarers and social security contributions. It also suggests that a compromise formula be found for the composition of crews of ships under the European flag with European and non-domiciled seafarers.

A SHIPPING POLICY CLASH WITHIN THE COMMISSION

The difficulties encountered within the Commission in relation to formulating its official policy proposals on the second stage of the Community's maritime policy were highlighted by the clash between Commissioners Narjes (Industry) and Clinton Davis (Transport) which became public in mid-July 1988.[13] The former, whose brief included shipbuilding, took the unusual step in producing his own internal paper which challenged the direction that the formulation of policy was taking in the Commission services directly responsible for shipping.

The Narjes paper identifies flagging out as the major problem that the Community faces and identifies four areas of action:

a) The introduction of a European Flag for Community ships,
b) Special tax regulations,
c) Adjustments in labour and insurance law,
d) Harmonisation of technical regulations.

The proposals in these areas of action are as follows:

(a) The establishment of a Community shipping register using the European flag, which could also be open to shipping companies from non-Community countries would aim at putting Community ships, crews and shipping companies on an equal footing with other international registers in a way to stop the flagging out trend. It could start as a parallel register for a transitional period. The existing ship registers of the Member States and the national legislations may stay untouched. The paper sees the advantages of the Euroregister as being: i) to hold in check the dangerous disintegration of the shipping laws of Member States caused by their own second registers, and ii) to give an incentive to harmonisation. It also states that the long term aim should be the transfer of the entire supervision and protective rights regarding ships flying the Community flag to a new European Register.

(b) The replacement of national tax rules with special rules regarding taxation of shipping under the Euroship Register. It proposes that a Community personal income tax tariff be established for seamen. It suggests that shipping companies might be taxed along the lines of the Greek tonnage tax.

(c) On labour matters it proposes that in any future Euroship Register, the running-crew will be composed of Community seafarers. Service crew could be non-Community seafarers. Shipping companies in the Community register should be dealing with a Uniform European Seafarers Union representing EC nationals. Non-domiciled seafarers should be represented by different national bodies. The social security of ships' crews must be covered by a uniform insurance scheme based on shipowners' and seafarers' contributions.

(d) In relation to technical matters it is stated that the Euroregister should lead to the harmonisation of regulations and standards for EC ships (eg. mutual recognition of equipment, certification and testing procedures). It is envisaged that the Euroregister is likely to need its own technical and legal staff and that it would adhere to the existing IMO and ILO Conventions' requirements.

The proposal involving the employment of non-domiciled seafarers as "service crews" in a future European Register brought an engry reaction from ITF general secretary. It is noteworthy in this respect that the position of Commissioner Clinton-Davis has been consistently in favour of the exclusive manning of the EC fleet by Community seafarers. This position was repeated in a speech delivered by Commissioner Clinton Davis to the Conference "Europe and the Sea" in Hamburg on September 27, 1988.[14] It also appears that the creation of a European

Register is not considered to be a priority in maritime policy formulation as fas as the Transport Commissioner and his services are concerned, contrary to what has been proposed by the Commissioner for Industry.

Instead, the latest information[15] suggests that the Directorate-General for Transport is working on a set of proposals that would recommend to Member States a favourable fiscal treatment for shipping activity, the reduction of social security costs and the reimbursement of repatriation costs for seafarers. It is envisaged that these proposals would also entail a set of guidelines on state aid to shipping within the Community, according to Articles 92 and 93 of the Treaty, so as to minimise distortions of competition.

These guidelines are unlikely to be strict bearing in mind that the Commission has very recently granted with ease approval of measures adopted by the Dutch government for strengthening the competitive position of its merchant fleet. These measures which will come in force on January 1st 1989 include an exemption from income tax of 35% of Dutch seafarers' income, so that the cost of pay faced by the shipowner can be decreased without a corresponding decrease in net pay. The fact that the Dutch government sought prior approval from the Commission for these fiscal measures confirms the widespread acceptance of the principle that the general provisions of the Treaty apply to international maritime transport irrespective of specific provisions taken under Article 84(2).

ASSESSMENT OF LIKELY FUTURE POLICY ORIENTATION

The above events demonstrate that policy formulation at Community level concerning the second stage of maritime policy is in a state of flux. This makes it very difficult to predict the likely course of future action in this area. There is strong pressure from the majority of European shipowners association for the adoption of favourable measures especially in the areas of taxation of shipping companies and labour costs. The adoption of such measures is also supported by the trade unions, who nevertheless link it to the exclusive employment of European seafarers. On the other hand, the Union of Greek Shipowners, representing a substantial percentage of Community tonnage, is keen to ensure the effective operation of existing legislation and is opposed to any Community harmonisation measures on the supply side that it considers will threaten the competitiveness of its members.

Governments of Member States appear to be sceptical about the whole exercise and some of them, notably Denmark, Germany and the Netherlands are finding national solutions to the problem of competitiveness of their fleets. These countries are likely to be indifferent to any optional harmonisation, such as the creation of a European Register in parallel to their national ones, and are likely to be inimical to any total harmonisation. Furthermore, governments are unlikely to accept special fiscal measures as an exceptional treatment for the shipping sector which might compromise their policies towards the implementation of the Single European Act and the 1992 White Paper. It must be remembered in this respect that the Single European Act still retains the requirement of unanimity in the Council on matters of taxation.[16] On top of that, the Commission has not managed so far to adopt a common position on the proposals to be submitted to the Council.

Nevertheless, the authors will not shy away from producing their own prediction on the likely course of future maritime policy at Community level: The Commission will finally produce proposals for the favourable fiscal treatment of maritime activity in the EC, and the granting of income tax concessions for seafarers. Given the lack of consensus at Council level the most likely instrument will take the form of a Commission Recommendation which will not be binding upon Member States. Finally, it is unlikely that in the foreseeable future any measures will be adopted leading to the creation of a European Register.

NOTES

1 See Chapter 11.

2 Commission of the EC "Progress Towards a Common Transport Policy; Maritime Policy" COM(85) 90 final.

3 See Chapter 7.

4 Lloyd's List, 31st March 1988.

5 Lloyd's List, 3rd June 1988.

6 See Chapter 6.

7 Reports respectively by Messrs H. Lewis General Secretary ITF, J. Saverys President of CAACE, and W. Hoffman German Ministry of Transport.

8 Lloyd's List, 8th May 1987.

9 See Chapter 3.

10 See Chapters 9 and 10.

11 These are also to be found in CAACE Annual Report 1987/1988.

12 European Parliament, Committee on Transport. Working Document in Preparation for the Report on a European Flag. Positive Action to Strengthen the Community's Shipping Companies Tabled by Mr M. Ebel, 25th April 1988, EN(88) 1120E. PE 123.188.

13 Lloyd's List, 15th July 1988.

14 Commission of the European Communities, Press Release IP(88) 572.

15 Lloyd's List, 29th November 1988.

16 Article 99 of the EEC Treaty as amended by article 17 of the Single European Act.

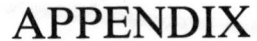

APPENDIX

I

(Acts whose publication is obligatory)

COUNCIL REGULATION (EEC) No 954/79

of 15 May 1979

concerning the ratification by Member States of, or their accession to, the
United Nations Convention on a Code of Conduct for Liner Conferences

THE COUNCIL OF THE EUROPEAN
COMMUNITIES,

Having regard to the Treaty establishing the European
Economic Community, and in particular Article 84 (2)
thereof,

Having regard to the draft Regulation submitted by
the Commission,

Having regard to the opinion of the European Parliament ([1]),

Having regard to the opinion of the Economic and
Social Committee ([2]),

Whereas a Convention on a Code of Conduct for
Liner Conferences has been drawn up by a Conference convened under the auspices of the United
Nations Conference on Trade and Development and
is open for ratification or accession ;

Whereas the questions covered by the Code of
Conduct are of importance not only to the Member
States but also to the Community, in particular from
the shipping and trading viewpoints, and it is therefore important that a common position should be
adopted in relation to this Code ;

Whereas this common position should respect the
principles and objectives of the Treaty and make a
major contribution to meeting the aspirations of developing countries in the field of shipping while at the
same same time pursuing the objective of the continuing application in this field of the commercial principles applied by shipping lines of the OECD countries
and in trades between these countries ;

Whereas to secure observance of these principles and
objectives, since the Code of Conduct contains no
provision allowing the accession of the Community as
such, it is important that Member States ratify or

accede to the Code of Conduct subject to certain arrangements provided for in this Regulation ;

Whereas the stabilizing role of conferences in
ensuring reliable services to shippers is recognized,
but it is nevertheless necessary to avoid possible
breaches by conferences of the rules of competition
laid down in the Treaty ; whereas the Commission
will accordingly forward to the Council a proposal for
a Regulation concerning the application of those rules
to sea transport,

HAS ADOPTED THIS REGULATION :

Article 1

1.   When ratifying the United Nations Convention
on a Code of Conduct for Liner Conferences, or when
acceding thereto, Member States shall inform the
Secretary-General of the United Nations in writing
that such ratification or accession has taken place in
accordance with this Regulation.

2.   The instrument of ratification or accession shall
be accompanied by the reservations set out in Annex
I.

Article 2

1.   In the case of an existing conference, each group
of shipping lines of the same nationality which are
members thereof shall determine by commercial negotiations with another shipping line of that nationality
whether the latter may participate as a national shipping line in the said conference.

If a new conference is created, the shipping lines of
the same nationality shall determine by commercial
negotiations which of them may participate as a
national shipping line in the future conference.

([1]) OJ No C 131, 5. 6. 1978, p. 34.
([2]) OJ No C 269, 13. 11. 1978, p. 46.

2. Where the negotiations referred to in paragraph 1 fail to result in agreement, each Member State may, at the request of one of the lines concerned and after hearing all of them, take the necessary steps to settle the dispute.

3. Each Member State shall ensure that all vessel-operating shipping lines established on its territory under the Treaty establishing the European Economic Community are treated in the same way as lines which have their management head office on its territory and the effective control of which is exercised there.

Article 3

1. Where a liner conference operates a pool or a berthing, sailing and/or any other form of cargo allocation agreement in accordance with Article 2 of the Code of Conduct, the volume of cargo to which the group of national shipping lines of each Member State participating in that trade or the shipping lines of the Member States participating in that trade as third-country shipping lines are entitled under the Code shall be redistributed, unless a decision is taken to the contrary by all the lines which are members of the Conference and parties to the present redistribution rules. This redistribution of cargo shares shall be carried out on the basis of a unanimous decision by those shipping lines which are members of the conference and participate in the redistribution, with a view to all these lines carrying a fair share of the conference trade.

2. The share finally allocated to each participant shall be determined by the application of commercial principles, taking account in particular of :

(a) the volume of cargo carried by the conference and generated by the Member States whose trade is served by it ;

(b) past performance of the shipping lines in the trade covered by the pool ;

(c) the volume of cargo carried by the conference and shipped through the ports of the Member States ;

(d) the needs of the shippers whose cargoes are carried by the conference.

3. If no agreement is reached on the redistribution of cargoes referred to in paragraph 1, the matter shall, at the request of one of the parties, be referred to conciliation in accordance with the procedure set out in Annex II. Any dispute not settled by the conciliation procedure may, with the agreement of the parties,

be referred to arbitration. In that event, the award of the arbitrator shall be binding.

4. At intervals to be laid down in advance, shares allocated in accordance with paragraphs 1, 2 and 3 shall be regularly reviewed, taking into account the criteria set out in paragraph 2 and in particular from the viewpoint of providing adequate and efficient services to shippers.

Article 4

1. In a conference trade between a Member State of the Community and a State which is a party to the Code of Conduct and not an OECD country, a shipping line of another Member State of the OECD wishing to participate in the redistribution provided for in Article 3 of this Regulation may do so subject to reciprocity defined at governmental or ship-owners' level.

2. Without prejudice to paragraph 3 of this Article, Article 2 of the Code of Conduct shall not be applied in conference trades between Member States or, on a reciprocal basis, between such States and the other OECD countries which are parties to the Code.

3. Paragraph 2 of this Article shall not affect the opportunities for participation as third country shipping lines in such trades, in accordance with the principles reflected in Article 2 of the Code of Conduct, of the shipping lines of a developing country which are recognized as national shipping lines under the Code and which are :

(a) already members of a conference serving these trades ; or

(b) admitted to such a conference under Article 1 (3) of the Code.

4. Articles 3 and 14 (9) of the Code of Conduct shall not be applied in conference trades between Member States or, on a reciprocal basis, between such States and other OECD countries which are parties to the code.

5. In conference trades between Member States and between these States and other OECD countries which are parties to the Code of Conduct, the shippers and ship-owners of Member States shall not insist on applying the procedures for settling disputes provided for in Chapter VI of the Code in their mutual relationships or, on a reciprocal basis, in relation to shippers and ship-owners of other OECD countries where other procedures for settling disputes have been agreed between them. They shall in parti-

cular take full advantage of the possibilities provided by Article 25 (1) and (2) of the Code for resolving disputes by means of procedures other than those laid down in Chapter VI of the Code.

Article 5

For the adoption of decisions relating to matters defined in the conference agreement concerning the trade of a Member State, other than those referred to in Article 3 of this Regulation, the national shipping lines of such State shall consult all the other Community lines which are members of the conference before giving or withholding their assent

Article 6

Member States shall, in due course and after consulting the Commission, adopt the laws, regulations or administrative provisions necessary for the implementation of this Regulation.

This Regulation shall be binding in its entirety and directly applicable in all Member States.

Done at Brussels, 15 May 1979.

For the Council
The President
R. BOULIN

ANNEX I

RESERVATIONS

When ratifying the Convention or when acceding thereto, Member States shall enter the following three reservations and interpretative reservation :

1. For the purposes of the Code of Conduct, the term 'national shipping line' may, in the case of a Member State of the Community, include any vessel-operating shipping line established on the territory of such Member State in accordance with the EEC Treaty.

2. (a) Without prejudice to paragraph (b) of this reservation, Article 2 of the Code of Conduct shall not be applied in conference trades between the Member States of the Community or, on a reciprocal basis, between such States and the other OECD countries which are parties to the Code.

   (b) Point (a) shall not affect the opportunities for participation as third country shipping lines in such trades, in accordance with the principles reflected in Article 2 of the Code, of the shipping lines of a developing country which are recognized as national shipping lines under the Code and which are :

   (i) already members of a conference serving these trades ; or

   (ii) admitted to such a conference under Article 1 (3) of the Code.

3. Articles 3 and 14 (9) of the Code of Conduct shall not be applied in conference trades between the Member States of the Community or, on a reciprocal basis, between such States and the other OECD countries which are parties to the Code.

4. In trades to which Article 3 of the Code of Conduct applies, the last sentence of that Article is interpreted as meaning that :

   (a) the two groups of national shipping lines will coordinate their positions before voting on matters concerning the trade between their two countries ;

   (b) this sentence applies solely to matters which the conference agreement identifies as requiring the assent of both groups of national shipping lines concerned, and not to all matters covered by the conference agreement.

———

ANNEX II

CONCILIATION REFERRED TO IN ARTICLE 3 (3)

The parties to the dispute shall designate one or more conciliators.

Should they fail to agree on the matter, each of the parties to the dispute shall designate a conciliator and the conciliators thus designated shall co-opt another conciliator to act as chairman. Should a party fail to designate a conciliator or the conciliators designated by the parties fail to reach agreement on the chairman, the President of the International Chamber of Commerce shall, at the request of one of the parties, make the necessary designations.

The conciliators shall make every endeavour to settle the dispute. They shall decide on the procedure to be followed. Their fees shall be paid by the parties to the dispute.

———

I

(Acts whose publication is obligatory)

COUNCIL REGULATION (EEC) No 4055/86

of 22 December 1986

applying the principle of freedom to provide services to maritime transport between Member States and between Member States and third countries

THE COUNCIL OF THE EUROPEAN COMMUNITIES,

Having regard to the Treaty establishing the European Economic Community, and in particular Article 84 (2) thereof,

Having regard to the draft Regulation submitted by the Commission,

Having regard to the opinion of the European Parliament ([1]),

Having regard to the opinion of the Economic and Social Committee ([2]),

Whereas the abolition, as between Member States, of obstacles to freedom of movement for services is laid down by Article 3 of the Treaty as one of the activities of the Community;

Whereas in accordance with Article 61 of the Treaty freedom to provide services in the field of maritime transport is to be governed by the provisions of the Title relating to transport;

Whereas the application of this principle within the Community is also a necessary condition for effectively pursuing, in relation to third countries, a policy aiming at safeguarding the continuing application of commercial principles in shipping;

Whereas Council Regulation (EEC) No 954/79 ([3]) preserves, *inter alia*, within conferences competitive access to that part of cargo liner shipping which is not covered by commitments to national shipping lines of third countries under the United Nations Convention on a Code of Conduct for Liner Conferences, when ratified by Member States;

([1]) OJ No C 255, 13. 10. 1986, p. 169.
([2]) OJ No C 172, 2. 7. 1984, p. 178.
([3]) OJ No L 121, 17. 5. 1979, p. 1.

Whereas, taking into account the fact that the Code of Conduct has not yet been ratified by all Member States and that certain third countries are not likely to ratify it, the Code is not yet applied in all Community trades nor is it likely to apply in the future in some of these trades;

Whereas the code of conduct applies only to liner conferences and the cargo carried by their members, and not to independent lines or to shipping companies operating in the field of bulk or tramp shipping, where the Community aims at maintaining a regime of fair and free competition;

Whereas the Community fully endorses Resolution No 2 adopted by the United Nations Conference of Plenipotentaries on a Code of Conduct for Liner Conferences and which states that in the interests of sound development of liner shipping services, non-conference shipping liners should not be prevented from operating as long as they adhere to the principle of fair competition on a commercial basis;

Whereas the Member States affirm their commitment to a freely competitive environment as being an essential feature of the dry and liquid bulk trades and are convinced that the introduction of cargosharing in these trades will have a serious effect on the trading interests of all countries by substantially increasing transportation costs;

Whereas Community shipowners are increasingly faced with new restrictions, imposed by third countries, on the freedom to provide maritime transport services for shippers established in their own country, in other Member States or in the third countries concerned, which may have harmful effects on Community trades as a whole;

Whereas some of the abovementioned restrictions are incorporated in bilateral agreements between third countries and some Member States, while other restrictions are reflected in similar provisions in the legislation or in administrative practices of some Member States;

Whereas therefore the principle of freedom to provide services should now be applied to maritime transport between Member States and between Member States and third countries so as progressively to abolish existing restrictions and prevent the introduction of new restrictions;

Whereas the structure of the Community shipping industry is such as to make it appropriate that the provisions of this Regulation should also apply to nationals of the Member States established outside the Community and to shipping companies established outside the Community and controlled by nationals of a Member State, if their vessels are registered in that Member State in accordance with its legislation;

Whereas provision should be made for reasonable transitional periods in accordance with the character of the type of transport concerned,

HAS ADOPTED THIS REGULATION:

Article 1

1.   Freedom to provide maritime transport services between Member States and between Member States and third countries shall apply in respect of nationals of Member States who are established in a Member State other than that of the person for whom the services are intended.

2.   The provisions of this Regulation shall also apply to nationals of the Member States established outside the Community and to shipping companies established outside the Community and controlled by nationals of a Member State, if their vessels are registered in that Member State in accordance with its legislation.

3.   The provisions of Articles 55 to 58 and 62 of the Treaty shall apply to the matters covered by this Regulation.

4.   For the purpose of this Regulation, the following shall be considered 'maritime transport services between Member States and between Member States and third countries' where they are normally provided for remuneration:

(a)   *intra-Community shipping services:*

the carriage of passengers or goods by sea between any port of a Member State and any port or off-shore installation of another Member State;

(b)   *third-country traffic:*

the carriage of passengers or goods by sea between the ports of a Member State and ports or off-shore installations of a third country.

Article 2

By way of derogation from Article 1, unilateral national restrictions in existence before 1 July 1986 on the carriage of certain goods wholly or partly reserved for vessels flying the national flag, shall be phased out at the latest in accordance with the following timetable:

— carriage between Member States by vessels flying the flag of a Member State: 31 December 1989

— carriage between Member States and third countries by vessels flying the flag of a Member State: 31 December 1991

— carriage between Member States and between Member States and third countries in other vessels: 1 January 1993

Article 3

Cargo-sharing arrangements contained in existing bilateral agreements concluded by Member States with third countries shall be phased out or adjusted in accordance with the provisions of Article 4.

Article 4

1.   Existing cargo-sharing arrangements not phased out in accordance with Article 3 shall be adjusted in accordance with Community legislation and in particular:

(a)   where trades governed by the United Nations Code of Conduct for Liner Conferences are concerned, they shall comply with this Code and with the obligations of Member States under Regulation (EEC) No 954/79;

(b)   where trades not governed by the United Nations Code of Conduct for Liner Conferences are concerned, agreement shall be adjusted as soon as possible and in any event before 1 January 1993 so as to provide for fair, free and non-discriminatory access by all Community nationals, as defined in Article 1, to the cargo-shares due to the Member States concerned.

2.   National action in pursuance of paragraph 1 shall be notified immediately to the Member States and the Commission. The consultation procedure established by Council Decision 77/587/EEC shall apply.

3.   Member States shall report to the Commission on progress made on the adjustments referred to in paragraph 1 (b), initially every six months and subsequently every year.

4.   When difficulties arise in the process of adjusting agreements to bring them into conformity with paragraph 1 (b), the Member State concerned shall inform the Council and the Commission. In cases where agreements are incompatible with paragraph 1 (b) and where the Member State concerned so asks, the Council shall, acting on a proposal from the Commission, take appropriate action.

Article 5

1.   Cargo-sharing arrangements in any future agreements with third countries are prohibited other than in those exceptional circumstances where Community liner shipping

companies would not otherwise have an effective opportunity to ply for trade to and from the third country concerned. In these circumstances such arrangements may be permitted in accordance with the provisions of Article 6.

2.   In cases where a third country seeks to impose cargo sharing arrangements on Member States in liquid or dry bulk trades, the Council shall take the appropriate action in accordance with Regulation (EEC) No 4058/86 concerning coordinated action to safeguard free access to cargoes in ocean trades (¹).

Article 6

1.   If a Member State's nationals or shipping companies, as defined in Article 1, paragraphs 1 and 2, are experiencing, or are threatened by, a situation where they do not have an effective opportunity to ply for trade to and from a particular third country, the Member State concerned shall inform the other Member States and the Commission as soon as possible.

2.   The Council, acting by qualified majority on a proposal of the Commission, shall decide on the necessary action. Such action may include, in the circumstances envisaged in Article 5 (1), the negotiation and conclusion of cargo-sharing arrangements.

3.   If the Council has not decided on the necessary action within six months of a Member State providing information under paragraph 1, the Member State concerned may take such action as may for the time being be necessary to preserve an effective opportunity to ply for trade in accordance with Article 5 (1).

4.   Any action taken under paragraph 3 shall be in accordance with Community law and provide for fair, free and non-discriminatory access to the relevant cargo shares by nationals or Community shipping companies, as defined in Article 1 (1) and (2).

5.   National action in pursuance of paragraph 3 shall be notified immediately to the Member States and the Commission. The consultation procedure established by Council Decision 77/587/EEC shall apply.

Article 7

The Council, acting in accordance with the conditions laid down in the Treaty, may extend the provisions of this Regulation to nationals of a third country who provide maritime transport services and are established in the Community.

Article 8

Without prejudice to the provisions of the Treaty relating to right of establishment, a person providing a maritime transport service may, in order to do so, temporarily pursue his activity in the Member State where the service is provided, under the same conditions as are imposed by that State on its own nationals.

Article 9

As long as restrictions on freedom to provide services have not been abolished, each Member State shall apply such restrictions without distinction on grounds of nationality or residence to all persons providing services within the meaning of Article 1 (1) and (2).

Article 10

Member States shall, before adopting laws, regulations or administrative provisions in implementation of this Regulation consult the Commission and shall communicate to the latter any such measures so adopted.

Article 11

The Council, acting in accordance with the provisions laid down in the Treaty, shall review this Regulation before 1 January 1995.

Article 12

This Regulation shall enter into force on the day following its publication in the *Official Journal of the European Communities*.

It shall be binding in its entirety and directly applicable in all Member States.

Done at Brussels, 22 December 1986.

For the Council
The President
G. SHAW

(¹) See page 21 in this Official Journal.

COUNCIL REGULATION (EEC) No 4056/86

of 22 December 1986

laying down detailed rules for the application of Articles 85 and 86 of the Treaty to maritime transport

THE COUNCIL OF THE EUROPEAN COMMUNITIES,

Having regard to the Treaty establishing the European Economic Community, and in particular Articles 84 (2) and 87 thereof,

Having regard to the proposal from the Commission,

Having regard to the opinion of the European Parliament ([1]),

Having regard to the opinion of the Economic and Social Committee ([2]),

Whereas the rules on competition form part of the Treaty's general provisions which also apply to maritime transport; whereas detailed rules for applying those provisions are set out in the Chapter of the Treaty dealing with the rules on competition or are to be determined by the procedures laid down therein;

Whereas according to Council Regulation No 141 ([3]), Council Regulation No 17 ([4]) does not apply to transport; whereas Council Regulation (EEC) No 1017/68 ([5]) applies to inland transport only; whereas, consequently, the Commission has no means at present of investigating directly cases of suspected infringement of Articles 85 and 86 in maritime transport; whereas, moreover, the Commission lacks such powers of its own to take decisions or impose penalties as are necessary for it to bring to an end infringements established by it;

Whereas this situation necessitates the adoption of a Regulation applying the rules of competition to maritime transport; whereas Council Regulation (EEC) No 954/79 of 15 May 1979 concerning the ratification by Member States of, or their accession to, the United Nations Convention on a Code of Conduct for Liner Conference ([6]) will result in the application of the Code of Conduct to a considerable number of conferences serving the Community; whereas the Regulation applying the rules of competition to maritime transport foreseen in the last recital of Regulation (EEC) No 954/79 should take account of the adoption of the Code;

whereas, as far as conferences subject to the Code of Conduct are concerned, the Regulation should supplement the Code or make it more precise;

Whereas it appears preferable to exclude tramp vessel services from the scope of this Regulation, rates for these services being freely negotiated on a case-by-case basis in accordance with supply and demand conditions;

Whereas this Regulation should take account of the necessity, on the one hand to provide for implementing rules that enable the Commission to ensure that competition is not unduly distorted within the common market, and on the other hand to avoid excessive regulation of the sector;

Whereas this Regulation should define the scope of the provisions of Articles 85 and 86 of the Treaty, taking into account the distinctive characteristics of maritime transport; whereas trade between Member States may be affected where restrictive practices or abuses concern international maritime transport, including intra-Community transport, from or to Community ports; whereas such restrictive practices or abuses may influence competition, firstly, between ports in different Member States by altering their respective catchment areas, and secondly, between activities in those catchment areas, and disturb trade patterns within the common market;

Whereas certain types of technical agreement, decisions and concerted practices may be excluded from the prohibition on restrictive practices on the ground that they do not, as a general rule, restrict competition;

Whereas provision should be made for block exemption of liner conferences; whereas liner conferences have a stabilizing effect, assuring shippers of reliable services; whereas they contribute generally to providing adequate efficient scheduled maritime transport services and give fair consideration to the interests of users; whereas such results cannot be obtained without the cooperation that shipping companies promote within conferences in relation to rates and, where appropriate, availability of capacity or allocation of cargo for shipment, and income; whereas in most cases conferences continue to be subject to effective competition from both non-conference scheduled services and, in certain circumstances, from tramp services and from other modes of transport; whereas the mobility of fleets, which is a characteristic feature of the structure of availability in the shipping field, subjects conferences to constant competition which they are unable as a rule to eliminate as far as a substantial proportion of the shipping services in question is concerned;

([1]) OJ No C 172, 2. 7. 1984, p. 178; OJ No C 255, 13. 10. 1986, p. 169.

([2]) OJ No C 77, 21. 3. 1983, p. 13; OJ No C 344, 31. 12. 1985, p. 31.

([3]) OJ No 124, 28. 11. 1962, p. 2751/62.

([4]) OJ No 13, 21. 2. 1962, p. 204/62.

([5]) OJ No L 175, 23. 7. 1968, p. 1.

([6]) OJ No L 121, 17. 5. 1979, p. 1.

Whereas, however, in order to prevent conferences from engaging in practices which are incompatible with Article 85 (3) of the Treaty, certain conditions and obligations should be attached to the exemption;

Whereas the aim of the conditions should be to prevent conferences from imposing restrictions on competition which are not indispensable to the attainment of the objectives on the basis of which exemption is granted; whereas, to this end, confernces should not, in respect of a given route, apply rates and conditions of carriage which are differentiated solely by reference to the country of origin or destination of the goods carried and thus cause within the Community deflections of trade that are harmful to certain ports, shippers, carriers or providers of services ancillary to transport; whereas, furthermore, loyalty arrangements should be permitted only in accordance with rules which do not restrict unilaterally the freedom of users and consequently competition in the shipping industry, without prejudice, however, to the right of a conference to impose penalties on users who seek by improper means to evade the obligation of loyalty required in exchange for the rebates, reduced freight rates or commission granted to them by the conference; whereas users must be free to determine the undertakings to which they have recourse in respect of inland transport or quayside services not covered by the freight charge or by other charges agreed with the shipping line;

Whereas certain obligations should also attached to the exemption; whereas in this respect users must at all times be in a position to acquaint themselves with the rates and conditions of carriage applied by members of the conference, since in the case of inland transports organized by shippers, the latter continue to be subject to Regulation (EEC) No 1017/68; whereas provision should be made that awards given at arbitration and recommendations made by conciliators and accepted by the parties be notified forthwith to the Commission in order to enable it to verify that conferences are not thereby exempted from the conditions provided for in the Regulation and thus do not infringe the provisions of Articles 85 and 86;

Whereas consultations between users or associations of users and conferences are liable to secure a more efficient operation of maritime transport services which takes better account of users' requirements; whereas, consequently, certain restrictive practices which could ensue from such consultations should be exempted;

Whereas there can be no exemption if the conditions set out in Article 85 (3) are not satisfied; whereas the Commission must therefore have power to take the appropriate measures where an agreement or concerted practice proves to have certain effects incompatible with Article 85 (3); whereas, in view of the specific role fulfilled by the conferences in the sector of the liner services, the reaction of the Commission should be progressive and proportionate; whereas the Commission should consequently have the power first to address recommendations, then to take decisions;

Whereas the automatic nullity provided for in Article 85 (3) in respect of agreements or decisions which have not been

granted exemption pursuant to Article 85 (3) owing to their discriminatory or other features applies only to the elements of the agreement covered by the prohibition of Article 85 (1) and applies to the agreement in its entirety only if those elements do not appear to be severable from the whole of the agreement whereas the Commission should therefore, if it finds an infringement of the block exemption, either specify what elements of the agreement are by the prohibition and consequently automatically void, or indicate the reasons why those elements are not severable from the rest of the agreement and why the agreement is therefore void in its entirety;

Whereas, in view of the characteristics of international maritime transport, account should be taken of the fact that the application of this Regulation to certain restrictive practices or abuses may result in conflicts with the laws and rules of certain third countries and prove harmful to important Community trading and shipping interests; whereas consultations and, where appropriate, negotiations authorized by the Council should be undertaken by the Commission with those countries in pursuance of the maritime transport policy of the Community;

Whereas this Regulation should make provision for the procedures, decision-making powers and penalties that are necessary to ensure compliance with the prohibitions laid down in Article 85 (1) and Article 86, as well as the conditions governing the application of Article 85 (3);

Whereas account should be taken in this respect of the procedural provisions of Regulation (EEC) No 1017/68 applicable to inland transport operations which takes account of certain distinctive features of transport operations viewed as a whole;

Whereas, in particular, in view of the special characteristics of maritime transport, it is primarily the responsibility of undertakings to see to it that their agreements, decisions and concerted practices conform to the rules on competition, and consequently their notification to the Commission need not be made compulsory;

Whereas in certain circumstances undertakings may, however, wish to apply to the Commission for confirmation that their agreements, decisions and concerted practices are in conformity with the provisions in force; whereas a simplified procedure should be laid down for such cases,

HAS ADOPTED THIS REGULATION:

SECTION I

Article 1

Subject-matter and scope of the Regulation

1. This Regulation lays down detailed rules for the application of Articles 85 and 86 of the Treaty to maritime transport services.

2. It shall apply only to international maritime transport services from or to one or more Community ports, other than tramp vessel services.

3. For the purposes of this Regulation:

(a) 'tramp vessel services' means the transport of goods in bulk or in break-bulk in a vessel chartered wholly or partly to one or more shippers on the basis of a voyage or time charter or any other form of contract for non-regularly scheduled or non-advertised sailings where the freight rates are freely negotiated case by case in accordance with the conditions of supply and demand;

(b) 'liner conference' means a group of two or more vessel-operating carriers which provides international liner services for the carriage of cargo on a particular route or routes within specified geographical limits and which has an agreement or arrangement, whatever its nature, within the framework of which they operate under uniform or common freight rates and any other agreed conditions with respect to the provision of liner services;

(c) 'transport user' means an undertaking (e.g. shippers, consignees, forwarders, etc.) provided it has entered into, or demonstrates an intention to enter into, a contractual or other arrangement with a conference or shipping line for the shipment of goods, or any association of shippers.

Article 2

Technical agreements

1. The prohibition laid down in Article 85 (1) of the Treaty shall not apply to agreements, decisions and concerted practices whose sole object and effect is to achieve technical improvements or cooperation by means of:

(a) the introduction or uniform application of standards or types in respect of vessels and other means of transport, equipment, supplies or fixed installations;

(b) the exchange or pooling for the purpose of operating transport services, of vessels, space on vessels or slots and other means of transport, staff, equipment or fixed installations;

(c) the organization and execution of successive or supplementary maritime transport operations and the establishment or application of inclusive rates and conditions for such operations;

(d) the coordination of transport timetables for connecting routes;

(e) the consolidation of individual consignments;

(f) the establishment or application of uniform rules concerning the structure and the conditions governing the application of transport tariffs.

2. The Commission shall, if necessary, submit to the Council proposals for the amendment of the list contained in paragraph 1.

Article 3

Exemption for agreements between carriers concerning the operation of scheduled maritime transport services

Agreements, decisions and concerted practices of all or part of the members of one or more liner conferences are hereby exempted from the prohibition in Article 85 (1) of the Treaty, subject to the condition imposed by Article 4 of this Regulation, when they have as their objective the fixing of rates and conditions of carriage, and, as the case may be, one or more of the following objectives:

(a) the coordination of shipping timetables, sailing dates or dates of calls;

(b) the determination of the frequency of sailings or calls;

(c) the coordination or allocation of sailings or calls among members of the conference;

(d) the regulation of the carrying capacity offered by each member;

(e) the allocation of cargo or revenue among members.

Article 4

Condition attaching to exemption

The exemption provided for in Articles 3 and 6 shall be granted subject to the condition that the agreement, decision or concerted practice shall not, within the common market, cause detriment to certain ports, transport users or carriers by applying for the carriage of the same goods and in the area covered by the agreement, decision or concerted practice, rates and conditions of carriage which differ according to the country of origin or destination or port of loading or discharge, unless such rates or condditions can be economically justified.

Any agreement or decision or, if it is severable, any part of such an agreement or decision not complying with the preceding paragraph shall automatically be void pursuant to Article 85 (2) of the Treaty.

Article 5

Obligations attaching to exemption

The following obligations shall be attached to the exemption provided for in Article 3:

1. *Consultations*

There shall be consultations for the purpose of seeking solutions on general issues of principle between transport users on the one hand and conferences on the other concerning the rates, conditions and quality of scheduled maritime transport services.

These consultations shall take place whenever requested by any of the abovementioned parties.

2. *Loyalty arrangements*

The shipping lines' members of a conference shall be entitled to institute and maintain loyalty arrangements with transport users, the form and terms of which shall be matters for consultation between the conference and transport users' organizations. These loyalty arrangements shall provide safeguards making explicit the rights of transport users and conference members. These arrangements shall be based on the contract system or any other system which is also lawful.

Loyalty arrangements must comply with the following conditions:

(a) Each conference shall offer transport users a system of immediate rebates or the choice between such a system and a system of deferred rebates:

— under the system of immediate rebates each of the parties shall be entitled to terminate the loyalty arrangement at any time without penalty and subject to a period of notice of not more than six months; this period shall be reduced to three months when the conference rate is the subject of a dispute;

— under the system of deferred rebates neither the loyalty period on the basis of which the rebate is calculated nor the subsequent loyalty period required before payment of the rebate may exceed six months; this period shall be reduced to three months where the conference rate is the subject of a dispute.

(b) The conference shall, after consulting the transport users concerned, set out:

(i) a list of cargo and any portion of cargo agreed with transport users which is specifically excluded from the scope of the loyalty arrangement; 100 % loyalty arrangements may be offered but may not be unilaterally imposed;

(ii) a list of circumstances in which transport users are released from their obligation of loyalty; these shall include:

— circumstances in which consignments are dispatched from or to a port in the area covered by the conference but not advertised and where the request for a waiver can be justified, and

— those in which waiting time at a port exceeds a period to be determined for each port and for each commodity or class of commodities following consultation of the transport users directly concerned with the proper servicing of the port.

The conference must, however, be informed in advance by the transport user, within a specified period, of his intention to dispatch the consignment from a port not advertised by the conference or to make use of a non-conference vessel at a port served by the conference as soon as he has been able to establish from the published schedule of sailings that the maximum waiting period will be exceeded.

3. *Services not covered by the freight charges*

Transport users shall be entitled to approach the undertakings of their choice in respect of inland transport operations and quayside services not covered by the freight charge or charges on which the shipping line and the transport user have agreed.

4. *Availability of tariffs*

Tariffs, related conditions, regulations and any amendments thereto shall be made available on request to transport users at reasonable cost, or they shall be available for examination at offices of shipping lines and their agents. They shall set out all the conditions concerning loading and discharge, the exact extent of the services covered by the freight charge in proportion to the sea transport and the land transport or by any other charge levied by the shipping line and customary practice in such matters.

5. *Notification to the Commission of awards at arbitration and recommendations*

Awards given at arbitration and recommendations made by conciliators that are accepted by the parties shall be notified forthwith to the Commission when they resolve disputes relating to the practices of conferences referred to in Article 4 and in points 2 and 3 above.

Article 6

Exemption for agreements between transport users and conferences concerning the use of scheduled maritime transport services

Agreements, decisions and concerned practices between transport users, on the one hand, and conferences, on the other hand, and agreements between transport users which may be necessary to that end, concerning the rates, conditions and quality of liner services, as long as they are provided for in Article 5 (1) and (2) are hereby exempted from the prohibition laid down in Article 85 (1) of the Treaty.

Article 7

Monitoring of exempted agreements

1. *Breach of an obligation*

Where the persons concerned are in breach of an obligation which, pursuant to Article 5, attaches to the exemption provided for in Article 3, the Commission may, in order to put an end to such breach and under the conditions laid down in Section II:

— address recommendations to the persons concerned;

— in the event of failure by such persons to observe those recommendations and depending upon the gravity of the breach concerned, adopt a decision that either prohibits them from carrying out or requires them to perform specific acts or, while withdrawing the benefit of the block exemption which they enjoyed, grants them an individual exemption according to Article 11 (4) or withdraws the benefit of the block exemption which they enjoyed.

2. *Effects incompatible with Article 85 (3)*

(a) Where, owing to special circumstances as described below, agreements, decisions and concerted practices which qualify for the exemption provided for in Articles 3 and 6 have nevertheless effects which are incompatible with the conditions laid down in Article 85 (3) of the Treaty, the Commission, on receipt of a complaint or on its own initiative, under the conditions laid down in Section II, shall take the measures described in (c) below. The severity of these measures must be in proportion to the gravity of the situation.

(b) Special circumstances are, *inter alia,* created by:

(i) acts of conferences or a change of market conditions in a given trade resulting in the absence or elimination of actual or potential competition such as restrictive practices whereby the trade is not available to competition; or

(ii) acts of conference which may prevent technical or economic progress or user participation in the benefits;

(iii) acts of third countries which:

— prevent the operation of outsiders in a trade,

— impose unfair tariffs on conference members,

— impose arrangements which otherwise impede technical or economic progress (cargo-sharing, limitations on types of vessels).

(c) (i) If actual or potential competition is absent or may be eliminated as a result of action by a third country, the Commission shall enter into consultations with the competent authorities of the third country concerned, followed if necessary by negotiations under directives to be given by the Council, in order to remedy the situation.

If the special circumstances result in the absence or elimination of actual or potential competition contrary to Article 85 (3) (b) of the Treaty the Commission shall withdraw the benefit of the block exemption. At the same time it shall rule on whether and, if so, under what additional conditions and obligations an individual exemption should be granted to the relevant conference agreement with a view, *inter alia,* to obtaining access to the market for non-conference lines;

(ii) If, as a result of special circumstances as set out in (b), there are effects other than those referred to in (i) hereof, the Commission shall take one or more of the measures described in paragraph 1.

Article 8

Effects incompatible with Article 86 of the Treaty

1.   The abuse of a dominant position within the meaning of Article 86 of the Treaty shall be prohibited, no prior decision to that effect being required.

2.   Where the Commission, either on its own initiative or at the request of a Member State or of natural or legal persons claiming a legitimate interest, finds that in any particular case the conduct of conferences benefiting from the exemption laid down in Article 3 nevertheless has effects which are incompatible with Article 86 of the Treaty, it may withdraw the benefit of the block exemption and take, pursuant to Article 10, all appropriate measures for the purpose of bringing to an end infringements of Article 86 of the Treaty.

3.   Before taking a decision under paragraph 2, the Commission may address to the conference concerned recommendations for termination of the infringement.

Article 9

Conflicts of international law

1.   Where the application of this Regulation to certain restrictive practices or clauses is liable to enter into conflict with the provisions laid down by law, regulation or administrative action of certain third countries which would compromise important Community trading and shipping interests, the Commission shall, at the earliest opportunity, undertake with the competent authorities of the third countries concerned, consultations aimed at reconciling as far as possible the abovementioned interest with the respect of Community law. The Commission shall inform the Advisory Committee referred to in Article 15 of the outcome of these consultations.

2.   Where agreements with third countries need to be negotiated, the Commission shall make recommendations to the Council, which shall authorize the Commission to open the necessary negotiations.

The Commission shall conduct these negotiations in consultation with an Advisory Committee as referred to in Article 15 and within the framework of such directives as the Council may issue to it.

3.   In exercising the powers conferred on it by this Article, the Council shall act in accordance with the decision-making procedure laid down in Article 84 (2) of the Treaty.

SECTION II

RULES OF PROCEDURE

Article 10

Procedures on complaint or on the Commission's own initiative

Acting on receipt of a complaint or on its own initiative, the Commission shall initiate procedures to terminate any infringement of the provisions of Articles 85 (1) or 86 of the Treaty or to enforce Article 7 of this Regulation.

Complaints may be submitted by:

(a) Member States;

(b) natural or legal persons who claim a legitimate interest.

Article 11

Result of procedures on complaint or on the Commission's own initiative

1.   Where the Commission finds that there has been an infringement of Articles 85 (1) or 86 of the Treaty, it may by decision require the undertakings or associations of undertakings concerned to bring such infringement to an end.

Without prejudice to the other provisions of this Regulation, the Commission may, before taking a decision under the preceding subparagraph, address to the undertakings or associations of undertakings concerned recommendations for termination of the infringement.

2.   Paragraph 1 shall apply also to cases falling within Article 7 of this Regulation.

3.   If the Commission, acting on a complaint received, concludes that on the evidence before it there are no grounds for intervention under Articles 85 (1) or 86 of the Treaty or Article 7 of this Regulation, in respect of any agreement, decision or practice, it shall issue a decision rejecting the complaint as unfounded.

4.   If the Commission, whether acting on a complaint received or on its own initiative, concludes that an agreement, decision or concerted practice satisfies the provisions both of Article 85 (1) and of Article 85 (3) of the Treaty, it shall issue a decision applying Article 85 (3). Such decision shall indicate the date from which it is to take effect. This date may be prior to that of the decision.

Article 12

Application of Article 85 (3) — objections

1.   Undertakings and associations of undertakings which seek application of Article 85 (3) of the Treaty in respect of agreements, decisions and concerted practices falling within the provisions of Article 85 (1) to which they are parties shall submit applications to the Commission.

2.   If the Commission judges an application admissible and is in possession of all the available evidence, and no action under Article 10 has been taken against the agreement, decision or concerted practice in question, then it shall publish as soon as possible in the *Official Journal of the European Communities* a summary of the application and invite all interested third parties and the Member States to submit their comments to the Commission within 30 days. Such publications shall have regard to the legitimate interest of undertakings in the protection of their business secrets.

3.   Unless the Commission notifies applicants, within 90 days from the date of such publication in the *Official Journal of the European Communities,* that there are serious doubts as to the applicability of Article 85 (3), the agreement, decision or concerted practice shall be deemed exempt, insofar as it conforms with the description given in the application, from the prohibition for the time already elapsed and for a maximum of six years from the date of publication in the *Official Journal of the European Communities.*

If the Commission finds, after expiry of the 90-day time limit, but before expiry of the six year period, that the conditions for applying Article 85 (3) are not satisfied, it shall issue a decision declaring that the prohibition in Article 85 (1) is applicable. Such decision may be retroactive where the parties concerned have given inaccurate information or where they abuse the exemption from the provisions of Article 85 (1).

4.   The Commission may notify applicants as referred to in the first subparagraph of paragraph 3 and shall do so if requested by a Member State within 45 days of the forwarding to the Member State of the application in accordance with Article 15 (2). This request must be justified on the basis of considerations relating to the competition rules of the Treaty.

If it finds that the conditions of Article 85 (1) and of Article 85 (3) are satisfied, the Commission shall issue a decision applying Article 85 (3). The decision shall indicate the date from which it is to take effect. This date may be prior to that of the application.

Article 13

Duration and revocation of decisions applying Article 85 (3)

1. Any decision applying Article 85 (3) taken under Article 11 (4) or under the second subparagraph of Article 12 (4) shall indicate the period for which it is to be valid; normally such period shall not be less than six years. Conditions and obligations may be attached to the decision.

2. The decision may be renewed if the conditions for applying Article 85 (3) continue to be satisfied.

3. The Commission may revoke or amend its decision or prohibit specified acts by the parties:

(a) where there has been a change in any of the facts which were basic to the making of the decision;

(b) where the parties commit a breach of any obligation attached to the decision;

(c) where the decision is based on incorrect information or was induced by deceit, or

(d) where the parties abuse the exemption from the provisions of Article 85 (1) granted to them by the decision.

In cases falling within (b), (c) or (d), the decision may be revoked with retroactive effect.

Article 14

Powers

Subject to review of its decision by the Court of Justice, the Commission shall have sole power:

— to impose obligations pursuant to Article 7;

— to issue decisions pursuant to Article 85 (3).

The authorities of the Member States shall retain the power to decide whether any case falls within the provisions of Article 85 (1) or Article 86, until such time as the Commission has initiated a procedure with a view to formulating a decision in the case in question or has sent notification as provided for in the first subparagraph of Article 12 (3).

Article 15

Liaison with the authorities of the Member States

1. The Commission shall carry out the procedures provided for in this Regulation in close and constant liaison with the competent authorities of the Member States; these authorities shall have the right to express their views on such procedures.

2. The Commission shall immediately forward to the competent authorities of the Member States copies of the complaints and applications, and of the most important documents sent to it or which it sends out in the course of such procedures.

3. An Advisory Committee on agreements and dominant positions in maritime transport shall be consulted prior to the taking of any decision following upon a procedure under Article 10 or of any decision issued under the second subparagraph of Article 12 (3), or under the second subparagraph of paragraph 4 of the same Article. The Advisory Committee shall also be consulted prior to the adoption of the implementing provisions provided for in Article 26.

4. The Advisory Committee shall be composed of officials competent in the sphere of maritime transport and agreements and dominant positions. Each Member State shall nominate two officials to represent it, each of whom may be replaced, in the event of his being prevented from attending, by another official.

5. Consultation shall take place at a joint meeting convened by the Commission; such meeting shall be held not earlier than fourteen days after dispatch of the notice convening it. This notice shall, in respect of each case to be examined, be accompanied by a summary of the case together with an indication of the most important documents, and a preliminary draft decision.

6. The Advisory Committee may deliver an opinion notwithstanding that some of its members or their alternates are not present. A report of the outcome of the consultative proceedings shall be annexed to the draft decision. It shall not be made public.

Article 16

Requests for information

1. In carrying out the duties assigned to it by this Regulation, the Commission may obtain all necessary information from the Governments and competent authorities of the Member States and from undertakings and associations of undertakings.

2. When sending a request for information to an undertaking or association of undertakings, the Commission shall at the same time forward a copy of the request to the competent authority of the Member State in whose territory the seat of the undertaking or association of undertakings is situated.

3. In its request, the Commission shall state the legal basis and the purpose of the request, and also the penalties provided for in Article 19 (1) (b) for supplying incorrect information.

4. The owners of the undertakings or their representatives and, in the case of legal persons, companies

or firms, or of associations having no legal personality, the person authorized to represent them by law or by their constitution, shall be bound to supply the information requested.

5. Where an undertaking or association of undertakings does not supply the information requested within the time limit fixed by the Commission, or supplies incomplete information, the Commission shall by decision require the information to be supplied. The decision shall specify what information is required, fix an appropriate time limit within which it is to be supplied and indicate the penalties provided for in Article 19 (1) (b) and Article 20 (1) (c) and the right to have the decision reviewed by the Court of Justice.

6. The Commission shall at the same time forward a copy of its decision to the competent authority of the Member State in whose territory the seat of the undertaking or association of undertakings is situated.

Article 17

Investigations by the authorities of the Member States

1. At the request of the Commission, the competent authorities of the Member States shall undertake the investigations which the Commission considers to be necessary under Article 18 (1), or which it has ordered by decision pursuant to Article 18 (3). The officials of the competent authorities of the Member States responsible for conducting these investigations shall exercise their powers upon production of an authorization in writing issued by the competent authority of the Member State in whose territory the investigation is to be made. Such authorization shall specify the subject matter and purpose of the investigation.

2. If so requested by the Commission or by the competent authority of the Member State in whose territory the investigation is to be made, Commission officials may assist the officials of such authority in carrying out their duties.

Article 18

Investigating powers of the Commission

1. In carrying out the duties assigned to it by this Regulation, the Commission may undertake all necessary investigations into undertakings and associations of undertakings.

To this end the officials authorized by the Commission are empowered:

(a) to examine the books and other business records;

(b) to take copies of or extracts from the books and business records:

(c) to ask for oral explanations on the spot;

(d) to enter any premises, land and vehicles of undertakings.

2. The officials of the Commission authorized for the purpose of these investigations shall exercise their powers upon production of an authorization in writing specifying the subject matter and purpose of the investigation and the penalties provided for in Article 19 (1) (c) in cases where production of the required books or other business records is incomplete. In good time before the investigation, the Commission shall inform the competent authority of the Member State in whose territory the same is to be made of the investigation and of the identity of the authorized officials.

3. Undertakings and associations of undertakings shall submit to investigations ordered by decision of the Commission. The decision shall specify the subject matter and purpose of the investigation, appoint the date on which it is to begin and indicate the penalties provided for in Article 19 (1) (c) and Article 20 (1) (d) and the right to have the decision reviewed by the Court of Justice.

4. The Commission shall take decisions referred to in paragraph 3 after consultation with the competent authority of the Member State in whose territory the investigation is to be made.

5. Officials of the competent authority of the Member State in whose territory the investigation is to be made, may at the request of such authority or of the Commission, assist the officials of the Commission in carrying out their duties.

6. Where an undertaking opposes an investigation ordered pursuant to this Article, the Member State concerned shall afford the necessary assistance to the officials authorized by the Commission to enable them to make their investigation. To this end, Member States shall take the necessary measures, after consulting the Commission, before 1 January 1989.

Article 19

Fines

1. The Commission may by decision impose on undertakings or associations of undertakings fines of from 100 to 5 000 ECU where, intentionally or negligently:

(a) they supply incorrect or misleading information, either in a communication pursuant to Article 5 (5) or in an application pursuant to Article 12; or

(b) they supply incorrect information in response to a request made pursuant to Article 16 (3) or (5), or do not supply information within the time limit fixed by a decision taken under Article 16 (5); or

(c) they produce the required books or other business records in incomplete form during investigations under Article 17 or Article 18, or refuse to submit to an investigation ordered by decision issued in implementation of Article 18 (3).

2. The Commission may by decision impose on undertakings or associations of undertakings fines of from 1 000 to one million ECU, or a sum in excess thereof but not exceeding 10 % of the turnover in the preceding business year of each of the undertakings participating in the infringement, where either intentionally or negligently:

(a) they infringe Article 85 (1) or Article 86 of the Treaty, or do not comply with an obligation imposed under Article 7 of this Regulation;

(b) they commit a breach of any obligation imposed pursuant to Article 5 or to Article 13 (1).

In fixing the amount of the fine, regard shall be had both to the gravity and to the duration of the infringement.

3. Article 15 (3) and (4) shall apply.

4. Decisions taken pursuant to paragraphs 1 and 2 shall not be of criminal law nature.

The fines provided for in paragraph 2 (a) shall not be imposed in respect of acts taking place after notification to the Commission and before its Decision in application of Article 85 (3) of the Treaty, provided they fall within the limits of the activity described in the notification.

However, this provision shall not have effect where the Commission has informed the undertakings concerned that after preliminary examination it is of the opinion that Article 85 (1) of the Treaty applies and that application of Article 85 (3) is not justified.

Article 20

Periodic penalty payments

1. The Commission may by decision impose on undertakings or associations of undertakings periodic penalty payments of from 50 to 1 000 ECU per day, calculated from the date appointed by the decision, in order to compel them:

(a) to put an end to an infringement of Article 85 (1) or Article 86 of the Treaty the termination of which it has ordered pursuant to Article 11, or to comply with an obligation imposed pursuant to Article 7;

(b) to refrain from any act prohibited under Article 13 (3);

(c) to supply complete and correct information which it has requested by decision taken pursuant to Article 16 (5);

(d) to submit to an investigation which it has ordered by decision taken pursuant to Article 18 (3).

2. Where the undertakings or associations of undertakings have satisfied the obligation which it was the purpose of the periodic penalty payment to enforce, the Commission may fix the total amount of the periodic penalty payment at a lower figure than that which would arise under the original decision.

3. Article 15 (3) and (4) shall apply.

Article 21

Review by the Court of Justice

The Court of Justice shall have unlimited jurisdiction within the meaning of Article 172 of the Treaty to review decisions whereby the Commission has fixed a fine or periodic penalty payment; it may cancel, reduce or increase the fine or periodic penalty payment imposed.

Article 22

Unit of account

For the purpose of applying Articles 19 to 21 the ECU shall be that adopted in drawing up the budget of the Community in accordance with Articles 207 and 209 of the Treaty.

Article 23

Hearing of the parties and of third persons

1. Before taking decisions as provided for in Articles 11, 12 (3) second subparagraph, and 12 (4), 13 (3), 19 and 20, the Commission shall give the undertakings or associations of undertakings concerned the opportunity of being heard on the matters to which the Commission has taken objection.

2. If the Commission or the competent authorities of the Member States consider it necessary, they may also hear other natural or legal persons. Applications to be heard on the part of such persons where they show a sufficient interest shall be granted.

3. Where the Commission intends to give negative clearance pursuant to Article 85 (3) of the Treaty, it shall publish a summary of the relevant agreement, decision or concerted practice and invite all interested third parties to submit their observations within a time limit which it shall fix being not less than one month. Publication shall have regard to the legitimate interest of undertakings in the protection of their business secrets.

Article 24

Professional secrecy

1. Information acquired as a result of the application of Articles 17 and 18 shall be used only for the purpose of the relevant request or investigation.

2.   Without prejudice to the provisions of Articles 23 and 25, the Commission and the competent authorities of the Member States, their officials and other servants shall not disclose information acquired by them as a result of the application of this Regulation and of the kind covered by the obligation of professional secrecy.

3.   The provisions of paragraphs 1 and 2 shall not prevent publication of general information or surveys which do not contain information relating to particular undertakings or associations of undertakings.

Article 25

Publication of decisions

1.   The Commission shall publish the decisions which it takes pursuant to Articles 11, 12 (3), second paragraph, 12 (4) and 13 (3).

2.   The publication shall state the names of the parties and the main content of the decision; it shall have regard to the legitimate interest of undertakings in the protection of their business secrets.

Article 26

Implementing provisions

The Commission shall have power to adopt implementing provisions concerning the scope of the obligation of communication pursuant to Article 5 (5), the form, content and other details of complaints pursuant to Article 10, applications pursuant to Article 12 and the hearings provided for in Article 23 (1) and (2).

Article 27

Entry into force

This Regulation shall enter into force on 1 July 1987.

This Regulation shall be binding in its entirety and directly applicable in all Member States.

Done at Brussels, 22 December 1986.

For the Council
The President
G. SHAW

COUNCIL REGULATION (EEC) No 4057/86

of 22 December 1986

on unfair pricing practices in maritime transport

THE COUNCIL OF THE EUROPEAN COMMUNITIES,

Having regard to the Treaty establishing the European Economic Community, and in particular Article 84 (2) thereof,

Having regard to the draft Regulation submitted by the Commission,

Having regard to the opinion of the European Parliament (¹),

Having regard to the opinion of the Economic and Social Committee (²),

Whereas there is reason to believe, *inter alia* on the basis of the information system set up by Council Decision 78/774/EEC (³), that the competitive participation of Community shipowners in international liner shipping is adversely affected by certain unfair practices of shipping lines of third countries;

Whereas the structure of the Community shipping industry is such as to make it appropriate that the provisions of this Regulation should also apply to nationals of Member States established outside the Community or cargo shipping companies established outside the Community and controlled by nationals of Member States, if their ships are registered in a Member State in accordance with its legislation;

Whereas such unfair practices consist of continuous charging of freight rates for the transport of selected commodities which are lower than the lowest freight rates charged for the same commodities by established and representative shipowners;

Whereas such pricing practices are made possible by non-commercial advantages granted by a State which is not a member of the Community;

Whereas the Community should be able to take redressive action against such pricing practices;

Whereas there are no internationally agreed rules as to what constitutes an unfair price in the maritime transport field;

Whereas, in order to determine the existence of unfair pricing practices, provision should therefore be made for an

appropriate method of calculation; whereas when calculating the 'normal freight rate' account should be taken of the comparable rate actually charged by established and representative companies operating within or outside conferences or otherwise of a constructed rate based on the costs of comparable companies plus a reasonable margin of profit;

Whereas appropriate factors relevant for the determination of injury should be laid down;

Whereas it is necessary to lay down the procedures for those acting on behalf of the Community shipping industry who consider themselves injured or threatened by unfair pricing practices to lodge a complaint; whereas it seems appropriate to make it clear that in the case of withdrawal of a complaint, proceedings may, but need not necessarily, be terminated;

Whereas there should be cooperation between the Member States and the Commission both as regards information about the existence of unfair pricing practices and injury resulting therefrom, and as regards the subsequent examination of the matter at Community level; whereas, to this end, consultations should take place within an Advisory Committee;

Whereas it is appropriate to lay down clearly the rules of procedure to be followed during the investigation, in particular the rights and obligations of the Community authorities and the parties involved, and the conditions under which interested parties may have access to information and may ask to be informed of the principal facts and considerations on the basis of which it is intended to propose the introduction of a redressive duty;

Whereas, in order to discourage unfair pricing practices, but without preventing, restricting or distorting price competition by non-conference lines, providing that they are working on a fair and commercial basis, it is appropriate to provide, in cases where the facts as finally established show that there is an unfair pricing practice and injury, for the possibility of imposing redressive duties on particular grounds;

Whereas it is essential, in order to ensure that redressive duties are levied in a correct and uniform manner, that common rules for the application of such duties be laid down; whereas, by reason of the nature of the said duties, such rules may differ from the rules for the levying of normal import duties;

Whereas open and fair procedures should be provided for the review of measures taken and for the investigation to be reopened when circumstances so require;

(¹) OJ No C 255, 15. 10. 1986, p. 169.
(²) OJ No C 344, 31. 12. 1985, p. 31.
(³) OJ No L 258, 21. 9. 1978, p. 35.

Whereas appropriate procedures should be established for examining applications for refund of redressive duties,

HAS ADOPTED THIS REGULATION:

Article 1

Objective

This Regulation lays down the procedure to be followed in order to respond to unfair pricing practices by certain third country shipowners engaged in international cargo liner shipping, which cause serious disruption of the freight pattern on a particular route to, from or within the Community and cause or threaten to cause major injury to Community shipowners operating on that route and to Community interests.

Article 2

In response to unfair pricing practices as described in Article 1 which cause major injury, a redressive duty may be applied by the Community.

A threat of major injury may only give rise to an examination within the meaning of Article 4.

Article 3

For the purposes of this Regulation:

(a) 'third country shipowner' means cargo liner shipping companies other than those mentioned under (d);

(b) 'unfair pricing practices' means the continuous charging on a particular shipping route to, from or within the Community of freight rates for selected or all commodities which are lower than the normal freight rates charged during a period of at least six months, when such lower freight rates are made possible by the fact that the shipowner concerned enjoys non-commercial advantages which are granted by a State which is not a member of the Community;

(c) the 'normal freight rate' shall be determined taking into account:

  (i) the comparable rate actually charged in the ordinary course of shipping business for the like service on the same or comparable route by established and representative companies not enjoying the advantages in (b);

  (ii) or otherwise the constructed rate which is determined by taking the costs of comparable companies not enjoying the advantages in (b) plus a reasonable margin of profit. This cost shall be computed on the

basis of all costs incurred in the ordinary course of shipping business, both fixed and variable, plus a reasonable amount for overhead expenses.

(d) 'Community shipowners' means:

— all cargo shipping companies established under the Treaty in a Member State of the Community;

— nationals of Member States established outside the Community or cargo shipping companies established outside the Community and controlled by nationals of Member States, if their ships are registered in a Member State in accordance with its legislation.

Article 4

Examination of injury

1. Examination of injury shall cover the following factors:

(a) the freight rates offered by Community shipowners' competitors on the route in question, in particular in order to determine whether they have been significantly lower than the normal freight rate offered by Community shipowners, taking into account the level of service offered by all the companies concerned;

(b) the effect of the above factor on Community shipowners as indicated by trends in a number of economic indicators such as:

— sailings,

— utilization of capacity,

— cargo bookings,

— market share,

— freight rates (that is depression of freight rates or prevention of freight rate increases which would normally have occurred),

— profits,

— return of capital,

— investment,

— employment.

2. Where a threat of injury is alleged, the Commission may also examine whether it is clearly foreseeable that a particular situation is likely to develop into actual injury. In this regard, account may also be taken of factors such as:

(a) the increase in tonnage deployed on the shipping route where the competition with Community shipowners is taking place;

(b) the capacity which is already available or is to become available in the foreseeable future in the country of the foreign shipowners and the extent to which the tonnage resulting from that capacity is likely to be used on the shipping route referred to in (a).

3. Injury caused by other factors which, either individually or in combination, are also adversely affecting Community shipowners must not be attributed to the practices in question.

Article 5

Complaint

1. Any natural or legal person, or any association not having legal personality, acting on behalf of the Community shipping industry who consider themselves injured or threatened by unfair pricing practices may lodge a written complaint.

2. The complaint shall contain sufficient evidence of the existence of the unfair pricing practice and injury resulting therefrom.

3. The complaint may be submitted to the Commission, or a Member State, which shall forward it to the Commission. The Commission shall send Member States a copy of any complaint it receives.

4. The complaint may be withdrawn, in which case proceedings may be terminated unless such termination would not be in the interest of the Community.

5. Where it becomes apparent after consultation that the complaint does not provide sufficient evidence to justify initiating an investigation, then the complainant shall be so informed.

6. Where, in the absence of any complaint, a Member State is in possession of sufficient evidence both of unfair pricing practices and of injury resulting therefrom for Community shipowners, it shall immediately communicate such evidence to the Commission.

Article 6

Consultations

1. Any consultations provided for in this Regulation shall take place within an Advisory Committee, which shall consist of representatives of each Member State, with a representative of the Commission as Chairman. Consultations shall be held immediately on request by a Member State or on the initiative of the Commission.

2. The Committee shall meet when convened by its Chairman. He shall provide the Member States, as promptly as possible, with all relevant information.

3. Where necessary, consultation may be in writing only; in such case the Commission shall notify the Member States

and shall specify a period within which they shall be entitled to express their opinions or to request an oral consultation.

4. Consultation shall in particular cover:

(a) the existence of unfair pricing practices and the amount thereof;

(b) the existence and extent of injury;

(c) the causal link between the unfair pricing practices and injury;

(d) the measures which, in the circumstances, are appropriate to prevent or remedy the injury caused by unfair pricing practices and the ways and means for putting such measures into effect.

Article 7

Initiation and subsequent investigation

1. Where, after consultation, it is apparent that there is sufficient evidence to justify initiating a proceeding the Commission shall immediately:

(a) announce the initiation of a proceeding in the *Official Journal of the European Communities;* such announcements shall indicate the foreign shipowner concerned and his country of origin, give a summary of the information received, and provide that all relevant information is to be communicated to the Commission; it shall state the period within which interested parties may make known their views in writing and may apply to be heard orally by the Commission in accordance with paragraph 5;

(b) so advise the shipowners, shippers and freight forwarders known to the Commission to be concerned and the complainants;

(c) commence the investigation at Community level, acting in cooperation with the Member States; such investigation shall cover both unfair pricing practices and injury resulting therefrom and shall be carried out in accordance with paragraphs 2 to 8; the investigation of unfair pricing practices shall normally cover a period of not less than six months immediately prior to the initiation of the proceeding.

2. (a) Where appropriate the Commission shall seek all the information it deems necessary and attempt to chheck this information with the shipowners, agents, shippers, freight forwarders, conferences, associations and other organizations, provided that the undertakings or organizations concerned give their consent.

(b) Where necessary the Commission shall, after consultation, carry out investigations in third countries, provided that the firms concerned give their consent and the government of the country in question has been officially notified and raises no objection. The Commission shall be assisted by officials of those Member States which so request.

3. (a) The Commission may request Member States:

  — to supply information,

  — to carry out all necessary checks and inspections, particularly amongst shippers, freight forwarders, Community shipowners and their agents,

  — to carry out investigations in third countries, provided the firms concerned give their consent and the government of the country in question has been officially notified and raises no objection.

  (b) Member States shall take whatever steps are necessary in order to give effect to requests from the Commission. They shall send to the Commission the information requested together with the results of all inspections, checks or investigations carried out.

  (c) Where this information is of general interest or where its transmission has been requested by a Member State, the Commission shall forward it to the Member States provided it is not confidential, in which case a non-confidential summary shall be forwarded.

  (d) Officials of the Commission shall be authorized, if the Commission or a Member State so requests, to assist the officials of Member States in carrying out their duties.

4. (a) The complainant and the shippers and shipowners known to be concerned may inspect all information made available to the Commission by any party to an investigation as distinct from internal documents prepared by the authorities of the Community or its Member States provided that it is relevant to the defence of their interests and not confidential within the meaning of Article 8 and that it is used by the Commission in the investigation. To this end, they shall address a written request to the Commission, indicating the information required.

  (b) Shipowners subject to investigation and the complainant may request to be informed of the essential facts and considerations on the basis of which it is intended to recommend the imposition of redressive duties.

  (c) (i) Requests for information pursuant to (b) shall:

    — be addressed to the Commission in writing,

    — specify the particular issues on which information is sought.

   (ii) The information may be given either orally or in writing, as considered appropriate by the Commission. It shall not prejudice any subsequent decision which may be taken by the Council. Confidential information shall be treated in accordance with Article 8.

   (iii) Information shall normally be given no later than 15 days prior to the submission by the Commission of any proposal for action pursuant to Article 11. Representations made after the information is given may be taken into consideration only if received within a period to be set by the Commission in each case, which shall be at least 10 days, due consideration being given to the urgency of the matter.

5. The Commission may hear the interested parties. It shall so hear them if they have, within the periods prescribed in the notice published in the *Official Journal of the European Communities,* made a written request for a hearing showing that they are an interested party likely to be affected by the result of the proceeding and that there are particular reasons why they should be given a hearing.

6. Furthermore, the Commission shall, on request, give the parties directly concerned an opportunity to meet, so that opposing views may be presented and any argument put forward by way of rebuttal. In providing this opportunity the Commission shall take account of the need to preserve confidentiality and of the convenience of the parties. There shall be no obligation on any party to attend a meeting and failure to do so shall not be prejudicial to that party's case.

7. (a) This Article shall not preclude the Council from reaching preliminary determinations or from applying measures expeditiously.

  (b) In cases in which any interested party refuses access to, or otherwise does not provide, necessary information within a reasonable period, or significantly impedes the investigation, findings, affirmative or negative, may be made on the basis of the facts available.

8. Proceedings on unfair pricing practices shall not constitute a bar to customs clearance of the goods to which the freight rates concerned apply.

9. (a) An investigation shall be concluded either by its termination or by action pursuant to Article 11. Conclusion should normally take place within one year of the initiation of the proceeding.

  (b) A proceeding shall be concluded either by the termination of the investigation without the imposition of duties and without the acceptance of undertakings or by the expiry or repeal of such duties or by the lapse of undertakings in accordance with Articles 14 or 15.

Article 8

Confidentiality

1. Information received in pursuance of this Regulation shall be used only for the purpose for which it was requested.

2. (a) Neither the Council, nor the Commission, nor Member States, nor the officials of any of these, shall reveal any information received in pursuance of this Regulation of which confidential treatment has been requested by its supplier, without specific permission from the supplier.

   (b) Each request for confidential treatment shall indicate why the information is confidential and shall be accompanied by a non-confidential summary of the information, or a statement of the reasons why the information is not susceptible of such summary.

3. Information will ordinarily be considered to be confidential if its disclosure is likely to have a significantly adverse effect upon the supplier or the source of such information.

4. However, if it appears that a request for confidentiality is not warranted and if the supplier is either unwilling to make the information public or to authorize its disclosure in generalized or summary form, the information in question may be disregarded.

The information may also be disregarded where such request is warranted and where the supplier is unwilling to submit a non-confidential summary, provided that the information is susceptible of such summary.

5. This Article shall not preclude the disclosure of general information by the Community authorities and in particular of the reasons on which decisions taken in pursuance of this Regulation are based, or disclosure of the evidence relied on by the Community authorities insofar as necessary to explain those reasons in court proceedings. Such disclosure must take into account the legitimate interest of the parties concerned that their business secrets should not be divulged.

Article 9

Termination of proceedings where protective measures are unnecessary

1. If it becomes apparent after consultation that protective measures are unnecessary, then, where no objection is raised within the Advisory Committee referred to in Article 6 (1), the proceeding shall be terminated. In all other cases the Commission shall submit to the Council forthwith a report on the results of the consultation, together with a proposal that the proceeding be terminated. The proceeding shall stand terminated if, within one month, the Council, acting by a qualified majority, has not decided otherwise.

2. The Commission shall inform the parties known to be concerned and shall announce the termination in the *Official Journal of the European Communities* setting forth its basic conclusions and a summary or the reasons therefor.

Article 10

Undertakings

1. Where, during the course of investigation, undertakings are offered which the Commission, after consultation, considers acceptable, the investigation may be terminated without the imposition of redressive duties.

Save in exceptional circumstances, undertakings may not be offered later than the end of the period during which representations may be made under Article 7 (4) (c) (iii). The termination shall be decided in conformity with the procedure laid down in Article 9 (1) and information shall be given and notice published in accordance with Article 9 (2).

2. The undertakings referred to under paragraph 1 are those under which rates are revised to an extent such that the Commission is satisfied that the unfair pricing practice, or the injurious effects thereof, are eliminated.

3. Undertakings may be suggested by the Commission, but the fact that such undertakings are not offered or an invitation to do so is not accepted, shall not prejudice consideration of the case. However, the continuation of unfair pricing practices may be taken as evidence that a threat of injury is more likely to be realized.

4. If the undertakings are accepted, the investigation of injury shall nevertheless be completed if the Commission, after consultation, so decides or if request is made by the Community shipowners concerned. In such a case, if the Commission, after consultation, makes a determination of no injury, the undertaking shall automatically lapse. However, where a determination of no threat of injury is due mainly to the existence of an undertaking, the Commission may require that the undertaking be maintained.

5. The Commission may require any party from whom an undertaking has been accepted to provide periodically information relevant to the fulfilment of such undertakings, and to permit verification of pertinent data. Non-compliance with such requirements shall be construed as a violation of the undertaking.

Article 11

Redressive duties

Where investigation shows that there is an unfair pricing practice, that injury is caused by it and that the interests of the Community make Community intervention necessary, the Commission shall propose to the Council, after the consultations provided for in Article 6, that it introduce a redressive duty. The Council, acting by a qualified majority, shall take a Decision within two months.

Article 12

In deciding on the redressive duties, the Council shall also take due account of the external trade policy considerations as well as the port interests and the shipping policy considerations of the Member States concerned.

Article 13

General provisions on duties

1. Redressive duties shall be imposed on the foreign shipowners concerned by regulation.

2. Such regulation shall indicate in particular the amount and type of duty imposed, the commodity or commodities transported, the name and the country of origin of the foreign shipowner concerned and the reasons on which the Regulation is based.

3. The amount of the duties shall not exceed the difference between the freight rate charged and the normal freight rate referred to in Article 3 (c). It shall be less if such lesser duty would be adequate to remove the injury.

4. (a) Duties shall be neither imposed nor increased with retroactive effect and shall apply to the transport of commodities which, after entry into force of such duties, are loaded or discharged in a Community port.

   (b) However, where the Council determines that an undertaking has been violated or withdrawn, the redressive duties may be imposed, on a proposal from the Commission, on the transport of commodities which were loaded or discharged in a Community port not more than 90 days prior to the date of application of these duties, except that in the case of violation or withdrawal of an undertaking such retroactive assessment shall not apply to the transport of commodities which were loaded or discharged in a Community port before the violation or withdrawal. These duties may be calculated on the basis of the facts established before the acceptance of the undertaking.

5. Duties shall be collected by Member States in the form, at the rate and according to the other criteria laid down when the duties were imposed, and independently of the customs duties, taxes and other charges normally imposed on imports of goods transported.

6. Permission to load or discharge cargo in a Community port may be made conditional upon the provision of security for the amount of the duties.

Article 14

Review

1. Regulations imposing redressive duties and decisions to accept undertakings shall be subject to review, in whole or in part, where warranted. Such review may be held either at the request of a Member State or on the initiative of the Commission. A review shall also be held where an interested party so requests and submits evidence of changed circumstances sufficient to justify the need for such review, provided that at least one year has elapsed since the conclusion of the investigation. Such requests shall be adressed to the Commission, which shall inform the Member States.

2. Where, after consultation, it becomes apparent that review is warranted, the investigation shall be re-opened in accordance with Article 7, where the circumstances so require. Such reopening shall not *per se* affect the measures in operation.

3. Where warranted by the review, carried out either with or without reopening of the investigation, the measures shall be amended, repealed or annulled by the Community institution competent for their adoption.

Article 15

1. Subject to paragraph 2, redressive duties and undertakings shall lapse after five years from the date on which they entered into force or were last amended or confirmed.

2. The Commission shall normally, after consultation and within six months prior to the expiry of the five year period, publish in the *Official Journal of the European Communities* a notice of the impending expiry of the measure in question and inform Community shipowners known to be concerned. This notice shall state the period within which interested parties may make known their views in writing and may apply to be given a hearing by the Commission in accordance with Article 7 (5).

Where an interested party shows that the expiry of the measure would again lead to injury or threat of injury, the Commission shall carry out a review of the measure. The measure shall remain in force pending the outcome of this review.

Where redressive duties and undertakings lapse under this Article the Commission shall publish a notice to that effect in the *Official Journal of the European Communities*.

Article 16

Refund

1.   Where the shipowner concerned can show that the duty collected exceeds the difference between the freight rate charged and the normal freight rate referred to in Article 3 (c) the excess amount shall be reimbursed.

2.   In order to request the reimbursement referred to in paragraph 1, the foreign shipowner may submit an application to the Commission. The application shall be submitted via the Member State within the territory of which the commodities transported were loaded or discharged and within three months of the date on which the amount of the redressive duties to be levied was duly determined by the competent authorities.

The Member State shall forward the application to the Commission as soon as possible, either with or without an opinion as to its merits.

The Commission shall inform the other Member States forthwith and give its opinion on the matter. If the Member States agree with the opinion given by the Commission or do not object to it within one month of being informed, the Commission may decide in accordance with the said opinion. In all other cases, the Commission shall, after consultation, decide whether and to what extent the application should be granted.

Article 17

Final provisions

This Regulation shall not preclude the application of any special rules laid down in agreements concluded between the Community and third countries.

Article 18

Entry into force

This Regulation shall enter into force on 1 July 1987.

This Regulation shall be binding in its entirety and directly applicable in all Member States.

Done at Brussels, 22 December 1986.

For the Council
The President
G. SHAW

COUNCIL REGULATION (EEC) No 4058/86

of 22 December 1986

concerning coordinated action to safeguard free access to cargoes in ocean trades

THE COUNCIL OF THE EUROPEAN COMMUNITIES,

Having regard to the Treaty establishing the European Economic Community, and in particular Article 84 (2) thereof,

Having regard to the draft Regulation submitted by the Commission,

Having regard to the opinion of the European Parliament ([1]),

Having regard to the opinion of the Economic and Social Committee ([2]),

Whereas an increasing number of countries resort to protecting their merchant fleets either unilaterally, through legislation or administrative measures, or through bilateral agreements with other countries;

Whereas certain countries, by virtue of measures they have adopted or practices they have imposed, have distorted the application of the principle of fair and free competition in shipping trade with one or more Community Member States;

Whereas in respect of liner trades the United Nations Convention on a Code of Conduct for Liner Conferences, which entered into force on 6 October 1983, grants certain rights to shipping companies which are members of a conference operating a pool;

Whereas, increasingly, third countries which are contracting parties or signatories to that Convention interpret its provisions in such a way as effectively to expand the rights given under the Convention to their companies both in liner and tramp trades, to the disadvantage of Community companies or companies of other OECD countries, whether conference members or not;

Whereas in respect of bulk trades there is an increasing tendency on the part of third countries to restrict access to bulk cargoes, which poses a serious threat to the freely competitive environment broadly prevailing in the bulk trades; whereas the Member States affirm their commitment to a freely competitive environment as being an essential feature of the dry and liquid bulk trades and are convinced

that the introduction of cargo-sharing in these trades will have a serious effect on the trading interests of all countries by substantially increasing transportation costs;

Whereas the restriction of access to bulk cargoes would adversely affect the merchant fleets of the Member States, as well as substantially increasing the transportation costs of such cargoes, and would thereby have a serious effect on the trading interests of the Community;

Whereas the Community should be enabled to provide for coordinated action by Member States if the competitive position of Member States' merchant fleets or Member States' trading interests are adversely affected by cargo reservation to shipping companies of third countries or if required by an international agreement;

Whereas Council Decision 77/587/EEC ([3]) provides, *inter alia*, for consultation on the various aspects of developments which have taken place in relations between Member States and third countries in shipping matters;

Whereas Council Decision 83/573/EEC ([4]) provides, *inter alia*, for concertation by Member States of any countermeasures they may take in relation to third countries and for the possibility of a decision on the joint application by Member States of appropriate countermeasures forming part of their national legislation;

Whereas it is necessary to elaborate and refine the machinery provided for in these Decisions with a view to providing for coordinated action by Member States in certain circumstances at the request of a Member State or Member States or on the basis of an international agreement,

HAS ADOPTED THIS REGULATION:

Article 1

The procedure provided for by this Regulation shall be applicable when action by a third country or by its agents restricts or threatens to restrict free access by shipping companies of Member States or by ships registered in a Member State in accordance with its legislation to the transport of:

— liner cargoes in Code trades, except where such action is taken in accordance with the United Nations Convention on a Code of Conduct for Liner Conferences;

— liner cargoes in non-Code trades;

— bulk cargoes and any other cargo on tramp services;

([1]) OJ No C 255, 15. 10. 1986, p. 169.
([2]) OJ No C 344, 31. 12. 1985, p. 31.

([3]) OJ No L 239, 17. 9. 1977, p. 23.
([4]) OJ No L 332, 28. 11. 1983, p. 37.

— passengers;

— persons or goods to or between offshore installations.

This procedure shall be without prejudice to the obligations of the Community and its Member States under international law.

Article 2

For the purposes of this Regulation:

— 'home-trader' means a shipping company of a third country which operates a service between its own country and one or more Member States;

— 'cross-trader' means a shipping company of a third country which operates a service between another third country and one or more Member States.

Article 3

Coordinated action may be requested by a Member State.

The request shall be made to the Commission; the latter shall make the appropriate recommendations or proposals to the Council within four weeks.

The Council, acting in accordance with the voting procedure laid down in Article 84 (2) or the Treaty, may decide on the coordinated action provided for in Article 4.

In deciding on coordinated action, the Council shall also take due account of the external trade policy considerations. as well as the port interests and the shipping policy considerations of the Member States concerned.

Article 4

1. Coordinated action may consist of:

(a) diplomatic representation to the third countries concerned, in particular where their actions threaten to restrict access to trade;

(b) counter-measures directed at the shipping company or companies of the third countries concerned or at the shipping company or companies of other countries which benefit from the action taken by the countries concerned, whether operating as a hometrader or as a cross-trader in Community trades.

Those countermeasures may consist, separately or in combination, of:

(i) the imposition of an obligation to obtain a permit to load, carry or discharge cargoes; such a permit may be subject to conditions or obligations;

(ii) the imposition of a quota;

(iii) the imposition of taxes or duties.

2. Diplomatic representations shall be made before countermeasures are taken.

Such countermeasures shall be without prejudice to the obligations of the European Community and its Member States under international law, shall take into consideration all the interests concerned and shall neither directly nor indirectly lead to deflection of trade within the Community.

Article 5

1. When deciding upon one or more of the countermeasures referred to in Article 4 (1) (b) the Council shall specify, as appropriate, the following:

(a) the developments which have caused countermeasures to be taken;

(b) the trade or range of ports to which the countermeasures are to apply;

(c) the flag or shipping company of the third country whose cargo reservation measures restrict free access to cargoes in the shipping area concerned;

(d) maximum volume (percentage, weight in tonnes, containers) or value of cargo which may be loaded or discharged in ports of Member States;

(e) maximum number of sailings from and to ports of Member States;

(f) amount or percentage and basis of the taxes and duties to be levied and the manner in which they will be collected;

(g) the duration of the countermeasures.

2. Where the countermeasures envisaged by paragraph 1 are not provided for by the national legislation of a Member State they may be taken in accordance with the Council Decision referred to in the third paragraph of Article 3 by the Member State concerned on the basis of this Regulation.

Article 6

1. If the Council has not adopted the proposal on coordinated action within a period of two months, Member States may apply national measures unilaterally or as a group, if the situation so requires.

2. However, Member States may, in cases of urgency, take the necessary national measures on a provisional basis, unilaterally or as a group, even within the two-month period referred to in paragraph 1.

3. National measures taken in pursuance of this Article shall be notified immediately to the Commission and to the other Member States.

Article 7

During the period in which the countermeasures are to apply, the Member States and the Commission shall consult each other in accordance with the consultation procedure established by Decision 77/587/EEC every three months or earlier if the need arises, in order to discuss the effects of the countermeasures in force.

Article 8

The procedure provided for by this Regulation may be applied when action by a third country or its agents restricts or threatens to restrict the access of shipping companies of another OECD country where, on a basis of reciprocity, it has been agreed between that country and the Community to resort to coordinated resistance in the case of restriction of access to cargoes.

Such country may make a request for coordinated action and join in such coordinated action in accordance with this Regulation.

Article 9

This Regulation shall enter into force on 1 July 1987.

This Regulation shall be binding in its entirety and directly applicable in all Member States.

Done at Brussels, 22 December 1986.

For the Council
The President
G. SHAW

GENERAL BIBLIOGRAPHY

A. Articles/Books

BAYER, N.J. - Antitrust comes to maritime transport in the European Economic Community. Federal Bar News & Journal, Vol. 34, N° 7, (September 1987) p. 299.

BERGESTRAD, S., DOGANIS, R. - The Impact of Soviet Shipping. Published by Allen of Unwin, 40 Museum Street, London XXIA ILU (1987).

BREDIMA, A. - The Common Shipping Policy of the EEC. Common Market Law Review (1981).

BREDIMA, A. - Methods of Interpretation and Community Law. European Studies in Law n° 6, North-Holland Publishing Co, Amsterdam (1978).

BREDIMA, A. - EEC/Liberalism or Protectionism in Maritime Transport?. Naftika Chronika (May 1984).

BREDIMA, A., TZOANNOS, J. - In search of a common shipping policy for the EC. Journal of Common Market Studies (1982).

CLOSE, G. - Article 84 EEC: the Development of Transport Policy in the Sea and Air Sectors. (1980) 5 E.L.R. 188.

ERDMENGER, J. - The European Community Transport Policy. Gower (1983) 155 pp.

GROENENDIJK, J. - The Shipping Industry in the Nineties. Kweek School voor de Zeevaart, Speech, Amsterdam (24/10/85).

LOS, M.D. - Les armateurs grecs et les transports maritimes internationaux de marchandises en vrac. Lausanne (1980).

RIBIERE, J. - Les projets de la Commission des CE en matiere de transport maritime. Journal de la Marine Marchande (28/8/86) p. 2095.

RIDLEY, N. - Speech at Propeller Club, Washington
    D.C. (14/2/86).

SINGH, N. - Maritime Flag and International Law.
    Sijthoff, Leyden (1978) 161 pp.

STURMEY, S.G. - The Code of Conduct and the Review
    Conference. Athens (1988) 218 pp.

TZOANNOS, J. - The EC Common Maritime Transport
    proposals and the liberalisation of world
    shipping markets. Presented at Conference, The
    International Maritime Policy of the EC,
    Steyning, West Sussex (11-13/4/86).

TZOANNOS, J. - The fiscal regime for shipowning
    firms in the EEC. Institute of Economic and
    Industrial Research, Athens (1980).

B. Documents

CAACE - For a common maritime transport policy.
    Report by Comite des Associations d'Armateurs des
    Communautes Européennes (1986).

COMMISSION OF THE EC - Progress Towards a Common
    Transport Policy-Maritime Transport. COM(85)90
    final (14/3/85).

ECONOMIC AND SOCIAL COMMITTEE OF THE EC - Opinion on
    the Progress Towards a Common Transport Policy-
    Maritime Transport. CES 1023/85 (27/11/85).

ECONOMIC AND SOCIAL COMMITTEE OF THE EC - Opinion on
    the Progress Towards a Common Transport Policy -
    Maritime Transport. 2nd Part, CES (21/5/86).

ECONOMIC AND SOCIAL COMMITTEE OF THE EC - Report on
    the Progress Towards a Common Transport Policy -
    Maritime Transport.

ECONOMIC AND SOCIAL COMMITTEE OF THE EC - Appendix
    to the Report 28/4/86. CES 657/85, Rapporteurs:
    K. Mols Sorensen, A. Bredima.

EUROPEAN PARLIAMENT - Committee on Transport. Report on the Memorandum n[o] 3 on Progress Towards a Common Transport Policy-Maritime Transport PE 103.029 (27/5/86). Rapporteur: G.Anastassopoulos.

EUROPEAN SHIPPERS'COUNCILS - Progress towards a Common Transport Policy-Maritime Transport. Views of the European Shippers' Councils (October 1985).

EUROPEAN SHIPPERS'Councils - Policy Paper of the European Shippers' Councils on rules for the application of Articles 85-86 of the Treaty of Rome to Maritime Transport, (8/2/84).

INTERNATIONAL TRANSPORT WORKERS FEDERATION (ITF) - Towards a common maritime transport policy. Report by International Transport Workers Federation (1985).

NETHERLANDS SCIENTIFIC COUNCIL FOR GOVERNMENT POLICY - The Unfinished European Integration. N[o] 28, The Hague (1986).

UK-HOUSE OF LORDS - European Maritime Transport Policy. 514-567 Hansard, Official Report (1/5/86).

UK-HOUSE OF LORDS - European Maritime Transport Policy. Select Committee on the European Communities, 9th Report (18/5/86).

"Les Transports Maritimes a l'heure communautaire", Institute Mediterraneen des Transports Maritimes, Marseille, Conferences on 10-12/10/79, 1-3/6/82, 9-11/10/87.

"The EEC and Shipping-Maritime Practice and Competition Law: Heading for a Collision?": Institute of Maritime Law, Conference, 11/2/1988, London.

"EEC Shipping Law": European Study Conferences Ltd, Conference, 4-5/2/1988, Rotterdam.

ABOUT THE AUTHORS

Dr. Anna Bredima-Savopoulou is an attorney at law and has obtained an LLB from Athens University, an LLM in Shipping Law from University College London, a certificate in EEC Law from the University of Paris and a Ph. D. in EEC Law from University College London. She is a legal advisor on EEC/International Affairs at the Union of Greek Shipowners, a member of the Economic and Social Committee of the European Communities and a member of the Board of Directors of the Comité des Associations d'Armateurs des Communautés Européennes (CAACE).

Professor John Tzoannos is Professor of Business Finance at the Athens School of Economics and Business Science, as well as head of the Maritime Research Department at the Institute of Economic and Industrial Research (IOBE) in Athens. He obtained a BA in Economics from the University of Manchester, an MSc. in economics and econometrics from the University of Southampton and a Ph. D. in industrial economics from the University of Birmingham. He is a member of the Board of Directors of the CAACE.